A THEOLOGY OF HEALTH

A THEOLOGY OF HEALTH

Wholeness and Human Flourishing

TYLER J. VANDERWEELE

University of Notre Dame Press

Notre Dame, Indiana

Copyright © 2024 by the University of Notre Dame
University of Notre Dame Press
Notre Dame, Indiana 46556
www.undpress.nd.edu

All Rights Reserved

Library of Congress Control Number: 2024937293

ISBN: 978-0-268-20833-2 (Hardback)
ISBN: 978-0-268-20835-6 (WebPDF)
ISBN: 978-0-268-20832-5 (Epub3)

Published in the United States of America

To my wife,

L I S A,

who sustains my flourishing and health

and that of our family in ways

too numerous to fully comprehend.

"Thou hast made us for thyself, O Lord, and our heart is restless until it finds its rest in thee."

(Augustine, Confessions, 1,1)

CONTENTS

	Preface	ix
PART I	**HEALTH AND WHOLENESS**	
	Introduction. Health as Wholeness	3
I.1	The Health of Persons and Human Flourishing	10
I.2	The Health of the Body	28
I.3	Health, Unity, and Goodness	44
I.4	Health and Community	52
I.5	Health and Spiritual Well-Being	70
I.6	Health and Responsibility	80
I.7	The Implications of Health as Wholeness	99
PART II	**ILL HEALTH AND SIN**	
	Introduction. Ill Health as the Absence of Wholeness	133
II.1	Agency, Sin, and Ill Health	137
II.2	Injustice and Ill Health	142
II.3	Fallenness and Ill Health	149
II.4	Sin and Death	155
II.5	Incapacity and Sin	159
II.6	Ill Health and Suffering	162
II.7	The Implications of Ill Health and Sin	172

PART III	**HEALING AND SALVATION**	
	Introduction. Healing as the Restoration of Wholeness	193
III.1	Healing of Persons and Healing from Sin	196
III.2	Healing and Love	200
III.3	Healing and Jesus Christ	215
III.4	The Church, Community, and Healing	229
III.5	The Limits of Healing	251
III.6	God, Resurrection, and Salvation	259
III.7	The Implications of Healing and Salvation	267

A Nontheological Postscript	293
Appendix *Propositional Outline*	307
A Brief Glossary Concerning Health and Illness	319
References	323
Index	353

PREFACE

The origin of this book came about in part through the repeated teaching of a course at Harvard University on the topic of religion and public health. While my teaching in this course focuses principally on the empirical research on the topic, I regularly try to interweave that material with questions of interpretation and implications, especially during times of open discussion. The empirical research on the topic has become increasingly sophisticated and rigorous in recent decades, generally suggesting mostly beneficial associations between religious participation and health and well-being. However, it has seemed to me that there has not been comparable progress in sophistication with regard to interpretation and exploration of the implications of this body of work. Proper interpretation of the results requires not only a nuanced understanding of the empirical research but also some understanding of the life of religious communities, their own internal ends, and how and in what ways these are, or are not, oriented toward health. Interpretation also requires a sense of what constitutes health, with regard to how both the public health community and religious communities understand health, and how these understandings may be similar or different. Much of the philosophical and conceptual literature on health has centered on critique, refinement, or occasionally defense of the World Health Organization's definition of health as "a state of complete physical, mental, and social well-being, and not merely the absence of disease or infirmity" (World Health Organization, 1946). Surprisingly little attention, it seemed, had been paid to how religious communities understand health and to the question of how health is to be understood from a theological or religious perspective. In my various searches, I had considerable difficulty locating works that explicitly addressed this topic—that is to say, that provided a theology of health.

There is a fairly sizable literature concerning the theology of health *care*, often centered on questions of what it means to be a good clinician or to provide good patient care, understood from a theological perspective. However, much less attention seems to have been paid as to how health itself was to be understood theologically. My initial inquiries and searches unveiled relatively little, and for some time I thought that there was no book-length treatment that addressed this question. A search for a book concerning the theology of health yielded no results. While certain works initially seemed promising and some offered some relevant material, most of these works quickly turned to matters of health care, giving only a cursory treatment of the concept of health itself. This included an entire series of books published by Crossroads in the 1980s on Health/Medicine and the Faith Traditions, each volume of which was devoted to a different religious tradition. These had relatively little material on the concept of health itself. What seemed to me at the time a lack of adequate consideration of the topic was puzzling, and at some point during 2016, I decided I would attempt some sort of contribution. This project seemed important in its own right, but I also wanted a fuller and more explicit understanding of health to guide my own future work and thinking. The formation of the Human Flourishing Program at Harvard, which I began in 2016, was in part prompted by and then further influenced my thinking around these questions of the scope of health and well-being.

In 2017, when I again taught the course on religion and public health at Harvard, I decided to conclude the course with a brief sketch of what I took to be a Christian understanding of a theology of health. While this material extended beyond what students might have reasonably expected from the course description, and perhaps especially so in a mostly secular and certainly pluralistic context, nevertheless, from what I could tell, the material was well received. The course was attended by students from a range of faith traditions and by those with no faith tradition. Although the presentation of this material was from an explicitly Christian theological perspective, I acknowledged that how health is understood will of course vary by religious or cultural tradition and that my own thinking was strongly shaped by my own faith tradition. I encouraged the students to reflect on their own understandings of health and how these were shaped by their own respective cultural and religious traditions and encouraged them to raise these more fundamental questions on the nature of and the meaning of health more frequently. I argued that it would be of benefit, even within a pluralistic context, to discuss these matters more explicitly and to understand how various perspectives were similar or different. I argued that doing so would allow us to clarify what we were aiming at in our work in public health, would help us better identify areas of agreement and consensus, and would make us all more aware of where there were disagreements or potential tensions or conflicts, thereby also hopefully enabling more satisfactory approaches to navigating them. I have continued to teach this material in subsequent iterations of the course and have altered the course's title to "Religion, Well-being, and Public Health" so as to emphasize potentially more expansive understandings of health.

Over the years, I have also tried to return to these questions again and again in my own thinking and work, and I began plans for writing a book on an explicitly Christian theology of health. In fact, I was to discover that works that addressed these questions directly did exist, although they were not titled *Theology of Health*. Jean-Claude Larchet's *Theology of Illness* approached these questions from an Eastern Orthodox perspective, drawing upon and weaving together theological reflections concerning health and illness, especially from the Church fathers. While illness is allegedly the focus of the book, it also offers an outline of a positive theology of health. Around the same time, I came across Neil Messer's book *Flourishing*, and although its title suggests a more expansive purview, it too offers an explicit theology of health, principally from a Christian Reformed perspective, though it also draws substantially upon the work of Aquinas. In contrast with Larchet's book, Messer's book also has a much a greater engagement with contemporary philosophical, clinical, and cultural perspectives on health and disease. These two books influenced my thinking substantially, and my indebtedness to them extends well beyond the various references to these books that appear in the pages that follow. It is difficult to speculate about what my understanding would have been without these works. As Christian theologies of health, both books are well worth reading. Somewhat later, I also came across Almut Caspary's *In Good Health*, which provides an outline of a number of historical theologies of health, including material from Tatian, Tertullian, Basil the Great, and especially Augustine, and brings these theologians into dialogue with contemporary philosophical debate and contemporary medicine. Taken together, these three books provided much of what I had been searching for. However, by the time I was aware of all three, I was already sufficiently deeply engaged in this project of trying to develop a book-length treatment of a Christian theology of health that I did not want to set it aside, in spite of the presence of these three other excellent texts. I also still felt that I had something further to contribute.

This book has a few distinctive features, and I hope that its contribution is not overly redundant with these other three books. First, while Larchet's book and Messer's book offer constructive theologies of health, Larchet's does so from an Eastern Orthodox perspective and Messer's principally from a Reformed perspective. The present book attempts to do so from a predominantly Catholic perspective. My own religious trajectory has been from the Presbyterian Church to the Anglican Church to the Roman Catholic Church, having been received therein during the summer of 2012. While I have tried to keep much of the content of the present book relatively ecumenical, it will be clear especially, for example, on matters of social teaching or on material concerning the understanding of the Church and the sacraments and their relation to health and well-being, that a Catholic understanding underlies much of what is written. The book also draws heavily on the thought of Thomas Aquinas. The present volume should arguably not be understood as a Thomistic theology of health; it does not devote sufficient attention to detailed exegesis of Aquinas's works to present it as such. Moreover, while the topic of bodily health comes up numerous times in Aquinas's writings, it is secondary to broader considerations of Aquinas concerning happiness, flourishing, and the final end of the human person.

The topic of happiness and flourishing brings me to another distinctive feature of this book. One of its central premises, running throughout the development, is that we have two concepts of health: the health of the body and the health of the person. Our narrower concept of the "health of the body" concerns the body's parts and systems being and functioning as normal so as to allow for the full range of characteristically human activities. The broader concept of the "health of the person" is essentially synonymous with "flourishing" or "complete human well-being." Both the narrower and the broader concepts of health arise in our ordinary language concerning health, and both can be manifest simultaneously, as in the sentence, "Every day he just sits in his room; he is physically healthy, but he is not a healthy person." I argue in the book that some of the conceptual confusions and puzzles around health arise from a failure to recognize these two distinct concepts of health and a failure to clarify which is in view in any particular context. The book provides a theology for both the health of the body and the health of the person. On the latter especially, Aquinas has a great deal to say, and the indebtedness of the book to his thought will be clear from even a cursory glance at the footnotes.

The footnotes are relatively extensive, occupying over one-quarter of the text. I have tried to relegate to the footnotes much of the technical material and my interaction with other parts of the relevant scholarly literature. Some of the footnotes simply provide more extensive sets of references; others provide greater engagement with related literature or slightly fuller expositions of the thought of various theologians or contributors. Some provide engagement with the empirical research on related topics; others offer more speculative proposals. I have tried to keep the primary text itself relatively readable and nontechnical. Determining what to include in the main text and what to assign to footnotes was difficult, and it is possible that too much has been placed in footnotes. As a small compensatory measure, the footnotes are indeed footnotes rather than endnotes, and so for the interested reader that material can be consulted immediately in the course of reading rather than having to turn to the back of the book.

However, as a result of this structure, there is perhaps somewhat less engagement with the contemporary philosophical and clinical literature in the main text than is the case with Messer's or Caspary's book, and I would strongly encourage turning to those texts for further theological engagement with other contemporary perspectives on health. In this book, much, though not all, of such engagement is to be found in footnotes. Also, while I have tried to engage with as much of the literature on the theology of health as I have been able to find, the same is not true with regard to the theology of health *care*. As noted above, that is a much larger literature. There is some engagement with this literature, especially in the implications sections that conclude each of the book's three parts, but it is far from exhaustive. The same is even more so the case with the literature on any given theological topic. There is some engagement, often selectively with Aquinas, the teachings of the Catholic Church, and other specific theologians and works, but on almost any given theological topic, only a very small fraction of the relevant literature is addressed. This was necessary given the numerous areas of theology the book draws upon. The main text is intended to be principally a constructive theology of health, and the relevant literature is drawn upon as needed to attempt to support this construction.

A few additional comments on the structure of the book perhaps merit mention. To facilitate easily accessible summaries of this material and to make clearer potential points of consensus and disagreement, the various sections and subsections are organized around a series of propositions. Each section and subsection begins with a proposition, and the material that then follows provides a more substantial exposition. In order to distinguish the propositions from the corresponding sections and subsections, references to the sections are prefaced by Roman numerals and references to the propositions are prefaced by Arabic numerals so that, for example, references would be made to "Proposition 3.2d" but to "Section III.2d." While the propositions always correspond to the analogous sections, there is more material in the sections than is contained in the propositions. All of the various propositions are also collected together in the appendix in the form of a propositional outline. This constitutes a concise summary of the book's contents. The appendix also provides a brief glossary of terms concerning health and illness as employed in the text.

The question of the intended audience of the book is a difficult one. The most straightforward answer would be that the primary audience is constituted by Christians in academic, biomedical, or public fields interested in a Christian understanding of health. This might include Christians working in medicine, public health, or public policy as well as Christian ethicists and theologians interested in questions of health and health care. While this would perhaps constitute the primary intended audience for the book, my hope for the book's readership is somewhat broader, including both more general Christian and non-Christian audiences, and I will consider each of these broader audiences in turn and comment on how these intended and hoped-for audiences have shaped the content and structure of the book.

My hope for Christian audiences is that the book may be of some interest to just about any Christian reader, for several reasons. First, pretty much everyone is at least partially concerned about their health. Nearly everyone would prefer to be healthy than unhealthy. What Christian traditions and teachings have to say about health is thus relevant. Second, the book attempts to offer not only a theology of bodily health but also a theology concerning the health of the person, or flourishing; and the pursuit of human well-being is certainly relevant to everyone. Much of the book in some sense tries to bridge theological understandings and more contemporary work concerning well-being. This bridge is attempted both with respect to thought, scholarship, and ideas and with respect to the language employed. The result certainly does not do full justice to either literature, but there is arguably value in at least trying to point to theology's contribution to our understanding of flourishing and also perhaps how contemporary discussions of well-being might shed light on theology. Third, the body and the human person, understood as part of God's creation, arguably has something to teach us about God. Although the title *Theology of Health*, with the ambiguous preposition "of," is principally to be understood along the lines of "theological perspectives on health" rather than "what we learn about God from the nature of health," the book has at least something to offer on this latter topic as well. The study of the health and wholeness of the body and of the person itself arguably offers a lens through which to understand how these matters reflect something of God's nature and being, unity and perfections, will and action, and creativity, goodness, and love. Finally, the book is arguably relevant to a more general Christian audience because of the Church's calling to care for those who are sick and in need and to provide both material and spiritual aid. Doing this well can be facilitated by a better understanding of health, of what it is that we are aiming for. It is my hope that the book might in some small way therefore be of service to the Church by providing additional insight into the nature of health, its relation to other goods and ends, the challenges and opportunities in potentially partnering with the institutions of public health and medicine and by pointing toward the powerful resources the Church has at its disposal in the promotion of health, including community life, forgiveness, love, healing, prayer, and a message of hope and salvation. In any case, it is in part because of this aspiration of a broader readership that I have tried to keep most of the exposition and discussion at a less specialized academic level, in the hope that the main text would be of interest to those outside the academic community. Only time will tell the extent to which I have succeeded at this.

Perhaps yet more aspirational, I also hope that some of the material in this book might be of interest to audiences who are not Christian, but who are directly engaged in public health or medicine, or in research and scholarship within these fields. I hope this for several reasons. First, as per the course I teach at Harvard, I hope that this material might give rise to more frequent conversations about what we mean by health and greater clarity about what ends we are seeking when we work to promote health. Even for those who may disagree—and perhaps disagree strongly—with some of the perspectives offered in this book, I hope it might prompt more regular and substantial reflection on how we understand health.

Second, while the book has been written from an explicitly Christian theological perspective, I believe that some of the insights arising from this perspective may be of interest, value, and relevance even to those who do not embrace the Christian faith. Some of the implications of the positions put forward, concerning, for example, community, forgiveness, and love as pathways to healing, do not necessarily require a distinctively theological perspective. I have made some effort throughout to structure arguments, where possible, in a more universally accessible manner and to only draw upon more distinctively theological and Christian presuppositions when the positions or material at hand seem to require it. But again, even when more theological material and arguments are being employed, I think some of the insights that arise may be of value to those from other traditions. Different cultures, traditions, and perspectives can offer their own distinctive insights that may be of relevance to those outside the traditions from which they arise. To that end, I conclude the book with a "nontheological postscript." In it, I attempt to briefly explore and describe what I see as the relevance and implications of the material in this book for those who do not embrace a Christian perspective on these topics, and I try to express what I see as some of the insights of this "theology of health" in nontheological terms. A reader from outside the Christian tradition might well begin, and possibly also end, there. Throughout this nontheological postscript, I have provided references to relevant and related nontheological (and often empirical) work on these topics, along with references to the relevant sections of the theological exposition of the book from which the insights were drawn. I hope that this material at least might be of interest to a considerably wider audience.

Third, my hope is that by making this material on a theology of health more explicit, there will be a greater understanding of how many Christians and Christian organizations around the world, perhaps somewhat implicitly, approach this topic of health and that such understanding might be of importance and of some interest even to those who are not Christian. For those working directly in public health and medicine, it will provide some insight into how some of the more than two billion Christians around the world potentially think about these topics. It will, I hope, provide insights that medical and public health professionals can use to better engage with many people on matters of health, illness, and healing, even if they reject the theological categories. It will thus perhaps allow for a broadening of cultural competence in serving the public health and health care needs of many throughout the world. Such understanding, I hope, may also help establish partnerships between public health institutions and religious organizations. As I discuss in part III of the book, I very much believe that there is much to be gained by greater partnerships between religious organizations and public health institutions. Many of these partnerships of the past have been successful; some have also faced conflicts and challenges. A well-developed conception of health and well-being requires an understanding of the human person, and on this topic there is no entirely neutral ground on which to stand. Conceptions of the health of the person, and arguably to some extent even health of the body, cannot be value neutral. As noted above, a greater understanding of distinctive positions might facilitate finding common ground and more clearly identifying the specific points of disagreement. One of the critical steps to navigating disagreements and tensions is understanding them and understanding the other's perspective more deeply. I hope the book can in some small way assist readers with this as well. My hope is that partnerships might be facilitated and challenges better confronted by increased understanding.

Finally, and related to the first point, I hope the book might prompt conversations on these topics, on questions of what matters most in life, on questions of the health of the person and not just on questions of the health of the body. My view is that a Christian understanding of these topics, of health and well-being, helps guide us in promoting these ends and corresponds in some way, as best as we have understood it, to God's intent, and that this Christian understanding points us to truth. Likewise, those who disagree with Christian perspectives on these topics or come from other cultural, religious, or philosophical traditions or ways of thinking will often believe that their own understanding will help guide efforts to promote health and will provide a vision for human life that is grounded, as best as possible, in their understanding of the truth. The visions and the truth claims are not always reconcilable. However, by discussion, dialogue, and exchange of ideas, we are each often led to greater clarity about our own positions and a greater understanding of the positions of others. We thereby also have a greater capacity to find consensus. In addition, hopefully each person can gradually come to a better understanding of what is true. Toward the end of the book (part III, section 3.7i), I discuss how different individuals and different communities will often have different visions of the good, but how there is also often considerable overlap. Complete consensus in this life will not be attainable, but a collective pursuit of truth together, being more aware of and refining our common understandings and our disagreements, can, I believe, be of potential benefit to all. That collective pursuit of truth together on the most important questions requires a more frequent and a more explicit discussion of these matters, of what is most important, of what truly constitutes well-being, of how we understand the human person, and of the most ultimate ends. It is in this spirit that I offer up the reflections in this book, and it is for this reason that I hope the material may in part be of some interest to those who do not share the perspective of the Christian faith.

I suspect that some of my colleagues in public health may be surprised by the publication of this book. My primary role at the School of Public Health at Harvard has been, and in large part continues to be, as an epidemiologic methodologist. Although I hold a degree in philosophy and theology and have continued to read on both topics, I am certainly not a theologian by vocation, nor was I hired as one. And while I have not in any way hidden my faith, my engagement of that faith with matters central to public health has certainly never been as explicit as it is in this book. Although some of my empirical research has considered associations between participation in religious community and subsequent health and well-being, that work has not been carried out with an explicitly Christian theological perspective.

In this book, I more explicitly come to some of the central questions of health and public health with a distinctively Christian viewpoint. As I have carried out the empirical research on religious communities over the past years, I have come back time and again to the question of what, from religious understanding in general and from Christian theology in particular, is most relevant to public health and to the understanding of health. Community—religious and otherwise—is of course critical, but this is not the only idea or concept from Christian theology that seems of importance to public health. Christian theology makes regular appeal to concepts such as love and forgiveness, sin and injustice, restoration and salvation. The book is an attempt to lay out, drawing upon prior work in the Christian tradition, what I see as being of greatest relevance to public health and our understanding of health and well-being from a Christian perspective. I believe that bringing all perspectives to the table, including more personal and faith-based ones, is ultimately the best way to understand one another and to help one another come to an understanding of truth.

I am indebted to many people and institutions that have enabled and facilitated the writing of this book. I am grateful for the sabbatical granted by the Harvard T. H. Chan School of Public Health during the 2019–2020 academic year that provided the time to formally begin working on this manuscript. I am grateful to Balliol College and the University of Oxford for hosting me and my family for the Eastman Professorship that academic year, during which I wrote a first draft of the book. I am grateful to the many colleagues at Harvard University and elsewhere, especially those at the Human Flourishing Program and the Initiative on Health, Spirituality, and Religion who have, over the years, helped shape my thinking on these matters. The present text is about twice the length of the draft I completed while at Oxford. The expansion is due in no small part to the work of the Human Flourishing Program. I had been unable to work on the manuscript during the 2020–2021 academic year due to administrative responsibilities as acting director of the Population Health Sciences doctoral program at the T. H. Chan School of Public

Health. However, this delay gave time for the Human Flourishing Program's work on love and on community to expand substantially, and the final text has been enriched considerably by the insights that have emerged from that work. My colleagues Michael Balboni, Tracy Balboni, Howard Koh, and others at the Initiative on Health, Spirituality, and Religion at Harvard have provided ongoing support, inspiration, partnership, and collaboration. Early conversations with Michael and Tracy began to make the need for this work clear to me. Their friendship, encouragement, and thoughtfulness over the years has been, and continues to be, invaluable. The relationships between this book and the Health, Spirituality, and Religion Initiative and the Human Flourishing Program have been constantly mutually enriching for me and have continually shaped and refined my understanding of the health of the body and the health of the person. The work of the Initiative on Health, Spirituality, and Religion and my colleagues at that initiative gave birth to the idea for this book. Pondering these matters with those colleagues both gave rise to, and has subsequently been informed by, the formation of the Human Flourishing Program.

I am grateful for the many readers who commented on the near-final draft of this manuscript, including Edward Brooks, Brendan Case, Dominic Doyle, Lydia Dugdale, Fr. John Grieco, Jeffrey Hanson, Patrick Kelly, Warren Kinghorn, Tim Lomas, Katelyn Long, Elias Nosrati, John Peteet, Matthew Potts, Fr. Michael Rozier, Xavier Symons, and Wylin Wilson, along with several anonymous reviewers. Their collective insights have strengthened and enriched the book considerably, have pointed me to new ideas and additional material, and have kept me from a number of errors and omissions. While the errors have at least been reduced, there are surely others that remain, and the omissions, while fewer than before, are certainly quite considerable still. For these I take responsibility and offer my apologies, and I will correspondingly be grateful for the corrections and refinements yet to come. I am also grateful for the many who have contributed to these various topics in ways that I have been unable to document in this book. In many ways, the work of theology is a collective enterprise, with insights over time drawing upon, building upon, and integrating and refining those of the past. I am grateful therefore for the rich theological traditions of the Church, along with my own formation in it. Most of the present text is merely a weaving together of prior theological content with a selection of materials oriented toward the relation of that content to an understanding of health. I am grateful for funding support from the John Templeton Foundation, the Lee Family Fund, and endowment funds from the Harvard T. H. Chan School of Public Health that provided support for the time needed to write and complete this book. Finally, I am grateful for the support of friends and family, and especially for my wife, Lisa, whose patience, love, partnership, long-suffering, insight, and faith have both enabled and provided the foundation for the writing of this book on a theology of health. It is to her that this book is dedicated.

    Tyler J. VanderWeele
    Chestnut Hill, Massachusetts

PART I

HEALTH AND WHOLENESS

"Thou hast made us for thyself, O Lord"
(Augustine, 400/1991, book 1, section 1)

Propositional Outline of Part I:
Health is wholeness as intended by God.

1.0. Health can be understood as wholeness, either of the body or of the person.
1.1. The health of the person is complete physical, mental, social, and spiritual well-being.
1.2. The health of the body is constitutive of and contributes to the health of the person.
1.3. The complete person, body and soul, was created good by God as an integrated whole.
1.4. The complete health of the person includes wholeness of one's community.
1.5. The complete health of the person includes communion with God.
1.6. Health is the responsibility of the individual and the community but depends also on circumstances beyond the control of either.
1.7. The implications of health as wholeness.

Introduction

Health as Wholeness

Proposition 1.0. Health can be understood as wholeness, either of the body or of the person.

The etymology of the English word "health" is derived from Old English "*hælþ*," or wholeness. This relation of health to wholeness or soundness is also present in other languages.[1] To be whole is to be intact, to have all of the parts together, to be functioning as a thing ought to, to not be missing something essential, to conform to what a thing characteristically is. If something has a purpose, then wholeness entails that the thing is functioning well. To what extent can the idea of wholeness be used to understand health?

The concept of health has been the topic of considerable dispute.[2] Some of the dispute centers on the breadth of the concept. The World Health Organization defines health as "a state of complete physical, mental, and social well-being, and not merely the absence of disease or infirmity."[3] Many criticize this definition of health as being too broad.

---

1. The Spanish "*salud*" and the Italian "*salute*" derive from the Latin "*salūtem*," the accusative singular of "*salūs*," which is related to "*salvus*," which is ultimately from the Proto-Indo-European "*solh*," meaning "whole, complete." The French "*santé*" derives from the Latin "*sānitātem*," the accusative of "*sānitās*," meaning "health, soundness." The Greek "*hygia*" means "health, soundness." The German "*Gesundheit*" and the related Dutch "*gezondheid*" derive from the Middle High German "*Gesunt*," from the Old High German "*Gisunt*," which comes from the Proto-West Germanic "*Gasund*," a prefixed form of "*Sund*," from the Proto-Germanic "*Sundaz*," which comes from the Proto-Indo-European root "*swen*," meaning "sound."

2. The use of the word "health" pertains principally to living things, whereas "wholeness" is often used of things that are not living. However, even "health" is sometimes used metaphorically of nonliving things, as in expressions such as "the health of a car's motor" and in more ambiguous cases of corporate entities such as the "health of a community," to which I will turn further below.

3. WHO (1946).

The criticisms of the this definition of health include that it extends beyond the purview of medicine or expands the scope of medicine too far, that it seems to concern all of human well-being or provides a standard that is too demanding, that it is impossible to operationalize, that there will not be consensus on what constitutes well-being, and that it may lead to endless expansion of what are considered rights.[4] Many thus prefer a narrower definition of health that focuses principally on the body.

However, our everyday language seems to suggest uses of the word "health" that extend beyond the health of the body. We might say, for example, "Every day he just sits in his room. He is physically healthy, but he is not a healthy person." Here "not healthy" is used to indicate that something is not right or whole about the person, even though his body may be intact and functioning well.

Some of the disputes around health can be resolved by simply acknowledging that the word "health" is used in two related but distinct senses.[5] There is the narrower conception of health that is focused on the health, or wholeness, of the body. And there is the broader conception of health that we might refer to as the health of the person, or the wholeness of the person. These two concepts of health are interrelated. As will be developed further below, the health of the person is in part constituted by the health of the body. Moreover, numerous aspects of the health of the person, such as psychological well-being, often have effects on the health the body.[6] The relations between health of the body and health of the person are perhaps especially complicated when it comes to questions of mental health. The relations and distinctions between these are also important when trying to understand the scope and limits of medicine. These issues will be discussed further in sections I.2 and I.7.

---

4. For example, see Breslow (1972) on extending beyond medicine; Callahan (1973) and Huber et al. (2011) on expanding the scope of medicine too far; Saracci (1997) and Messer (2013) on extending to all well-being; Huber et al. (2011) and Garner (1979) on providing too demanding a standard; Bice (1976) on the absence of consensus on the meaning of well-being; Huber et al. (2011) on being impossible to operationalize; and Saracci (1997) on the endless expansion of rights.

5. Fagerlind et al. (2010); VanderWeele et al. (2019a).

6. For recent reviews of the empirical evidence of the effects of psychological well-being on physical health, see Martín-María et al. (2017), Hernandez et al. (2018), Trudel-Fitzgerald et al. (2019), and Steptoe (2019).

Rather than disputing whether "health" should be used in just one or the other of these broader or narrower senses, it can be acknowledged that in our ordinary language we use "health" in both of these senses, in different contexts. Greater clarity can be attained by acknowledging both uses, and then specifying, when relevant, whether the broader sense (health of persons) or narrower sense (health of bodies) of the concept of health is in view.[7]

However, even if we grant these distinctions, more questions and disputes about the definition of health arise. Some definitions are based on conformity to or lack of deviation from normality,[8] while others are based on some notion of functionality or the ability to achieve goals.[9] The former definitions are often viewed as more objective or value neutral than the latter.[10] Both approaches, however, confront challenges. Definitions based on normality face the difficulty of defining what such normality means or how one goes about determining it.[11] Definitions based on functionality must contend with the complexity of how the body or the person is to function. Whether objective standards for functionality exist or whether functionality is simply to be understood as the capacity to function as one desires or to achieve whatever goals one

---

7. Some of the proliferation of definitions of health are arguably attributable to trying to correctly place the concept of health somewhere along a spectrum between health of the body at one end and health of the person at the other. Various proponents argue that each end of the spectrum is too extreme for a definition of health, and proposals subsequently abound for more expansive conceptions of health that extend beyond health of the body while "avoiding the excesses of the WHO definition" (Messer, 2013, 11), i.e., the other end of the spectrum, the health of the person. Of course, countless proposals can be put forward that lie somewhere between these two ends of the spectrum (e.g., Fulford, 1993; Nordenfelt, 1995; Law and Widdows, 2008; Huber et al., 2011; Messer, 2013).

8. Boorse (1975) is considered the standard account of health defined in terms of "biostatistical normality." He also refers to the contribution of normality to the functions of survival and reproduction, but these functions are to be understood in a value-neutral way.

9. Kass (1975); Fulford (1993); Nordenfelt (1995); Law and Widdows (2008).

10. See Messer (2013) and Caspary (2010) for review, discussion, and critique from a theological perspective of some of the definitions and understandings of health that have been proposed in the philosophical, medical, and public health literatures. See also Brickenbach (2017) for discussion of these approaches within the context of the WHO definition of health.

11. Amundson (2000); Gammelgaard (2000).

decides upon is a contested issue.[12] The relation of values to functionality likewise continues to be an important issue of dispute, along with whether these values are objectively or subjectively grounded.[13]

Neither of these approaches to defining health is adequate without an account of what the human body or the human person is meant to be; that is, without some conception of its nature. Some of the disputes around the definition of health thus likely also pertain to competing understandings of human nature.

Theology has provided its own accounts of what constitutes human nature. Such accounts in Christian theology are grounded in God's intent for the human person and the human body in God's creation of it.[14] In such accounts, the wholeness of the human body or the wholeness of the human person concerns its conformity to God's intent.[15] That intent is constituted in part by the intended end, or purpose or goal, sought for its own sake, of the human body and human person. That end is God himself—as persons we are ultimately to be aiming for union with God. In the words of St. Augustine, "Thou hast made us for thyself, O Lord, and our heart is restless until it finds its rest in thee."[16]

---

12. Engelhardt (1974); Schramme (2007); Kovács (1998); Nordenfelt (2001).

13. Messer (2013); Mordacci (1995); Fedoryka (1997); Megone (1998); Wakefield (2000).

14. See, for example, chapter 3 of the *Compendium of the Social Doctrine of the Church* (Catholic Church, 2004) for an outline of one such account.

15. God's intent is not to be understood as something arbitrary or capricious, but rather as something rational and grounded in God's very being. God's intent for the human person can be discerned at least in part by reason and what follows from the nature of the human person. That which can be made evident by reason concerning the conduct of the human person is sometimes referred to as "natural law." The *Compendium of the Social Doctrine of the Church* describes natural law as "the light of intellect infused within us by God [by which] we know what must be done and what must be avoided" (Catholic Church, 2004, 140). It also notes that there is a relation between the natural law and God's being: "This law has been given by God to creation. . . . It consists in the participation in his eternal law, which is identified with God himself" (Catholic Church, 2004, 140).

16. Augustine (400/1991, book I, chapter 1). The rendering of Augustine's Latin "*fecisti nos ad te et inquietum est cor nostrum, donec requiescat in te*" as "Thou hast made us for thyself, O Lord, and our heart is restless until it finds its rest in thee" is common in many popular books and on websites but does not seem to appear in any major published translation of the *Confessions*. It is perhaps a conflation of Edward Bouverie Pusey's translation, "for Thou madest us for Thyself, and our heart is

In subsequent sections, an understanding from Christian theology of God's intent for the human person and the human body will be developed in greater detail. This section's focus is on the meaning of health, or wholeness. The grounding of the notion of health, of wholeness, in God's intent arguably resolves some of the aforementioned difficulties. It grounds normality in God's intent, since at some level, that intent is the same across persons, although, as discussed further below, discerning that intent is not necessarily straightforward. It provides content to what constitutes a well-functioning person, grounded principally in movement toward the person's final end in God. It furthermore provides some relation between normality-based and functionality-based notions of health: both are grounded in conformity to God's intent. These ideas will be developed further in the sections that follow.

The distinction between the health of the body and the health of the person helps us understand the persistence of conceptions of health that are conceived of as more objectively grounded, value-neutral accounts of health as those pertaining to the health of the body, and the accounts of health that are more value-laden concerning functionality and goals as those pertaining to the health of the person. We can see how understandings of the health of the person may vary by social and cultural context and even by individual circumstances.[17] However, from the perspective of Christian theology, even with health of a person, there is an objective reality to wholeness and to a person's final end, grounded in God's intent. That conformity to God's intent is also sometimes referred to in Christian theology as holiness.[18] Understood theologically, to be healthy is to be whole, to be in perfect conformity with God's intent.[19]

---

restless, until it repose in Thee," and Henry Chadwick's translation, "you have made us for yourself, and our heart is restless until it rests in you," with "O Lord" inserted for context.

17. Nordenfelt (2001).

18. Both "holy" and "wholeness" derive from the Proto-Indo-European "*kailo*," "whole, uninjured." Likewise, "health" derived from the Old English "*hælþ*," which derived from the Proto-Germanic "*hailitho*," from the Proto-Indo-European "*kailo*," "whole, uninjured" (see Hoad, 1986).

19. See also Pargament et al. (2022) for discussion, drawn principally from the psychological literature, on how wholeness and related notions of holiness form the foundation of religion's contributions to human flourishing.

Health as a perfect state of wholeness is an ideal, and, as will be discussed below and in part II, one that at present is only partially ever attained in this life. Health is always relative to that ideal. This too is reflected in our language. Although "health" in its primary sense refers to a state of wholeness, we also use "health" in a derivative sense to refer to the condition of a thing with respect to an ideal state of wholeness.[20] The use of "health" in its primary sense is reflected in statements such as "health is the consequence of a good diet." The use of "health" concerning the condition of a thing with respect to the ideal is reflected in statements such as "his health is poor" or "he is in good health." Although we desire the ideal state of perfect wholeness, it is only partially attained here and now. The relation between our experience here and now and the fulfillment of wholeness as God's ultimate intent is taken up in part III of the book.[21]

Propositional Summary 1.0: Health can be understood as wholeness, either of the body or of the person.

1.0a. Etymologically, the word "health" is related to wholeness.

1.0b. Wholeness is to be understood as a thing being as it is meant to be.

---

20. See, for example, the first two entries for "health" in the *Oxford English Dictionary*.

21. We might thus distinguish between God's intent for the human body and the human person in God's creation and God's ultimate intent for the human body and the human person. In many contexts, we might think of "health" as wholeness of the body or of the person as God intended in creation, here and now. And here and now, health is always imperfect, relative to the ideal. However, as part III of this book will discuss, from the perspective of Christian theology, God's intent is that eventually this wholeness will be brought to perfection and fulfillment and that it will be fulfilled in a way that extends even beyond God's initial creation. God's grace, or favor, ultimately will fulfill and perfect the human nature that was established in creation. This is captured well in Aquinas's often-cited phrase in the opening of the *Summa Theologica*, "grace does not destroy nature but perfects it" (Aquinas (1274/1920, I.1.8.ad 2; see also I.II.109.3, I.II.109.5, I.II.110.1). As discussed in part II of the book, that our wholeness here and now is imperfect even relative to God's intent in creation is because we have been created free and we can, and have, used that freedom in ways contrary to God's intent. However, we have been created free in order to be able to freely love. As discussed in part III of the book, the restoration and fulfillment of our wholeness comes from God's love and from an empowering of our capacity to love God and to love others. That God's grace allows for a perfecting and fulfillment of nature as established in creation enables us to more fully experience God's love.

1.0c. We have two distinct concepts of health: health or wholeness of the body and health or wholeness of the person.
1.0d. An understanding of wholeness requires some conception of the nature of a thing.
1.0e. In a theological understanding, the nature and end of the body and of the person are found in God's intent; health of the body and of the person are thus constituted by wholeness of the body and the person as intended by God.
1.0f. Health is always relative to an ideal.
1.0g. God's intent for wholeness may be understood with respect to the current created order or with respect to God's final intent.

I.1. The Health of Persons and Human Flourishing

Proposition 1.1. The health of the person consists of complete physical, mental, social, and spiritual well-being.

1.1a. The health of persons includes physical, mental, social, and spiritual well-being.

Health is wholeness, understood as wholeness of the person or as wholeness of the body. We will consider health understood in its narrower sense of wholeness of the body in the next section. Here we will consider health in its broader sense, the health or wholeness of the person.

Health or wholeness of a person might be understood theologically as wholeness in conformity with God's intent as to who and how that person should be. Attempting to discern God's intent is in no way straightforward and is in part the work of theology. It is the Christian belief that in the course of history, and most definitively in the person of Jesus Christ, God has communicated something of that intent and moreover that God's revelation of that intent, and God's self-communication, is contained in the Scriptures and in the transmission of and interpretation of God's revelation in the life of the Church. Theology then provides reflection upon the Christian Scriptures and the traditions of the Church, making use of reason and interpreting experience to try to make sense of reality and of God's intent.[1] There are of course also limits to such

---

1. This task of theology is in no way straightforward, and many theological questions remain open to dispute. It is the position of the Catholic Church (Catholic Church, 2000, 33–141) and of many Christian traditions that certain matters of theological doctrine are effectively settled, having been made clear by the writings of sacred Scripture and by the consistent teaching and theological reflection of the Church. This requires an understanding of Scripture and a belief that the theological reflection derived from it and from the transmission of Christian teachings are

reasoning and a need for humility in trying to discern that intent. There will always remain an element of mystery.²

The creation narratives the Scriptures begin with are an important source for discerning God's intent for the human person. There it seems that God's intent for each person and for all creation is that all aspects of being should be good.³ At the completion of the first creation narrative in Genesis, we read, "God saw everything that he had made, and indeed, it was very good" (Genesis 1). God's intent, actualized in creation, was that it would be good.⁴ As will be discussed in greater detail in part II of the

---

authoritative. However, even with such a stance, various other theological questions are open to dispute. Not all of theology and theological reflection is definitive doctrine, although reflection and systematic accounts of theology have informed and continue to inform the development of doctrine. One of the most comprehensive and systematic accounts of theology was Thomas Aquinas's *Summa Theologica* (Aquinas, 1274/1920) because of its extensive engagement both with Scripture and with a vast range of prior theological reflection. The account given here of a theology of health will engage extensively with, and draw heavily upon, Aquinas's *Summa Theologica*, although other sources will be used as well.

2. Although the *Summa Theologica* provides an extraordinary synthesis of theology, it also acknowledges mystery. The very first question in that work acknowledges that man's end in God "surpasses the grasp of his reason" (Aquinas, 1274/1920, I.1.1), that "we cannot know in what consists the essence of God" (Aquinas, 1274/1920, I.1.7.ad 1), and that "while [Scripture] describes a fact, it reveals a mystery" (Aquinas, 1274/1920, I.1.10). Yet the work defends theology and sacred doctrine as a science (Aquinas, 1274/1920, I.1.2–3). However, theology, as reasoned discourse about God, will always contain an element of mystery. God's nature and God's intent is far beyond full human understanding. Theology's task is to try to make sense, as best as possible with our limited understanding, of what we might say or know about God. An account of Aquinas's life comments that toward the end of his life, "St. Thomas Aquinas was celebrating Mass when he received a revelation that so affected him that he wrote and dictated no more, leaving his great work the 'Summa Theologiae' unfinished. To Brother Reginald's expostulations he replied, 'The end of my labors has come. All that I have written appears to be as so much straw after the things that have been revealed to me'" (Thurston and Attwater, 1990, 510). This conclusion, especially in light of the extraordinary synthesis of theology that he provided, points to the humility with which one is to approach the understanding of God's intent. Some degree of understanding is possible, but it must be kept in mind that our understanding in this life will always only ever be partial.

3. Aquinas (1274/1920, I.19.2, I.20.2).

4. In Aquinas's understanding (Aquinas 1274/1920) and other scholastic discussions of "transcendentals," being itself is good. All being has goodness insofar as it is created by God. Being and goodness coincide but differ in aspect, with goodness

book, that original goodness can be, and has been, disrupted by free actions contrary to God's intent. However, the intent was that all aspects of life and being would be good.

In some sense, the definition of health provided by the World Health Organization points toward a state in which all aspects of a person's life are good. As noted above, the World Health Organization's definition of health is "a state of complete physical, mental, and social well-being, and not merely the absence of disease or infirmity." The definition is broad and includes a person's well-being in its physical, mental, and social dimensions. Although the definition is sometimes critiqued for being too broad, the definition is not broad enough from a theological standpoint. It does not explicitly include any notion of spiritual well-being. If the health of a person is to include all aspects of one's being, then from the standpoint of Christian theology, this should include spiritual well-being. Several authors in considering the definition of health have thus also proposed a broadening of the World Health Organization's definition of health to include spiritual well-being, so that the health of a person would be understood as a "state of complete physical, mental, social, and *spiritual* well-being."[5] For all aspects of one's life to be good, one's relation to God—one's spiritual well-being—must also be good. The health of persons arguably includes their physical, mental, social, and spiritual well-being.[6]

---

constituted by being under the aspect of desirableness (Aquinas 1274/1920, I.5.1). Although beauty and goodness in a thing are fundamentally identical, beauty concerns a perception of goodness as due proportion by the cognitive faculties (Aquinas 1274/1920, I.5.4). All being has a beauty, although our capacity to recognize it may be limited.

5. Peng-Keller et al. (2022, 46), my emphasis; Larson (1996); Cloninger et al. (2010); VanderWeele (2017c). This expanded definition of health (of a person) as "complete physical, mental, social, and spiritual well-being" might be referred to as the "WHO+ definition" of health (VanderWeele and Lomas, 2023).

6. Lomas and VanderWeele (n.d.) proposed defining "well-being" as "a desirable state of quality." This might pertain to a person's physical, mental, social, or spiritual dimensions of existence and it thus becomes appropriate to speak of physical well-being as a "desirable physical state of quality," of "mental well-being" as a "desirable mental state of quality," etc. Complete human well-being could then be understood as a desirable state of quality with regard to all physical, mental, social, and spiritual dimensions of existence. Lomas and VanderWeele (n.d.) proposed defining health as "the attainment or realization of well-being" in any or all of these

1.1b. Health in its broadest sense, the wholeness of the person, is human flourishing, which can be understood as living in a state in which all aspects of a person's life are good.

That God's intent for the human person and for all creation was goodness suggests a way to understand the wholeness of the human person. Wholeness is attained when all aspects of a person's life are good. When the person is living in a state in which all aspects of their life are good, we might refer to that state as human flourishing.[7] This is effectively a state of complete health, or wholeness, of a person—a state of complete physical, mental, social, and spiritual well-being.[8] "Human flourishing"

---

dimensions, i.e., "the attainment or realization of a desirable state of quality." Lomas and VanderWeele (n.d.) proposed these definitions with the intent of trying to attain consensus outside a specific theological context. In these definitions, there is an intentional ambiguity in the notion that something is "desirable," which might be understood in a purely subjective sense (as to what is actually desired) or in an objective sense (as something that, from some ethical or metaphysical stance, is good or ought to be desired, irrespective of whether people actually desire it or not). The ambiguity was intentional to allow for both subjective and objective notions of well-being. These definitions also work within a Christian theological context if "desirable" is interpreted as "as intended or willed by God" and "quality" is used synonymously with "goodness." The definitions of Lomas and VanderWeele (n.d.), interpreted in an objective Christian theological context, then become, for well-being, "a state of goodness intended by God" and for health "the attainment or realization of a state of goodness intended by God," which can have, as its principal objects, either bodies or persons.

7. More precisely, flourishing, as an abstract noun, might be understood as "the state in which all aspects of a person's life are good" (VanderWeele, 2017b); flourishing, as a gerund or present participle, might be understood as "*living* in a state in which all aspects of a person's life are good" (VanderWeele, 2020c).

8. Although the terms "human flourishing" and "human well-being" are often used synonymously, one might draw a distinction between the two with the former term being somewhat more all-encompassing (VanderWeele and Lomas, 2023). If human flourishing constitutes "a state in which all aspects of a person's life are good," then this arguably includes the broader conditions and contexts that sustain such flourishing over time (see also sections I.4 and I.6 concerning the notion that flourishing also includes the concept that one's community is whole or good). One might then contrast human well-being, as "a state in which all aspects of a person's life are good *as they pertain to that individual*," with human flourishing, as "a state in which all aspects of a person's life are good (including the contexts in which that person lives)." Well-being concerns the individual; flourishing concerns both the individual and his or her context and community along with the conditions that sustain well-being. If a

might thus be understood synonymously with "complete health of a person." Such complete health of a person is an ideal and is at present only partially attainable. However, such a state of flourishing is God's intent.

This definition of health of a person or human flourishing as "a state in which all aspects of a person's life are good" could arguably be employed across traditions and need not be considered specific to the Christian faith.[9] However, how goodness is understood will of course vary across traditions, to some extent at least.

In this section and in the sections that follow, an understanding of flourishing or the health of a person that derives from a Christian understanding of goodness and of God's intent for the human person will be developed further. Goodness will be understood as attaining that which God intends. Thus, from a Christian perspective, human flourishing might be understood as living in "a state in which all aspects of a person's life are as intended by God." However, attention will also be given below to those aspects of the health of a person and to the domains of flourishing that are manifest as shared values across various religious and cultural traditions.[10] We will now turn to the question of what might

---

person is doing well within a corrupt system or an impoverished environment, we might say that although they have attained a certain degree of well-being, they are not fully flourishing. The term "flourishing" suggests a consonance between the person and the conditions, the community, and the environment in which he or she lives. In some sense, the distinction rests on how one interprets "social well-being," whether this is understood only as it pertains to that individual or with respect to the community as a whole and the conditions that sustain the entire community. Parallels might also be drawn here with the distinctions sometimes made between "individual" and "person" in personalist philosophy (Maritain, 1947; Burgos, 2018). See section I.4 for further discussion of how these distinctions relate to the common good. If one wanted to use the term "well-being" and also preserve these distinctions, then complete human well-being could be used synonymously with human flourishing, which would include social well-being understood in its broader sense, and the simpler term "human well-being" (i.e., not prefaced by "complete") might be used in reference to contexts in which social well-being is being understood in its narrower sense.

9. I originally put forward the definition of human flourishing, or complete human well-being, as a "state in which all aspects of a person's life are good" outside a theological context in a paper attempting to shape consensus on which aspects of well-being to focus on and measure in pluralistic contexts (VanderWeele, 2017a), although of course what precisely is understood by goodness will vary somewhat across traditions.

10. The commonalities in understandings of human flourishing might be understood as deriving in part from the "natural law"; i.e., the understanding from reason

be included in the expansive notion of flourishing in which all aspects of a person's life are good.

1.1c. Human flourishing consists in part in attaining happiness, bodily health, meaning, virtue, close relationships, good community, and spiritual well-being.

Numerous domains of human life are embedded in this conception of the health of a person, or human flourishing, as a state in which all aspects of a person's life are good. We might begin to understand these various domains of flourishing by considering the nature of the human person. Various domains of human flourishing may be understood as domains in which various aspects of a person's life are good. In the creation narrative, and in reflection upon the human experience, it seems that the human person was created by God to be (1) physical and embodied, (2) rational; (3) affective, with desire and emotion; (4) free and capable of action; (5) social and relational; and (6) spiritual. Goodness in life with respect to a person's being embodied might be described as bodily *health*. Goodness with respect to emotion and desire might be understood as *happiness*. Goodness with respect to a rational understanding of the world gives rise to an understanding of life's *meaning*. Goodness with respect to the will and free action constitutes *virtue*. Goodness with respect to the human person being a social creature manifests itself in *close relationships* and *good community*. And goodness with respect to the human person being a spiritual creature is constituted by a friendship with God, or *spiritual well-being*. We will briefly consider each of these in turn.

---

and from human nature itself, embedded to some degree in the thought of all people about what is right and wrong and what human life ought to consist of. Regarding its universality and thus also its potential to give rise to shared understandings of human flourishing, the *Compendium of the Social Doctrine of the Church* (Catholic Church, 2004, 140–142) notes, "The law is called 'natural' because the reason that promulgates it is proper to human nature. It is universal, it extends to all people insofar as it is established by reason. . . . Even when it is rejected in its very principles, it cannot be destroyed or removed from the heart of man. It always rises again in the life of individuals and societies. . . . Its precepts, however, are not clearly and immediately perceived by everyone."

Certainly, human flourishing, or health of the person, would include health of the body.[11] We are embodied, and the health of the person thus includes that the body is healthy. As described in the next section, the health of the body entails absence of disease and injury and that the body's parts and systems are intact and functioning so as to allow for the full range of activities characteristic of the human body. Although bodily health is undoubtedly a part of human flourishing, so also are numerous aspects of mental health. Mental health is sometimes understood as the absence of mental disorder and malfunction potentially related in certain ways to the brain, and in section I.2 below these relations will be considered in greater detail. The brain is of course itself a part of the body. However, the notion of complete mental well-being arguably includes not only the absence of mental distress and malfunction but also positive aspects of mental well-being.

Positive aspects of mental well-being include, among other things, happiness, including the experience of a certain goodness with respect to one's emotion and desires. Aristotle and Aquinas speak of happiness as the final end that all persons seek: happiness is that which is sought most of all for its own sake.[12] Aquinas understood happiness as a satisfaction

---

11. Many measures and conceptions of psychological well-being that have been put forward do not include physical health (VanderWeele, 2017a) and thus, while they may be reasonable approaches to *psychological* well-being, they should not be considered as capturing *human* well-being or flourishing more generally. See also section I.7h on psychological conceptions of well-being.

12. Aquinas (1274/1920, I.II.1.7); Aristotle (4th C BCE/1925, book I, chapter 7). Happiness in this more classical sense, as, say, a complete satisfaction of the will, encompasses but extends beyond happiness as conceived of in much of the psychology literature, which is arguably more akin to consistent experience of what Aquinas refers to as "delight" (Aquinas 1274/1920, I.II.31). Much of the psychology literature on happiness concerns either hedonic forms of feeling happy or evaluative forms of happiness that concern judgments that one has a happy or satisfying life (National Research Council, 2013). Unlike happiness as classically understood, not all action is necessarily aimed at attaining happiness in these narrower senses of hedonic and evaluative happiness. A more expansive understanding, arguably keeping in line with (although pushing the boundaries of) happiness as understood in psychology, might be taken as the *experience* of any state of quality or goodness (Lomas and VanderWeele, 2023). However, even this is arguably narrower than happiness as classically conceived. Happiness understood as the *complete* satisfaction of the will, as the ultimate and final end of life, toward which all other human action is oriented (Aquinas 1274/1920, I.II.1.6) is still greater in scope.

of the will and perfect happiness as the complete satisfaction of the will.[13] We can at present attain only an imperfect happiness in this life. When we attain something we desire, the will is satisfied and we are happy,

---

13. Aquinas (1274/1920, I.II.1.5). There is perhaps some resemblance between the view of perfect happiness constituted by the complete satisfaction of the will and desire-fulfillment theories of well-being (see Parfit, 1984), at least with respect to *perfect* well-being and *complete* satisfaction of the will. In Aquinas, the only way the will can be completely satisfied is by vision of the divine essence (Aquinas 1274/1920, I.II.3.8; Pieper, 1998). However, the fulfillment of desires more generally does not necessarily constitute well-being, since desires can be disordered. Fulfillment of properly ordered desires by rightly ordered means would contribute to one's well-being, as this would indeed be what is intended by God. Desire-fulfillment theories of well-being that refer to the desires a person would have if they were fully rational and fully informed (Brandt, 1979; Sidgwick, 1981; Railton, 1986) would come closer to the notion of flourishing from a Christian perspective, provided that those "fully rationally informed" desires were to be understood as deriving from God's perspective, i.e., having desires in alignment with God's intent. If this were so, all good as intended by God would be desired, and the fulfillment of those desires would be the attaining of the good intended by God. However, even then what makes the fulfillment of rationally informed desires constitute well-being is not principally the fulfillment of one's desire but the fulfillment of God's intent, and thus objections to even such knowledge-modified desire-fulfillment theories (e.g., Murphy, 1999) as not adequately describing what *grounds* well-being would arguably still pertain. Moreover, in the absence of perfectly formed desire, something could in principle be ultimately good for someone and in accord with God's intent without its being desired by that person. This is contrary to so-called hybrid theories (cf. Lauinger, 2013), which require that the good desired be constitutive of one's well-being. Nevertheless, as discussed further below with respect to character and virtue, having properly ordered desires is itself an important constitutive part of well-being. In the explanatory-enumerative categories employed by Fletcher (2013), perfectly rationally informed desire-fulfillment theories would thus be a correct enumerative theory of well-being that describes its content, but it would still not be a correct explanatory theory of well-being that provides the grounds of something being good. Both rightly ordered desires and the fulfillment of those desires are a part of the *content* of well-being. In contrast, conformity to God's intent is ultimately both what formally grounds well-being and what substantively specifies the content of well-being; it is both an explanatory and an enumerative theory. Well-being understood as the extent of conformity to God's intent might therefore also be understood as a type of, or perhaps rather as encompassing, a perfectionist theory of well-being (Hurka, 1993). Such perfectionist theories conceptualize well-being in terms of that which perfects an individual's nature. In the context of the theological understanding of flourishing given here, such perfection of human nature would be that in conformity with God's intent, although conformity to God's intent arguably pertains not just to human nature but also to various external goods such as adequate food or relationships.

temporarily at least. However, that happiness is often fleeting, as the desire for other things returns. Perfect happiness, Aquinas thought, was ultimately attainable only in relation to God.[14] Full flourishing—a state in which all aspects of one's life are good—however, would include happiness and ultimately also a complete satisfaction of the will, a perfect happiness, that we can only aspire to in this life. But that complete happiness is what we are ultimately seeking and what we achieve to an imperfect degree in this life. However, human flourishing includes the happiness we can attain in this life.

Understood in its broadest sense, complete mental well-being would also include having understanding and knowledge. An understanding of the ends we are pursuing (i.e., the goals sought for their own sake) and how we may attain them is important in attaining God's intent for the human person. In more contemporary terms, an understanding of one's end and the relation of oneself to that end and an understanding of the means to attain that end is sometimes referred to as having a sense of the meaning of life. An understanding of the significance of one's own activities in relation to that end is sometimes referred to as having a sense of meaning in life. The experience of the actual pursuit of that end and of the structuring of goals, actions, and identity so as to attain that end is sometimes referred to as having a sense of purpose. These various aspects of meaning and purpose are sometimes referred to as coherence for cognitive aspects, as significance for affective and evaluative aspects, and as purpose or direction for volitional aspects.[15] The health of a person includes having a sense of meaning and purpose.

From a Christian perspective, an understanding of God, of one's end in God, and how God's intent shapes one's understanding of life, the world, and all else would be a part of this system of meaning. For a person to be as intended by God, the person's cognitive, affective, and volitional orientation should be directed by and directed toward God.[16] For

---

14. Aquinas (1274/1920, I.II.3–5).

15. For a description of the emerging consensus within psychology on conceiving of meaning in these cognitive, affective, and volitional dimensions, see Martela and Steger (2016); George and Park (2016); and Hanson and VanderWeele (2021).

16. From the standpoint of Christian theology, coherence arguably finds its theological analogue in faith, purpose in hope, and significance in charity or love, the theological virtues discussed further below. However, the categories of coherence,

all aspects of a person's life to be good, a person's understanding and orientation must be good as well. The absence of such meaning and purpose will pose impediments to achieving one's end. Meaning might itself be understood as those aspects of knowledge that relate to one's origin and end and the relation of the world and one's activities to this.[17] Within Christian theology, that origin and end is God.[18]

If flourishing is understood as a state in which all aspects of a person's life are good, then for someone to be fully flourishing, their character should be good as well. Aristotle thought that happiness or flourishing consisted of action in accord with virtue,[19] virtue effectively being understood as habits in accord with reason to attain the good. Such habits would include those of the intellect, the will, one's behavior, and one's emotions. All of these are to be governed by reason to attain what is good, and from a Christian perspective, intended by God. In much of the Western philosophical work concerning virtue, four virtues in particular were thought to form the foundation of all other moral virtues. These four, sometimes called the cardinal virtues, were prudence, or practical wisdom; justice; fortitude, or courage; and temperance, or moderation.[20] These virtues were to rightly direct reason, the will and action, and emotion and desire.

---

purpose, and significance are conceptually broader than the theological virtues because these categories of coherence, purpose, and significance need not have God as their object.

17. It has been argued that the use of "meaning of life" with respect to the deepest and most fundamental questions of life is of relatively recent origin, arising in part because of the perceived loss of the sources of such meaning in abandoning traditional religious frameworks (Young, 2014). Prior to the introduction of the term "meaning of life" to refer to an understanding of life's most fundamental questions, this notion had sometimes been seen as the result of wisdom, or the habit of being concerned with the conclusions and ends of all knowledge, the setting in order of all of knowledge with respect to the highest cause; that is, God (Aquinas 1274/1920, I.II.57.2, II.II.45.1).

18. Aquinas (1274/1920, I.II.5).

19. Aristotle (4th C BCE/1925, book I, chapters 7–9).

20. Plato (4th C BCE/2004, book IV; wisdom 8:7); Pieper (1990); Aquinas, Albert, and Philip the Chancelor (2004). The origin of the concept of the cardinal virtues is generally traced to Plato and was adapted to the Christian tradition by Ambrose, Augustine, Aquinas and others. Ambrose is generally thought to have introduced the term "cardinal virtues," with the word "cardinal" deriving from "hinge." See Aquinas, Albert, and Philip the Chancelor (2004) for a brief history of ideas concerning the cardinal virtues from Plato through the medieval period.

Although precise definitions vary in nuance, an example of definitions of these four virtues from the catechism of the Catholic Church is as follows: "Prudence is the virtue that disposes practical reason to discern our true good in every circumstance and to choose the right means of achieving it.... Justice is the moral virtue that consists in the constant and firm will to give their due to God and neighbor.... Fortitude is the moral virtue that ensures firmness in difficulties and constancy in the pursuit of the good.... Temperance is the moral virtue that moderates the attraction of pleasures and provides balance in the use of created goods."[21]

Within Christian moral teaching, these four cardinal virtues are supplemented by the three so-called theological virtues—faith, hope, and love. These theological virtues direct a person to God; they perfect the intellect and the will, or desire; and they direct all other virtues to their final end of communion with God.[22] We will consider these theological virtues further in section I.5. However, if flourishing is living in a state in which all aspects of one's life are good, then this will entail good character and virtuous action as well.

God also intended human people to be relational. In the creation stories of Genesis, we read God's pronouncement that "it is not good that... man should be alone" (Genesis 2). For all aspects of one's life to be good, one's relationships should be good also. Thus, flourishing is constituted in part by good relationships. Good relationships require each person to understand the other, to appreciate the other's being, to take time to be with the other, and to seek the good of the other. This should pertain to individual relationships, but social well-being is also such that a person's relations with and in various communities should themselves be good. As will be discussed further below in section I.4, God's intent for the human person effectively extends beyond the person as an individual and toward that person being embedded in communities that are themselves good. God's intent for the person concerns who that person is, but it also concerns the person's relationship with the community and even the broader creation. If all aspects of a person's life are to be good, then one's community should be good or whole as well.

---

21. Catholic Church (2000, 1806–1809).
22. Aquinas (1274/1920, I.II.62; II.II.23).

In Christian theology, the importance of relationships and community can also be seen in the emphasis given to love. Love is given a central place not only in relationships but also with respect to moral teaching. Jesus summarized the whole of the law as "You shall love the Lord your God with all your heart, and with all your soul, and with all your mind. This is the greatest and first commandment. And a second is like it: You shall love your neighbor as yourself" (Matthew 22). Likewise, in St. Paul's Epistle to the Galatians, he writes, "For the whole law is summed up in a single commandment, 'You shall love your neighbor as yourself'" (Galatians 5:14). And in his first Epistle to the Corinthians, he writes, "If I give away all my possessions . . . but do not have love, I gain nothing" (1 Corinthians 13). Love here, and in the Christian tradition more generally, is understood not as a sentimental feeling but as a seeking of the good of the other, both the good for the other and the good that is constituted by the other, by being with the other.[23] This centrality of love points to the centrality of relationships in flourishing. Good relationships are necessary for a state of wholeness in which all aspects of a person's life are good.

The centrality of love, understood in the Christian sense, pertains not only to relationships with others but also to relationship with God. "You shall love the Lord your God with all your heart, and with all your soul, and with all your mind" (Matthew 22:37). A state of full health, of wholeness, of flourishing, in which all aspects of one's life are good, entails right relation with God. That relation with God, described sometimes as communion or love or charity or friendship with God, is central to human well-being.[24] God's intent is that we would be in communion with him. This too is part of the wholeness of a person, and indeed, from the perspective of Christian theology it is the most central. Within the Christian tradition, the final end of the human person is often described as some form of communion with God.[25]

We might thus describe the health of the person, or *human flourishing*, as a state in which all aspects of a person's life are good, which from the perspective of Christian theology might be understood as all aspects

---

23. Aquinas (1274/1920, I.II.26.4); Stump (2006).
24. Aquinas (1274/1920, II.II.23).
25. Aquinas (1274/1920, I.II.1–5); Westminster Assembly (1647/2014); Catholic Church (2000).

of a person's life being as intended by God. *Eternal flourishing*, or perfect well-being, understood as the attainment of the final end of the human person, is complete communion with God. *Spiritual well-being* in this life might be understood as a state in which one's life is oriented toward eternal flourishing or as a state in which all aspects of a person's life are good with respect to his or her final end in God. Temporal well-being, or *temporal flourishing*, might then be understood as concerning all aspects of human flourishing that pertain to the goods in this life, including happiness and life satisfaction, physical and mental health, meaning and purpose, character and virtue, and close social relationships and good community.[26]

Thus understood, full human flourishing encompasses both spiritual and temporal well-being, with spiritual well-being, from a Christian perspective, being most central—that which brings a person to his or her final end of communion with God. Although spiritual well-being leading to eternal flourishing might thus be understood as the highest or most important good,[27] other goods, such as health and meaning and social relationships, also constitute their own distinct ends. They are perhaps also means to attaining the highest end, but they are also ends in and of themselves.[28] God's original intent was that the human person would flourish both in this life and more fully eternally with God. However, as discussed in section I.5 below and in parts II and III of this book in greater detail, because of sin and fallenness, these aspects of temporal and eternal flourishing can now come into conflict.[29] From the perspective

---

26. I have discussed these proposed definitions and their interrelations at greater length elsewhere (VanderWeele, 2020c), and these issues will also be considered further in subsequent sections of the book.

27. Sometimes referred to as "a superordinate good"; Aquinas (1274/1920, I. II.1.5, 3.8, 5.8); cf. Oderberg (2004).

28. Aquinas argues that health and other aspects of flourishing are to be directed to their final end in contemplation: "Likewise to this act [of contemplation] all other human activities seem to be directed as to their end. For to the perfection of contemplation there is requisite health of body; and all artificial necessaries of life are means to health. Another requisite is rest from the disturbing forces of passion: that is attained by means of the moral virtues and prudence. Likewise rest from exterior troubles, which is the whole aim of civil life and government" (Aquinas 1265/2014, 1.3.37).

29. From the standpoint of perfectionist explanatory theories of well-being (Hurka, 1993), wherein well-being is conceptualized in terms of that which perfects

of Christian theology, spiritual well-being and the pursuit of eternal flourishing are to be prioritized.[30] However, all other aspects of life are relevant and important for an account of human well-being and temporal flourishing. Human flourishing consists in part of attaining happiness, bodily health, meaning, virtue, close relationships, good community, and spiritual well-being.

1.1d. Various domains of human flourishing in fact constitute shared values across different traditions.

We have considered various aspects of flourishing, or the health of a person, including bodily health, happiness, meaning and purpose, character and virtue, close relationships, good community, and spiritual well-being.[31] These domains of flourishing are, for the most part, present in other religious and cultural traditions. Although the understanding of spiritual well-being will perhaps vary most dramatically across traditions, this may be less so with the various other domains. The other aspects of flourishing considered here—including happiness, health, meaning, virtue, and relationships—arguably are also shared by other traditions, religions, and cultures. Each of these various domains of human life arguably constitutes its own end. Flourishing in each of these domains is also almost universally desired. There can thus perhaps be considerable consensus around the pursuit of these ends.[32] The implications of the potential consensus that can be attained concerning human

---

an individual's nature, there can be conflict with respect to the perfecting of that nature from the temporal versus eternal standpoints. As discussed further in parts II and III, suffering and the loss of certain temporal goods can be a means to greater spiritual perfection. Even the intentional giving up of pleasures, honors, and material stability can be a means to greater spiritual perfection (Aquinas 1274/1920, I. II.108.4).

30. See also section I.5a.

31. As per section I.1a, we might understand human flourishing as consisting of a person's physical, mental, social, and spiritual well-being. Physical well-being is partially constituted by bodily health. Mental well-being might be subdivided into well-being concerning the heart, the will, and the intellect, which are themselves respectively partially constituted by happiness, virtue, and meaning. Social well-being is constituted by good relationships and good community, and spiritual well-being is constituted by good relationship with God.

32. VanderWeele (2017a).

flourishing are explored further in section I.7. How meaning and purpose or virtue are precisely understood may of course vary across traditions, but there is also considerable common ground as well, and that they are important is nearly universally recognized.[33] In contrast, the understanding of spiritual well-being is more differentiated across various religious or spiritual traditions.[34]

The wholeness of a person, or human flourishing, understood as a state in which all aspects of life are good, is expansive in scope. We have touched upon several central dimensions or domains of flourishing here, including happiness, bodily health, meaning, character, relationships, good community, and spiritual life. The list is not exhaustive. Other aspects could be included as well, such as aesthetic experience or knowledge considered more broadly. Attempts have been made to provide exhaustive lists[35] of the basic goods of human life.[36] Many of these basic

---

33. Dahlsgaard et al. (2005).

34. Although many of the world's religious and cultural traditions give importance to some notion of spiritual well-being, this will often be understood in ways that are different from one another and different from the Christian understanding. Traditions such as Buddhism in which a deity is not in general part of the understanding of the tradition's various practices and ends will certainly not conceive of spiritual well-being, or of the end of the human person, as the pursuit and attainment of communion with God. The present book is intended to develop a Christian theology of health, and while it is hoped that a considerable part of the development will be applicable across traditions, spiritual well-being is one domain of flourishing for which consensus will be less substantial, although there may be some common ground across traditions.

35. Finnis (2011), for example, gives as a list practical reflection, life, knowledge, play, aesthetic experience, sociability (friendship), practical reasonableness, and religion. Murphy (2001) gives a similar but slightly different list: life, knowledge, aesthetic experience, excellence in play and work, excellence in agency, inner peace, friendship and community, religion, and happiness. See Oderberg (2004) for a description and evaluation of additional lists from natural law theorists; see Alkire (2005) for a variety of lists from various other disciplines (principally social science) with varying levels of theoretical underpinning. It should be noted that the category of objects these various lists describe is not always identical and includes, e.g., "basic goods" (Oderberg, 2004) or "basic forms of human good" (Finnis, 1980), "central human capabilities" (Nussbaum, 2001), "dimensions of well-being" (Narayan, 2000), "domains of flourishing" (VanderWeele, 2017a), "human values" (Schwartz, 1994), and "axiological categories" (Max-Neef, 1992).

36. So-called objective list theorists concerning the concept of well-being characteristically conceive of well-being as the attaining of some list of goods that are

goods have been touched upon in the previous section as well, although sometimes with different terminology.[37] However, a difficulty with the claim that a list is exhaustive concerns adequate coverage of the conceptual space related to *all aspects* of a life being good.[38] It is arguably not possible to exhaustively enumerate all of the potential goods that might be included within the concept of human flourishing. The list of domains of human life considered above—happiness and life satisfaction, mental and physical health, meaning and purpose, character and virtue, close social relationships, good community, and spiritual well-being—is not intended to be exhaustive. Rather, the list includes various important aspects of physical, mental, social, and spiritual well-being that are important and around which some consensus could be attained owing to their being ends sought for their own sake and the fact that they

---

viewed as objectively good; see Fletcher (2015) for an overview of such accounts. Likewise, natural law theory often attempts to ground morality in terms of the pursuit of what is sometimes considered an exhaustive list of basic goods (Finnis, 1980; Murphy, 2001).

37. One difficulty with attempts to make exhaustive lists of objective goods for human flourishing is determining what is included in each domain or within the purview of each basic good and how exactly to categorize them. This pertains both to potentially overlapping content among the goods considered and to how finely to divide the categories. Are "life" and "health" the same basic good or are they distinct? Does "health" as a basic good include mental health or is mental health more akin to happiness or emotional well-being? Does having a sense of meaning fall under knowledge or is it something different? Should knowledge or the virtue of "science" (Aquinas 1274/1920, I.II.57.2) be considered a part of virtue or as a separate category? Should the moral and intellectual virtues be divided from one another? Should meaning and purpose be distinguished from one another? Some of these questions are taken up further in sections I.2 and I.6. However, there are arguably different ways to divide the conceptual space, and it is challenging to do so in a way that includes all aspects of well-being. Arguably for an objective list theory of well-being to be fully adequate—to correspond to *all* aspects of a person's life being good—the list in question would have to be infinite or include categories that are effectively infinite in scope. Any finite list would only ever constitute a partial characterization, although perhaps one that from a practical standpoint is mostly adequate.

38. Alternatively, one could simply define flourishing as attainment of a specific list of basic goods, but difficulties arise with respect to different lists employed by different authors and the possibility that the list of goods will be attained by someone who claims that they are not fully flourishing because some other aspect of life is not good.

are nearly universally desired.[39] These two criteria of being an end and being nearly universally desired might be used to help shape consensus across cultures and traditions about what to jointly pursue in the context of a pluralistic society.[40]

---

39. Arguably, discrepancies across different lists arise in part from different criteria being employed with respect to deriving lists of "basic goods." The criteria of being universally desired and constituting an end (VanderWeele, 2017a) were originally proposed to help broaden consensus about which aspects of well-being to promote and measure in pluralistic contexts. However, different criteria concerning what might be considered "basic goods" will of course give rise to different lists. Oderberg (2004), for example, also considers a criterion of the use of a particular human faculty and a criterion of intrinsic goodness, something being "good in itself." Thus, while knowledge of truth cannot be bad in itself (although it can be used for bad purposes or acquired by bad means), one might have bad purposes. Of course, one could embed this requirement of being "good in itself" into the description of the basic goods. Thus, friendship, conceived in an Aristotelean sense of "friendship of virtue" (Aristotle, 4th C BCE/1925, book VIII) is good by definition. Likewise, one could, in principle, specify basic goods, or domains of flourishing, as "good purposes" or "good character" or "good relationships," etc.

40. These criteria of being nearly universally desired and being an end, along with the five domains of happiness, health, meaning, character, and relationships, were initially put forward to try to broaden consensus around what to promote and measure with respect to well-being (VanderWeele, 2017a). A brief empirical assessment of well-being was proposed with two questions asked in each of these five domains, along with a two-question assessment of financial and material stability as important means to sustain these other ends over time. The questions were drawn primarily from those already in widespread use in the well-being literature with some degree of empirical validation. The measure has been employed in numerous cross-cultural contexts (Węziak-Białowolska et al., 2019; Höltge et al., 2023). Concerning assessment, arguably what is important to evaluate is not simply purpose, character, and relationships but also good purposes, good character (e.g., virtue), and good relationships, as per the prior footnote. Conceptions of what constitutes such goodness, for character, say, may of course vary across traditions, but there is also considerable common ground (Dahlsgaard et al., 2005). In the empirical assessments, the idea that purpose or character were in fact *good* was at least indirectly present in the wording of some of the questions. Of course, accurate evaluation of whether character, purposes, or relationships are good requires a certain practical wisdom or capacity for judgment, and there are thus limitations to self-reporting in evaluating these matters accurately. However, even in domains such as character and virtue, which may seem particularly problematic to self-assess, self-reported assessments of character are reasonably well correlated with other types of assessments (Fowers, 2014) and also highly predictive of other aspects of subsequent flourishing (Weziak-Bialowolska et al., 2021).

In summary, the health of a person in its broadest sense can be defined as human flourishing, a state in which all aspects of one's life are good. This entails complete physical, mental, social, and spiritual well-being. Such human flourishing is an ideal, and the scope of the notion is vast. It includes but is not limited to happiness, bodily health, meaning, virtue, close relationships, good community, and spiritual life.

Propositional Summary 1.1: The health of the person is complete physical, mental, social, and spiritual well-being.
- 1.1a. The health of persons includes physical, mental, social, and spiritual well-being.
- 1.1b. Health in its broadest sense, the wholeness of the person, is human flourishing, which can be understood as living in a state in which all aspects of a person's life are good.
- 1.1c. Human flourishing consists in part in attaining happiness, bodily health, meaning, virtue, close relationships, good community, and spiritual life.
- 1.1d. Various domains of human flourishing in fact constitute shared values across different traditions.

I.2. The Health of the Body

Proposition 1.2. The health of the body is constitutive of and contributes to the health of the person.

1.2a. Bodily health is constituted by the body's parts and systems being and functioning as normal so as to allow for the full range of activities characteristic of the human body.

In the previous section, we considered the health or wholeness of the human person. Here we will focus on health in its narrower sense—the health or wholeness of the body—but will also consider its relation to the health or wholeness of the person.

A healthy body, understood as the wholeness of the body, a body that is intact, is functioning, and is fulfilling its intended purpose. From a theological standpoint, a healthy or whole body is the body as God intends, but understanding that intent for the body is perhaps a more subtle question than the question of God's intent for the person as a whole. Grounding the definition of "health of the body" in terms of wholeness as intended by God in some sense resolves various conceptual problems concerning health, such as defining normality, by referring to God's intent as the objective standard, but this does not resolve the epistemic problem of knowing precisely what that intent is. This we can arrive at only through some combination of inference, which might include, for example, theology and teleology and empirical study (anatomy and physiology, for example). God created the human person as a physical material being. God's intent for the body can perhaps be inferred in part indirectly by repeated observation of what the body is characteristically capable of and how it characteristically operates.

We might conceive of health or wholeness of the body as being constituted by *the body's parts and systems being and functioning as normal so as to allow for the full range of activities characteristic of the human body*. As noted in the introductory section above, many definitions of health emphasize either normality[1] or functioning[2] or both. Normality and functioning are both important parts of the definition just provided. They are essentially referenced twice, first with regard to the normal function of the body's systems and parts and second with regard to what the body is characteristically capable of.

For the body to be whole, its systems and parts need to be intact and be functioning as they ordinarily do. Characterizing those systems and their function is part of the aim of the disciplines of anatomy and physiology. Through the study of bodily systems over time and with many individuals, the characteristic operation and function of those systems can be discerned. Whether a particular part or system is normal or intact depends in part on understanding its function and the consistency of that function across different individuals. A consistency of being and of proper function in part constitutes what is normal. One aspect of normality within this conceptualization of bodily health is this normality of the bodily systems and parts and their functions. These systems should be coordinated and operational in such a way that the body is capable of the range of functions and activities that are characteristic of the human body. Discernment of the typical range is formed from repeated observations across time and across many individuals. Importantly, for health or wholeness of the body, it must be the case both that its systems and parts are normal and functioning and that the body is capable of the range of functions it characteristically has.

A departure from normality of the systems and parts or restriction of the characteristic range of activities of the body constitutes a departure from full bodily health. Thus, a person who is not diseased or injured and whose systems are, for the time being, operating as they ought to but who has eaten too much and is obese and whose movements are severely restricted would not be considered to be in a state of full bodily health. This is not simply because the person's risk of future disease is higher but because of the limits to physical function. Conversely, someone who, unknown to him or her, is at the very earliest stages of colon cancer but whose physical function and activities are still effectively

---

1. Boorse (1975).
2. Kass (1975); Fulford (1993); Nordenfelt (1995); Law and Widdows (2008).

wholly unrestricted would still not be considered to be in a state of full bodily health because even though the person's body is entirely functional, the incipient disease is already present. Wholeness of the body requires both normality, including good function of the body's systems and parts, and the good functioning of the body as a whole.

Health, understood as wholeness of the body, entails that the body's physical systems and the body as a coordinate whole are functioning as they ought to. This is different from *persons* functioning as they ought to, or as they would like to. The body's functioning can be an important element for the person's functioning, but neither of the two is reducible to the other. The body can be whole, but the person may still be lonely. Conversely, even someone who is crippled or struggling with cancer may be functioning reasonably well, all things considered, as a person in the circumstances.[3]

Disease or injury, however, is a departure from the body's proper functioning and a departure from normality. This necessarily implies that the body is not entirely whole. As will be discussed further in part II, a deviation from normality in the proper functioning of systems can be the result of external pathogens that disrupt function, an internal malfunction of cellular processes, or external injury. A disease or an injury *of the body* as experienced *by the person* is what is referred to as illness or an injury *for the person*. The absence of disease does not necessarily imply the health or wholeness of the person, as indeed the WHO definition of health makes clear. However, disease or injury does not necessarily imply that the person is not generally well-functioning; again, it only indicates at least some lack of wholeness with regard to the body and the person.

As will be discussed in greater detail in section I.2f, part of normal function of the human body is reproductive in nature. The reproductive system is one of the many systems of the human body; its purpose is

---

3. Disability perspectives on health (Amundson, 2000; Merriam, 2009; Sulmasy, 2009) in some sense rightly insist that it is possible to attain relatively full flourishing (health as a person) even in the presence of physical impairment and that the capacity to be able to do so is in part shaped both by society's structuring of life and by its preconceptions and perceptions about the nature of disability. See Messer (2013) for helpful theological evaluation of disability perspectives on health; see also section I.7k for further discussion.

procreation. Although the reproductive functions of the body for men and for women differ, they operate in unison in their capacity to reproduce. What is healthy, what is normal, and what constitutes proper function for the body will thus differ for men and women. Both the differences and the union and coordination are important in understanding the health or wholeness of the body. Reproduction is the one bodily function for which such coordination across persons is necessary. The differences, potential union, and necessary coordination all also point to the social nature of the human person, which will be considered further in section I.4.

1.2b. The health of the body constitutes and contributes to the health of the person, or human flourishing.

The health of the body is an important aspect of human flourishing, of the health or wholeness of the person. If all aspects of a person's life are to be good, a person's bodily health must also be good. Human flourishing is constituted in part by physical health. It would be odd to say that someone were fully flourishing if they were bedridden or physically incapacitated by disease. Such a person may still be flourishing in various other ways, but they would not be fully flourishing physically. The health of the body thus constitutes one important dimension of the health of the person.

Moreover, bodily health also contributes to human flourishing causally. It can enable flourishing. Full bodily health gives the person a capacity to carry out a variety of activities and pursuits, to move about freely, to pursue various purposes, to be with and interact with others and form relationships.[4] When the body is functioning well, it gives what some authors have called a vitality, a plenitude, or "strength for life" to the person.[5] In some sense, this might be viewed as the contribution of the health of the body to the health of the person.

Various other important goods and ends can be, and are, pursued even with imperfect or severely impaired bodily health, but such poor bodily health will, in general, constitute an impediment. In general, good

---

4. Aquinas argues that "the perfections that preserve a thing in its species, as health and nutrition, though they perfect the animal, are not the end of its existence, but rather the other way about" (Aquinas, 1265, 1.3.26).

5. Barth (1961); Mordacci (1995); Messer (2013).

bodily health allows more easily for the pursuit of other goods and ends. As will be discussed at greater length in parts II and III of the book, important exceptions arise wherein poor bodily heath may in fact facilitate the formation of character or strengthen relationships or clarify one's most important purposes. Approached in the right manner, ill health or suffering may have such effects, perhaps even often.[6] However, in most cases, and as initially intended by God, bodily health enables human flourishing, the pursuit of the state in which all aspects of a person's life are good.

Not infrequently, we neglect to fully appreciate the important role bodily health plays in human flourishing. We often take physical health for granted and think of it more regularly only in its absence or when it is threatened. We sometimes become especially aware or cognizant of the body only when we are ill or in pain.[7] However, bodily health, the wholeness of the body, was the state in which God created man and woman. It is God's intent for the body, and it constitutes and enables human flourishing.

1.2c. Bodily health includes the health of the brain, which shapes, though does not fully encompass, mental health—the wholeness of the mind.

Bodily health includes the health of the brain: one that is intact, is functioning as it ought to, and enables the body to function as it ought to. The brain is part of the nervous system, one of the central physical systems that allows the human body to function. A healthy body requires a well-functioning brain. The brain also powerfully influences other aspects of the health of persons. Its functioning shapes the physical, mental, social, and spiritual life of an individual. We will return to some of these mutual influences further in section I.3.

However, as will be discussed below, complete mental health arguably extends beyond the health of the brain and bodily health. If health is to be understood as wholeness, then mental health might be understood as wholeness of the mind, which may be understood either in a narrow

---

6. We might thus distinguish between God's original intent for the body and the intent for the body under the circumstances of sin and the fall, which will be taken up in parts II and III of the book.

7. Gadamer (1996, chapter 5).

sense, as pertaining to the proper functioning of the brain, or in a broad sense, as pertaining to the wholeness of the person. However, even in its narrower sense, mental health arguably extends beyond the health of the brain. It is strongly influenced by the health of the brain but not identical to it.

The distinctions between the mind and brain and between mental health and the health of the brain are reflected in the differing language we use concerning the body versus the person. The body is understood as constituted by all physical aspects of the person, all of the bodily systems and parts. The person is understood as constituted by the entirety of an individual's being. It is the person who acts, who feels, who thinks. The body and the brain may be essential in those processes, but we do not generally speak of *bodies* acting. Our language preserves these distinctions.[8] For example, when speaking of the body, we might say, "His arm went up," but when speaking of the person, we would say, "He raised his arm." These are the same events, but the first is a description of a movement of the body; the second of an act of a person. We do not ascribe agency to bodies in the same way that we do to persons. It would be odd, for example, to say, "His body raised his arm." A materialist who thought that there was nothing beyond the physical world might nevertheless still grant the distinction; it is embedded in our language. Even if all mental processes were ultimately entirely dependent upon physical processes, our speech is still such that we employ these different descriptions. Analogously, it is the person, rather than the body, that thinks and feels.

The mental might be seen as being constituted by the range of descriptions that do not apply to physical entities and processes. The mind might be understood as the nonmaterial aspect of the human person. The soul of a person is sometimes spoken of in a similar manner, as the nonmaterial aspect of the human person or sometimes as the "form of the body."[9] Sometimes the words "soul" and/or "spirit" are used specifically with reference to those aspects of the human person that pertain to relations with God. There is considerable variation in the theological literature, and elsewhere, in how these terms are employed.[10] What can be

---

8. Hacker (1996); Kenny (1976); Wittgenstein (1953).

9. Aquinas (1274/1920, I.75.5); Catholic Church (2004, 129).

10. In Aquinas, the soul is the first principle of life and the form of the body (see Aquinas 1274/1920, I.75–76). The relation between body and the mind or soul has

affirmed is that certain distinctions can be drawn between the body and mind, but also that there is an integrated whole, the human person.[11] This unity of the human person will be discussed further in section I.3.

What seems clear is that bodily health includes the health of the brain. The health of the brain affects mental health as understood in its broad sense, as pertaining to human persons, and in its narrower sense, as wholeness of the mind pertaining to the proper functioning of the brain. As a bodily organ, the brain is central to bodily health and powerfully shapes mental health and other aspects of a person's life. These relations and distinctions will be developed further in the following section.

1.2d. Mental health may be understood as the wholeness of the mind, either in a narrower sense, as pertaining to the proper functioning of the brain, or in a broader sense, as pertaining to the wholeness of persons.

The concept of mental health, like health more generally, is subject to a number of different understandings. Some, although not all, of the disputes over the concept of mental health may arise in part because not just one but perhaps several distinct concepts may be in play in the different contexts in which the term "mental health" is used, depending in part on to what extent health is understood as referring to the body.

If health is to be understood as wholeness, then mental health might be understood as wholeness of the mind—the mind's being and functioning as it ought to. Viewed as such, this would be the expansive concept of complete mental well-being.[12] Mental health, understood in an

---

been a perennial question in philosophical and theological writings. Different Christian authors envision the human person either in more unitary or more dualistic terms (or even occasionally in tripartite terms, distinguishing between the soul and/or the spirit).

11. See also Fulford et al. (2006) and Moreira-Almeida et al. (2018) for discussions of mind-body questions as they relate to mental health and psychiatry.

12. In what follows, the term "mental health" (in the broad sense, as pertaining to the person) will be used synonymously with "mental well-being" as a state in which all aspects of a person's mental life are good. The term "mental ill health" (in its broad sense) will be used to refer to any lack of mental well-being. However, below, distinctions will be made between such mental ill health and more severe mental illness.

unqualified sense as the wholeness of the mind, would then arguably include all aspects of psychological well-being and various aspects of social and spiritual well-being. It would not include all aspects of flourishing because it would not include all aspects of physical health (or of social or spiritual well-being), but its conceptual coverage would be broad. This is a broader conception of mental health than is often employed in clinical contexts.

We might contrast this broader understanding of mental health with a narrower understanding of mental health as wholeness of the mind as it pertains to the right functioning of the brain.[13] The concern here is still with the wholeness of the mind—whether the mind is in some sense operating as it ought to—but now restricted to wholeness (or the lack thereof) that might arise from proper functioning (or malfunctioning) of the brain.[14] Delineating the boundaries of such a conception of mental health as pertaining to functioning of the brain is no doubt complex. However, the scope of such a conception is clearly considerably narrower than the broader conception of complete mental well-being considered above.

Bereavement presents an interesting case when contrasting these broader and narrower conceptions of mental health. In the normal course of bereavement, it might take a person many months to substantially

---

13. More precisely, we will define mental health (in the narrow sense, as it pertains to the body) as "no lack of wholeness of the mind arising from malfunction of the brain." As will be discussed below, in some sense, much lack of wholeness of the mind in fact can come from a well-functioning brain, one that perceives what is negative in one's environment and responds accordingly. This would still constitute having good mental health in its narrower sense of no lack of wholeness of the mind arising from malfunction of the brain, but not mental health in the broader sense of unqualified complete wholeness of mind; i.e. of mental well-being.

14. So-called normative or constructivist perspectives on mental illness understand mental disorders more as value-laden constructs, whereas naturalist or objectivist perspectives see them more as biological phenomena; see Kendler (2016) for further discussion. There is an analogy here to the normality versus functionality views of health discussed in sections I.0 and I.2a. Both are arguably relevant (cf. Wakefield, 1992, on "harmful dysfunction"). See also Stein et al. (2021) for further discussion of how both psychobiological malfunction or dysfunction and "harm" (negative mental experience) are relevant in considering mental disorders, along with discussion of a number of exemplar cases in which these considerations are relevant.

adjust to the loss, say, of a spouse. There will be times of intense sadness, perhaps sometimes a sense of meaninglessness, routines will be disrupted, energy levels and interest in life's ordinary activities may be low, and there may be moments of extreme anguish. Understood from the context of the person, we might say the grieving widow or widower is not in a good state of mental health. However, viewed from the perspective of the proper operation of the body and brain, we might say that the brain is indeed properly functioning: there has been a real loss and change and the neurological processes are in fact helping bring about a new understanding, a new equilibrium, and a new way of life for the individual and helping them accommodate what have been dramatic changes. The brain's operation is facilitating, not impeding, this process. This is not depression; it is bereavement. Sadness or suffering need not indicate pathology. It is a normal process. This is not mental illness, even though the person may be intensely sad and distressed; the brain is operating as it ought to. Bereavement may thus fall under poor mental health only in the first broader but not in the second narrower conception of mental health.[15]

Of course, there may be debates about how long bereavement might be expected to normally last, and it is possible that the mental and neurological patterns formed during this process of bereavement will become ingrained so that they perpetuate a sense of depression long after they are serving any function to help the person find a new equilibrium or patterns and routines in life. To the extent that the brain is contributing to this in ways that deviate from its normal functioning, we might then also talk about lack of mental health in the second, narrower sense. However, often bereavement does not result in such malfunctioning, and in such cases, while the person's mental well-being may be low, their mental health, understood from the narrower perspective of the proper functioning of the brain, may be perfectly normal.

When focusing on the narrower conception of mental health, questions might be raised as to whether this ought to be referred to as "mental health" at all or whether it might be preferable to refer to "health of the

---

15. See Zachar et al. (2017) for a history of the debates about the removal of the bereavement exclusion from depression in the fifth edition of the *Diagnostic and Statistical Manual of Mental Disorders*. See also Pies (2014) for discussion of the practical implications and potential value of that removal but the need to continue to exercise careful judgment in distinguishing depression from normal bereavement.

brain" and "diseases of the brain."[16] Brain health might then be seen as yet just another aspect of bodily health. However, a distinction can again be drawn between the mind and the brain. Their relations are complex and integrated, but the mind and brain are not conceptually identical, just as disease and illness are not conceptually identical. Disease concerns the body; illness concerns the human person. Likewise, while the brain is part of the body, the mind concerns the human person. Mental health fundamentally concerns the human person, even if the definition is restricted to those aspects of mental health that arise from malfunction of the brain.[17] One can further restrict attention to brain health, but mental health, even in the narrower sense considered above, extends beyond the health of the brain.

As discussed in section I.2a, illness is the human experience of bodily disease. Mental illness (understood in a narrower sense as illness arising from the brain) is likewise the human *experience* of a malfunction of the brain. In its narrower sense, mental illness is contingent upon some malfunction of the brain, but it concerns the fuller human mental *experience* of that malfunction, ranging from intense human emotion to negative thoughts to somatic consequences of emotion, thoughts, and neurological activity. Thus, even taken in this narrower sense (requiring some malfunction of the brain), mental illness still cannot be understood apart from the mental experience of the *person*. However, just as not all feelings of sickness (e.g., motion sickness) constitute illness and disease, so also not all negative mental experiences arising from an anomalous functioning of the brain constitute mental *illness*. We might refer to any feeling of sickness as some form of ill health but not as disease or illness. Likewise, we might refer to any negative mental experience as some form of mental ill health[18] (in the

---

16. Szasz (1976).

17. When considering mental health as conceptualized here, even in its narrow sense, we must confront issues such as what is constituted by wholeness of the mind; i.e., by mental well-being. This inevitably leads to philosophical questions of the nature of the mind and what constitutes a life well lived with respect to the mind. This will vary across traditions, and it is arguably in part this fact that also gives rise to different cultural understandings of what constitutes mental health and mental illness (Szasz, 1976; Sadler, 2005).

18. Mental ill-health in its broader sense might be understood as any lack of mental wholeness; i.e., any lack of mental well-being. In terms of language ordinarily

broader sense of lack of mental well-being) but not as mental illness, which arguably requires both some malfunction of the brain and other, more stringent criteria regarding severity.[19] We might refer to a

---

employed, however, the term "mental illness" is generally reserved for relatively extreme forms of mental ill-health that in some way also depend on some malfunction of the brain. One might follow Wakefield's definition of mental illness or disorder "as harmful dysfunction" (Wakefield, 1992) but add the qualification "of sufficient severity." See also the following footnote. In the discussion here, I will restrict the use of "mental illness" to this narrower sense and use "mental ill-health" for lack of mental wholeness or lack of mental well-being when the broader conception of mental health (of the person) is in view. See also the Brief Glossary in the Appendix for further delineation of the definitions proposed here.

19. For a negative mental experience to constitute mental illness in the narrow sense of arising from the malfunction of the brain, we might require additional criteria indicative of a certain severity: (1) that the mental experience be out of proportion with the circumstances, (2) that it be sufficiently intensely negative, (3) that it have a certain persistence, and (4) that the negative experience be outside the control of the person. If a negative persistent mental experience is proportionate to the circumstances (as in the case of bereavement), so that condition 1 is not satisfied, we might still refer to this as suffering or mental ill-health or lack of mental well-being, but not as mental illness. In the absence of condition 2, intensity, if what was repeatedly experienced was somewhat out of proportion but sufficiently mild so as to barely affect the individual, we would not typically refer to this as mental illness. In the absence of condition 3, persistence, even if the mental experience were intensely negative and out of proportion but only momentary, we might refer to it as a mental anomaly or disturbance but not as mental illness. With respect to condition 4, lack of control, one might conceive of circumstances in which a person freely chose, perhaps out of a sense of calling, say, exposure to stimuli that repeatedly provoked a response that was negative and out of proportion. However, given the control the person ultimately had over exposure to such stimuli, we would not ordinarily, it seems, refer to this as a case of mental *illness* (because of the person's control over the experience). However, intensely negative persistent mental experience that is out of proportion with circumstances and that the person does not have control over arguably constitutes what we characteristically refer to as mental illness. Stein et al. (2021) discuss the criteria of "symptom severity, excessiveness, and duration," and First and Wakefield (2013) discuss the criteria of "persistence . . . intensity of a symptom . . . disproportionality," although none of these authors explicitly discuss lack of control. Of the four additional criteria proposed here, the first, the criterion of being out of proportion with the circumstances, may be such that the contexts in which this criterion is met are most open to disagreement, perspective, and interpretation. In some sense, it can be judged only within a system of values and cultural practices. This may likewise in part give rise to the difficulty of defining specific mental illnesses. It might also be disputed as to whether mental experience needs to be *negative* in order to constitute mental illness. Should an excessive experience of mania and excitement

particular type of mental illness specified in terms of characteristic patterns of severe negative mental experience as a particular type of mental disorder.[20]

---

that is persistent, is out of proportion with reality, and is out of a person's control be considered mental illness, even if it is not undesired by a person? In the conceptualization proposed here, "negative" is to be understood not simply as undesired but also as objectively undesirable or as pertaining to the loss or absence of some objective good. Understood as such, persistent disproportionate mania, even if it is not undesired by the person, could still constitute mental illness in its lack of proportion with reality and consequently in its accompanying lack of rationality. Of course, such an understanding also requires an understanding of what constitutes objective goods, which will vary by philosophical or religious tradition.

20. The conceptualization of mental illness (in its narrow sense) presented here requires some form of malfunction of the brain in addition to the criteria in the prior endnote. Nevertheless, it is conceivable that those mental experiential criteria of being (1) out of proportion, (2) sufficiently intensely negative, (3) persistent, and (4) outside of the person's control may indeed indicate sufficient severity such that it is not possible that this would arise without some malfunction of the brain. If this were so, it would be possible to identify mental illness purely in terms of mental experience. However, in principle, it may be possible to identify mental illness either with respect to the activity of the brain or by reference to mental experience. First and Wakefield (2013) discuss the use of the "pathosuggestiveness of symptoms" to effectively infer internal dysfunction, given the present lack of knowledge concerning psychological and biological processes. However, the *definition* of specific mental illnesses arguably cannot be carried out independent of mental experience, since, as defined here, mental illness requires lack of wholeness of the mind of sufficiently severe degree. If it is the case that any mental experience that qualifies as mental illness must manifest itself through certain patterns of brain activity, it may be conceivable that mental illnesses could be subsequently identified and classified, either with respect to mental experience or with respect to activity of the brain. When classification is made with respect to patterns of brain activity, we might refer to this as a "brain disorder" or a "brain disease." (In the understanding and use of the terms presented here, the term "mental disease" would be a category mistake, although this could perhaps still be understood as, with only slight abuse of the proposed terminology, a disease of the body or brain that gives rise to the corresponding negative mental consequences.) Our scientific understanding of these processes and their relation to mental experience is at present sufficiently limited that current classification efforts rely almost exclusively upon mental experience, although they not infrequently take into account somatic conditions as well (American Psychiatric Association, 2013). See also Kendler and Parnas (2012) and Zachar and Kendler (2017) for a discussion of the philosophical issues around nosology and Kendler (2009) and Aftab and Ryznar (2021) for a description of the historical evolution of nosology.

As is clear from the discussion above, the phenomenon of mental illness cannot be understood apart from the interplay between body and mind.[21] Moreover, as will be discussed further in part II, dysfunction in a given system has diverse causes that extend beyond the system itself. It may well be the case that the eventual malfunction of the brain arose from a sequence of negative thoughts arising from some external circumstance. Likewise, as is clear from various forms of cognitive behavioral, existential, and psychoanalytic therapy, mental changes in cognition and understanding can go on to alter and correct various workings of the brain. The mind and the body are deeply interwoven. However, it is also the case that mental illness can sometimes be addressed through more direct physical means such as pharmacological agents. Mental health can be amenable to change and improvement accomplished principally through alteration in the brain, even though mental health itself, even understood in its narrow sense, extends beyond bodily health.[22]

---

21. Identifying mental illness and the interplay of malfunction and negative mental experience becomes more complex in the context of multiple forms of mental ill health. In principle, a physical anomaly could give rise to brain activity, making a person more susceptible to negative thoughts that might eventually culminate in depression. These negative thoughts might give rise to further fear and eventually to abnormal persistent and uncontrollable anxiety. It is conceivable that the brain could be functioning normally with respect to anxiety even though the content of the depressive negative thoughts were irrational and out of proportion, in part arising from the malfunction of the brain. In this case, we might refer to mental illness both with respect to depression and anxiety. However, the underlying brain anomaly effectively concerns making the person more susceptible to depressive negative thoughts. The brain might thus be operating properly in terms of anxiety, conditional on the negative thoughts, so that the brain would still be functioning well from a physical perspective concerning the anxiety but not the depression. It is also conceivable, however, that persistent anxiety arising from irrational negative thoughts would eventually lead to changes in brain activity that render the person abnormally susceptible to anxiety, even in the context of rational thoughts.

22. As footnotes 18–20 discuss, mental illness involves both dysfunction and negative mental experience (cf. Wakefield, 1992; Stein et al., 2021). This duality is part of the challenge of studying, classifying, and addressing mental illness. Different approaches and methodologies are arguably better suited to either malfunction or dysfunction or to negative mental experience. Dysfunction is perhaps better categorized by etiology, whereas mental experience is better categorized by description. The former will often aim at more objective criteria, with regard to the latter, while seemingly objective criteria can be put forward there will always be some reliance on subjective states. In principle, taxonomies of mental illness and disorder could

If we are to grant the distinction between mental health, understood as the wholeness of the mind, as it pertains to the person versus as it pertains to the body and brain, a complex question that arises is the proper scope of psychiatry. We will return to this question again in section I.7. However, it seems clear that in practice, many (though perhaps not all) psychiatrists see themselves as attending to certain aspects of mental health in the broader conception.

I.2e. God's intent for the body is to empower our capacity to love and to be united to others and to God.

We began this section with some consideration of what might be meant by bodily health and discussed its relation to the body's parts and systems being and functioning as normal and to the body's having the full range of activities characteristic to it. It was noted that in some ways, this was an exercise in inference, an attempt to infer what being normal or intact was for the body's systems or parts by observing many individuals over time and examining the consistency of their functioning. A similar exercise of inference is likewise also required to understand the characteristic range of activities the human body allows in which all of its parts and systems coordinate. God's intent may in some sense be implicit in the consistent functioning of the body and its systems. It would seem that God's intent for the body was for it to allow for a range of activities in which the human person could freely choose to engage in the pursuit of various ends. Such an understanding arguably arises simply from the examination of the consistency and functioning of the human body. However, theologically, one can arguably attain a deeper understanding of God's intent for the body either through further examination of human relations or from God's revelation of that intent.

---

perhaps be categorized by either etiology or mental experience. Treatment of mental disorders using cognitive and behavioral approaches might be best carried out based on taxonomies from mental experience. Pharmacological treatment of mental disorders might be best carried out using taxonomies of etiology, although both etiological and experiential insights and descriptions are likely to be relevant for understanding the other and for informing treatment. Understanding the relations and mappings between malfunction and negative mental experience and between different taxonomies will likely be critical in better understanding and treating mental illness.

In John Paul II's *Theology of the Body*, the meaning of the body is described as a gift for the donation of the self to the other in love—the body gives us various capacities to love. That love is often expressed in actions toward others.[23] This is true in human interactions in general and specifically within the context of marriage. The biblical creation stories speak of God creating human persons as man and woman. The bodies, their differences, and their capacity for union indicate that they were created for one another. In the creation story in Genesis 2–3, God declares that "it is not good that . . . man should be alone" and the creation of woman follows. Man and woman were created for one another. The human person is meant to be in relationship. The capacity of the body for giving of self is found in relationships in general and in marriage more specifically. In marriage, the man and the woman commit to one another in love and give themselves to each other bodily in love, which in turns allows for procreation, the bringing forth of new life, the extension of the family. The two are said to become one flesh (Genesis 2). That love and union is part of God's intent for the body, but it also points to the ultimate end of the human person in union with God. The marriage and union of man and woman points to the union of Christ and the Church (Ephesians 5), which will be discussed further in part III of the book.

That final end of the human person is depicted in the Bible and in Christian theology as also one in which, in union with God, there will be no marriage or giving in marriage (Matthew 22). Rather, the body will be transformed and infused by the Spirit of God. The human body in a state of or calling to celibacy points to that final end of the human body in God in a way that complements the human body within marriage pointing to the union of Christ and the Church. The meaning of the body in celibacy and in marriage complement one another. Celibacy points to our final state in union with God; marriage points to the meaning of the body in loving, and in reflecting God's love for us and in the union of Christ and the Church. The body's meaning is thus found in love; God's intent for the body is an empowering of the capacity to love. The body is to be cared for in its own right, and also to enable the pursuit of many activities, including our loving others.

---

23. John Paul II (2006); cf. Hogan (2006).

Propositional Summary 1.2: The health of the body is constitutive of and contributes to the health of the person.
- 1.2a. Bodily health is constituted by the body's parts and systems being and functioning as normal so as to allow for the full range of activities characteristic of the human body.
- 1.2b. The health of the body constitutes and contributes to the health of the person, or human flourishing.
- 1.2c. Bodily health includes the health of the brain, which itself shapes, though does not fully encompass, mental health—the wholeness of the mind.
- 1.2d. Mental health may be understood as the wholeness of the mind, either in a narrower sense, as pertaining to the proper functioning of the brain, or in a broader sense, as pertaining to the wholeness of persons.
- 1.2e. God's intent for the body is to empower our capacity to love and to be united to others and to God.

I.3. Health, Unity, and Goodness

Proposition 1.3. The human person, body and soul, was created good by God as an integrated whole.

1.3a. The human person was created good and the human body was created good.

The creation stories in Genesis affirm the goodness of the human body and the human person. "God saw everything that he had made, and indeed, it was very good" (Genesis 1). God made man and woman with bodies; creation was physical and material and the goodness of this is likewise affirmed. The human person is good. The human body is good. The material aspect of God's creation was part of God's intent.

In part II, we will discuss at greater length Christian theology concerning the fall and sin and their relation to health and the fact that the body is now subject to ill health. There was disruption to the body: "in pain you shall bring forth children . . . in toil . . . by the sweat of your face you shall eat bread" (Genesis 3). Nevertheless, the body and its eventual restoration to wholeness and transformation in salvation and resurrection are still affirmed as God's intent (1 Corinthians 15). A restoration of the body to goodness is part of God's intent. The body was created good and the goodness of the body, even in its present fallen state, is to be restored.

1.3b. The natural state of the human body as created by God is health.

Part of the goodness of the body is the fact that for most persons, its natural state is health through much of life. As will be discussed in greater detail in part II, with the fallenness and brokenness of the world, some people are born with significant health difficulties or severe bodily malformation. However, for many, health is the natural state. For much of life, the body's systems and parts are intact and functional and allow for the normal range of human activity.[1] The person's body is healthy. The body also often and effectively heals minor injuries naturally over time, and often the body will recover from disease by its normal operations as well. The body has a certain capacity for restoration.[2] Nature itself seems to play a role in healing and health.[3] This capacity of the body for healing and restoration is such that medicine is sometimes effective by following what the body itself normally or naturally accomplishes or by restoring its capacity to do so.[4] The natural state of the body as healthy and the body's capacity for restoration to health are part of the goodness of the body.

From a Christian perspective, this capacity of the body to restore itself is also understood as God's care and providence—God's ordering of and sustaining of the world. Part of that providence is the capacity of the body for health and healing. God himself is the first cause of all things, including the body, its health, and its capacity to restore health.[5] Aging and disease eventually limit this capacity, which, as will be discussed in part II of the book, occur within the context of the brokenness of the human person in ways that are contrary to God's intent. However, in most cases, health is the natural state of the human body. Health in some sense was, and is, God's intent.

---

1. Thus, while we might speak of "attaining" a state of mental health or well-being or of social or spiritual health or well-being, this language of "attaining" is often not as appropriate for physical health, since that is often present, at least at younger ages, without any particular effort on the part of the individual. We might instead thus speak of "experiencing" or "realizing" or "being in" a state of physical health. See also section I.1, footnote 27.

2. Aquinas (1265/2014, 1.3.157).

3. Gadamer (1996, chapter 8).

4. Aquinas argues that "many are healed by the operation of nature without the art of medicine. In these things that can be done both by art and nature, art imitates nature" (1265/2014, 1.2.75). Likewise, Gadamer (1996, chapter 2) argues that the work of the physician is to restore something, namely health, to its natural state and that nature itself assists in this process.

5. In the words of Augustine, "Nothing but the will of God is the prime cause of health and sickness, of rewards and punishments, of graces and recompenses." (Augustine 417/2019, III; cf. Aquinas 1265/2014, 1.3.97).

1.3c. The good of health presupposes the good of life, and life itself is to be respected from conception until death.

The health of the body and the health of the person presuppose life. We do not speak of the health of something when it is dead. Life is conceptually prior to health. Health is a good only within the context of life. The good of health presupposes the good of life. From a Christian perspective, life results from the act of God's creation. Life is a gift. As such, life is to be respected. Life is not in general to be intentionally ended. The act of intentionally ending the life of another is wrong in almost all contexts. The very nature of the act is contrary to God's will and God's intent.[6] It is a rejection of the gift of life and a rejection of God's intent. It is a cessation of and a denial of the goodness of the person and of the body. The goodness of the body, of the person, and of life is thus what lies behind the Christian prohibition[7] against abortion, euthanasia, and suicide, and it places substantial restrictions on capital punishment and war.[8] The

---

6. Aquinas (1275/1948, II.II.64).
7. May (2008); Koritansky (2012); Catholic Church (2000, 2258–2330).
8. Aquinas argues that while it is always wrong for a private individual to intentionally take the life of another (1274/1948, II.II.64.3), it is lawful for a public authority, in certain cases, to put a criminal to death for the sake of the common good (1274/1948, II.II.64.2,3, 65.1); and likewise a legitimate authority can engage in war under a just cause such as self-defense with right intent constituted by the preservation of the common good and the restoration of peace (1274/1948, II.II.40). With respect to capital punishment, in Aquinas's understanding there is strict restriction to those offenses that "inflict an irreparable harm, . . . as contain some horrible deformity" (1274/1948, II.II.66.6.ad 2) and "which conduce to the grave undoing of others" (1274/1948 II.II.103.ad 2). See also Koritansky (2012). Drawing on these principles, the catechism of the Catholic Church (2000; section 2267) stated, "Assuming that the guilty party's identity and responsibility have been fully determined, the traditional teaching of the Church does not exclude recourse to the death penalty, if this is the only possible way of effectively defending human lives against the unjust aggressor. . . . Today, in fact, as a consequence of the possibilities which the state has for effectively preventing crime, by rendering one who has committed an offense incapable of doing harm—without definitely taking away from him the possibility of redeeming himself—the cases in which the execution of the offender is an absolute necessity 'are very rare, if not practically non-existent.'" Following an address by Pope Francis (2017), this section (2267) was subsequently revised: "Recourse to the death penalty on the part of legitimate authority, following a fair trial, was long considered an appropriate response to the gravity of certain crimes and an acceptable, albeit extreme, means of safeguarding the common good. Today, however, there is an

respect for life, from the moment of conception until natural death, is an affirmation of the goodness of God's creation, the goodness of life, the goodness of the body, and the goodness of the person, as created and sustained by God.

1.3d. The human person is an integrated whole, and what occurs to one aspect of the person will affect the entire person.

The human person is an integrated whole. The soul and the body are not independent. The dependence of mental life on the body and on the activity of the brain were given some attention in sections I.2c and I.2d. The relations between various aspects of a person's life are both conceptual and causal. The health or wholeness of the person entails that all aspects of a person's life are good, including their bodily health. Lack of wholeness or ill functioning of the body implies some lack of wholeness of the person. Lack of wholeness of the mind likewise implies some lack of wholeness of the person.

However, the various aspects of the person are related to one another not only conceptually and constitutively but also causally. What happens to one aspect of the person can also affect other aspects of the person's life, directly or indirectly. The perception of a lack of wholeness of the body can sometimes give rise to a lack of peace, or a lack of wholeness of mind. Lack of wholeness of mind can sometimes disturb or disrupt bodily functioning, sleep, or other physical processes. The health of the mind and the health of the body are mutually interdependent. Mental health may affect physical health; physical health may affect mental health and aspects of social and spiritual well-being. The various aspects

---

increasing awareness that the dignity of the person is not lost even after the commission of very serious crimes. In addition, a new understanding has emerged of the significance of penal sanctions imposed by the state. Lastly, more effective systems of detention have been developed, which ensure the due protection of citizens but, at the same time, do not definitively deprive the guilty of the possibility of redemption. Consequently, the Church teaches, in the light of the Gospel, that 'the death penalty is inadmissible because it is an attack on the inviolability and dignity of the person,' and she works with determination for its abolition worldwide." Although cases of capital punishment do not themselves constitute murder, in light of the present circumstances, the Catholic Church teaches that this now never constitutes the right way forward.

of a person's life are interconnected. The various dimensions of health impenetrate one another, causally and conceptually.[9]

Lack of mental health, understood in either its broader or narrower sense, may adversely affect bodily health.[10] Some of this may be due to the neglect of practices that contribute to physical health. Someone experiencing intense sadness or depression may neglect exercise or eat too much, or not enough, or consume foods that are not healthy or drink excessively. They may be less likely to seek medical care, and their adherence to treatments may decrease. Lack of mental health constituted by intense anxiety, depression, or anger can adversely affect the body more directly. This might occur in part through the body's nervous system, through stress exerting its effects on the cardiovascular system, and through processes of inflammation and immune suppression.[11] The mind and one's mental health affects the body. These relations between mental health and bodily health are present also within Christian theology. In his apostolic letter *Salvifici doloris*, John Paul II noted that in treating the human person as a psychological whole, the Old Testament links moral suffering with the pain of specific parts of the body.[12] Psychological suffering appears to have a physical element. Again, the human person, mind and body, is an integrated whole.

Poorer mental health can likewise sometimes adversely affect relationships. Depression, anxiety, and mental distress can interfere with both the giving and the receiving of love. It has the potential to lead to problematic patterns of behavior that threaten the health of relationships. Declines in social connection and social support can result in poorer bodily health, both through less physical and material support available from these relationships but also through the effects that loneliness, stress, and sadness can more directly exert on bodily systems and function.[13]

---

9. See also Tillich (1981) for discussion of the similar dynamics and the overlapping aspects of various dimensions of health. See Smith (2015) on the interconnectedness of human action, personhood, subjective experience, and all of society with regard to flourishing.

10. For empirical summaries and meta-analytic evidence, see, for example, Roest et al. (2010); Wei et al. (2019); Martin-Maria et al. (2017); Trudel-Fitzgerald et al. (2019).

11. See Roest et al. (2010); Wei et al. (2019); Steptoe (2019).

12. John Paul II (1984, 6).

13. Holt-Lunstad et al. (2015).

Character and purpose likewise affect bodily health and other aspects of well-being. Lack of purpose and meaning can give rise to depression, despair, or neglect of the body.[14] A strong sense of purpose can help a person through times of trial; meaning can help a person better make sense of suffering. Character similarly can contribute to various aspects of health and well-being. Temperance can preserve bodily health. Fortitude can help a person through times of great difficulty and help them achieve various life goals.[15] Specific virtues such as hope or gratitude or forgiveness may orient a person toward what is good and protect against psychological distress, potentially also thereby affecting the health of the body.[16] Good character and virtue, understood as habits in accord with reason in order to obtain the good for oneself and others, can likewise help improve the health and well-being of others, improving not only their lives but also their relationships.[17] The various aspects of a person's life are deeply interrelated.

---

14. See, for example, Chen, Kim, et al. (2019a) and Kim, Nakamura, et al. (2022) for comprehensive empirical assessments of the effects of purpose in life on subsequent health and well-being. See Cohen et al. (2016) for a meta-analysis of the protective effects of purpose on all-cause mortality.

15. Although it is imperfect, the closest analogue to fortitude in the empirical literature may be assessments of grit, which has been studied principally in educational contexts and manifests in longitudinal associations with academic outcomes (Alan et al., 2019).

16. See Wade et al. (2014), Chen, Harris, et al. (2019b), and Ho et al. (2024) for empirical evidence concerning the effects of forgiveness on various aspects of health and well-being; Long, Kim, et al. (2020a) for the effects of hope; Emmons and McCullough (2003) and Davis et al. (2016) for the effects of gratitude; Seligman et al. (2005) and Schutte and Malouff (2019) for the use of character strengths; and Węziak-Białowolska et al. (2021) for the effect of the general disposition to do good on subsequent health and well-being. See also VanderWeele (2022a, 2022b) for reviews of the longitudinal and experimental literature on the effect of character on health and well-being.

17. If virtue is considered as a habit in accord with reason to obtain the good, then that good may be the good of oneself or the good of another. When a virtue such as compassion or love aims principally at the good of another, the seeking of that good may, at least at times, entail sacrifice and suffering with respect to oneself. The virtue of fortitude may require facing painful difficulties and challenges in fulfilling one's commitments and obligations for the service of the broader community. The virtue of generosity may require sacrificial giving to help those in need, giving rise to the potential that one's own material well-being is more likely to be compromised. Each of these and other virtues, by aiming at the good of the other, has the potential to bring about hardship and potentially greater psychological distress for oneself.

Conversely, lack of bodily health can adversely affect mental and spiritual health. Disease or injury may be a source of an intense anxiety and depression. A lack of energy may lead one to neglect relationships and spiritual practices. Physical disruption such as lack of sleep, hormonal abnormalities, or poor nutrition can give rise to depression. As noted above, however, illness and suffering can also sometimes lead to spiritual renewal or provide opportunities to work toward attaining a greater mental, social, and spiritual well-being. But depending on the person's response to illness and suffering, it is similarly possible that such lack of bodily health will adversely affect mental, social, and spiritual well-being.

As will be discussed in greater detail in section I.6, spiritual health arguably requires proper use of and care for the body and bodily health. Health and the body are gifts from God that are to be used rightly. In St. Paul's letter to the Corinthians, the body is pictured as a temple of the Holy Spirit received from God (1 Corinthians 6). As such, the body is to be honored; it is to be respected and treated rightly and not used for wrongdoing. Although the pursuit of God and one's final end of communion with God in some sense relativizes the importance of bodily health, bodily health is still a good.[18] It is something that is to be preserved to the extent possible and while respecting other goods and commitments. That this is so is integrally connected to one's spiritual life.

This has implications for empirical research as well (VanderWeele, 2022a, 2022b). The effects of character on the well-being of other individuals in one's communities or on the community itself, has been less frequently studied. This is problematic if virtue promotes the well-being of others and the well-being of the community and the common good. Given the small number of empirical studies on this topic to date, we may be substantially missing the importance of the effects of character on well-being. The standard design of current social science research practices, even rigorous longitudinal studies, is to collect data on a set of focal individuals over time and then to assess outcomes for those same individuals but not for other individuals in that person's community. Future research would benefit from examining the effects of the character on the health and well-being of others in the community.

18. In Aquinas (1265/2014, 3.143), "The chief good and final end of man is happiness: the higher good for him then is that which comes nearer to this end. Coming nearest to it of all is virtue, and whatever else advances man to good acts leading to happiness: next is a due disposition of reason and of the powers subject to it: after that, soundness of bodily health, which is necessary to unfettered action: lastly, exterior goods, as accessory aids to virtue."

One's body and entire being are to be treated as a gift and should be directed toward the love of others and of God. The body itself is to be loved and cared for out of love for God.[19]

> *Propositional Summary 1.3: The human person, body and soul, was created good by God as an integrated whole.*
> 1.3a. The human person was created good and the human body was created good.
> 1.3b. The natural state of the human body as created by God is health.
> 1.3c. The good of health presupposes the good of life, and life itself is to be respected from conception until death.
> 1.3d. The human person is an integrated whole, and what occurs to one aspect of the person will affect the entire person.

---

19. Aquinas (1274/1948, II.II.25.5).

I.4. Health and Community

Proposition 1.4. The complete health of the person includes a flourishing community.

1.4a. The complete wholeness of a person entails the wholeness of his or her community.

There is a deep relation between wholeness of the person and wholeness of the community. We are social, relational, and communal by nature.[1] For an individual to fully flourish, they must have a flourishing community. This is so for several reasons. First, as a social creature, a person requires relationships and a community to live fully as God intended. Second, a person's community influences various other aspects of a person's well-being. This takes place through the interactions a person has with others in the community, through the importance of the community in the person's development, through the resources the community provides, and through the experience of the community itself.[2] Complete wholeness of a person entails complete wholeness of the person's community.

The importance and centrality of community to human life is emphasized throughout the biblical account and its interpretation. The nature of God is presented as a Trinity, as God being three persons and yet one God.[3] Thus, within the unity of God there is community: God the Father, God the Son, and God the Holy Spirit. Community

---

1. Aristotle referred to the human person as a "political animal" (Aristotle, 4th C BC/1980, book I, chapter II). Likewise, Aquinas, in *On Kingship*, wrote, "it is natural for man, more than for any other animal, to be a social and political animal, to live in a group" (Aquinas, *On Kingship*, as translated in Crofts (1973, 156).
2. Maritain (1947); Phillips and Wong (2017); VanderWeele (2019a).
3. Matthew 28:19; John 10:30

and relationship are manifest in the very nature and source of all being.[4] The creation stories likewise point toward community: God created human persons as male and female, as relational, and the nature of the relations between man and woman is such as to generate community, children, and ultimately the family as the central community of human life.[5] In the account of the fall in Genesis 3, the consequences of departing from God's will affected not only the man and the woman but also childbearing, once again with consequences with regard to relational and communal life. The story of Cain and Abel that immediately follows is likewise an account of the consequences of sin in family, in community life. Family continues to be emphasized in the narratives of the book of Genesis and beyond. The history of God's presence with human persons given in the Old Testament is principally the history of a community, that of the people of Israel. Jesus himself is born into the context of a family, the family of Mary and Joseph. In his life and ministry, Jesus forms a community of disciples around himself.

There is also in the Christian theological and biblical tradition a strong sense of corporate solidarity. As will be discussed in greater detail in part II, while sin has an important individual aspect there is also a corporate aspect wherein all of humanity shares in original sin. Conversely, as will be discussed further in part III, salvation from sin through Jesus Christ has an important corporate aspect. The biblical picture of salvation involves a strong corporate element: it is described metaphorically as a marriage between Christ and the entire church (see Ephesians 5). God's intent for restoration is a communal intent.

The coming of the Spirit takes place in the context of the gathering of the community of Jesus's disciples that was formed out of Jesus's preaching and ministry and his giving of himself. The community that arose out of Jesus's disciples is the Church.[6] As described further in part III of this book, the community that is the Church has a central role as the means of healing, restoration, and salvation. However, the Church is not just the means of this salvation but is also in some sense its end. Many of the visions in the book of Revelation of the final restoration that

---

4. Cf. Maritain (1947); Catholic Church (2000, 254–255, 1693).
5. Cf. Catholic Church (2004, 146–148, 209–214).
6. Catholic Church (2000, 763–768).

God will accomplish are corporate in nature. This manifests the corporate nature of wholeness, of health, of healing, of salvation. Community is central to the well-being of the person both as a means and as an end.

1.4b. A community involves a common good, and this implies that the flourishing of one person ultimately depends on the well-being of others in the community.

The importance of the community in an individual's flourishing is also seen in Christian teachings on the common good.[7] The common good has been conceived of as "the sum of those conditions of social life which allow social groups and their individual members relatively thorough and ready access to their own fulfillment."[8] The common good might also be understood as the common end of a community.[9] The goal of a community is for its members to flourish in various ways and for the community to flourish *as a community*. The flourishing of a community thus unquestionably includes the flourishing of individuals. But for the community to flourish *as a community* it must also have good relationships, leadership, structures, practices, and unity in order to fulfill its purpose or mission, whether the community is a family, a

---

7. See, for example, Catholic Church (2004, 164–170); and Maritain (1947).
8. Paul VI (1965, 26); cf. John XXIII (1961, 74).
9. Aquinas (1274/1948, I.II.90.2.ad 2). Barbieri (2001) notes that the expression "common good" is ambiguous and has been used to denote the common purpose of a community, or alternatively the means that promote the good within the community, giving rise also to the criterion by which action concerning the good of the community is assessed. The definition given above in *Gaudium et Spes* (Paul VI, 1965, 26), "the sum of those conditions of social life which allow social groups and their individual members relatively thorough and ready access to their own fulfillment" primarily emphasizes the means or conditions of promoting the common good. This definition is presented in similar form in the *Compendium of the Social Doctrine of the Church* (Catholic Church, 2004, 164), although there, reference is also made to a "universal common good" constituted by God as "the ultimate end of his creatures" (Catholic Church, 2004, 170). There is a certain complementarity between means and ends insofar as sufficient means entail the relevant ends and the ends cannot be achieved without sufficient means. See also Keys (1995) for some discussion of how the common good understood as means versus end might help reconcile differing Thomistic interpretations and positions (those of Maritain and de Koninck) on the common good.

workplace, a voluntary organization, or the state. Although all communities aim to promote certain aspects of human flourishing or at least some perceived good, they differ in breadth, in the means of promoting flourishing, and in the specific aspects of flourishing that is their primary focus.[10]

A fully flourishing community also requires that all members of the community flourish.[11] Because each person is part of the community, their own flourishing is in part dependent on the community and on its other members, who are also flourishing. One cannot say that all aspects of a person's life are good if one's community and the life of its members are not good.[12] This creates a certain dependence of each person on the other. This dependence is reflected theologically in the fact that "the human person cannot find fulfilment in himself, that is, apart from the fact that he exists 'with' others and 'for' others."[13] For full flourishing, we need relationships; we need community; we need love. We cannot fully flourish unless we are flourishing with others, unless we are flourishing as a community.

---

10. Although much of the discussion of the common good specifically concerns the state, or the *political* common good, other communities have a common good and common ends that are pursued together. However, the state continues to be the primary focus of most discussions of the common good because its breadth encompasses the entirety of a nation, and because it has, in principle, the means to support the pursuit of flourishing for all its citizens. In *Gaudium et Spes* (Paul VI, 1965, 26), the common good in this context is understood as "the sum of those conditions of social life which allow social groups and their individual members relatively thorough and ready access to their own fulfillment." With increasing recognition of the interdependence of that common good across nations, though, the notion has been extended in various ways to a global or supranational common good (Barbieri, 2001) that continues in the most recent papal encyclicals (Francis 2015, 2020) and earlier ones.

11. Aquinas, for example, writes, "Now it is evident that all who are included in a community, stand in relation to that community as parts to a whole; while a part, as such, belongs to a whole, so that whatever is the good of a part can be directed to the good of the whole. It follows therefore that the good of any virtue, whether such virtue direct man in relation to himself, or in relation to certain other individual persons, is referable to the common good" (1274/1948, II.II.58.5).

12. The common good extends beyond the sum of the good of each individual in that it requires that each person be interested in the well-being of others for the other's sake (see Finnis, 1998, IV.3; Aquinas, 1272a, book VIII, chapter 5.1605).

13. Catholic Church (2004).

We might understand the common good of a community as the shared end of the community along with the means to attain that end,[14] means that require the members of the community to care for the well-being of one another.[15] The well-being of each member of the community is partially dependent on the well-being of the other members in order that the community can achieve its shared purpose. The common good both creates this interdependence and is reflective of the nature of human persons as relational and communal creatures.

The flourishing of a community includes the conditions that make such flourishing possible. The common good cannot be attained and

---

14. One might distinguish between a community's *general* common good and a community's *particular* common good. A community's general common good might be understood as the flourishing of the community as a community, the flourishing of its members, and the means to sustain such flourishing. The attaining of the community's general common good might then be understood as synonymous with the community flourishing, or a state in which all aspects of a community's life are good. In contrast, the *particular* common good might be understood as the shared aspects of flourishing that are particular to that community and the means needed to attain those aspects. The general common good of, say, a chess club, would include the flourishing of its members, and is thus considerably broader than its particular common good, of being a good community in which to play chess. In contrast, a nation's particular common good (or the *political* common good; see footnote 10 above) is much closer in scope to its general common good. However, from the standpoint of Christian theology, the particular common good and the general common good of a nation are not identical because, in pluralistic contexts at least, the attainment of the fullest possible spiritual well-being would not generally be understood as part of the particular shared end of the nation itself. From the standpoint of Christian theology, the general common good would include spiritual well-being and the means to one's final shared end in God, even though that is not a part of the nation's particular common good. That final shared end in God might be referred to as the *universal* common good of the whole of creation (Catholic Church, 2004, 170). In all cases, the particular common good of any community should contribute to and will be partially constitutive of the general common good, which itself is both constitutive of and also a means to the universal common good defined as the shared end in God. A general definition of "common good" that encompasses these various broader or narrower notions of the general, particular, or universal common good might thus be "the common shared end of a community, possibly including the broader flourishing of the community and its members, and possibly also including the means to attain the relevant end or ends."

15. The well-being of a community's members (and thus the necessity of willing the well-being of others in love as God intended) is needed constitutively for the community's general common good and is needed at least to some extent instrumentally for a community's particular common good.

safeguarded without coordinated effort of the community and it is the responsibility of each person to contribute to it. It requires each member to constantly seek the good of others as though it were their own good.[16] In his encyclical *Sollicitudo rei socialis*, John Paul II gave an account of the virtue of solidarity and our need for it. He defined this virtue as "a firm and persevering determination to commit oneself to the common good; that is to say to the good of all and of each individual, because we are all really responsible for all."[17] A person's well-being depends on the well-being of the community because there is a shared common good and purpose. This requires that a person's character, which is constitutive of their well-being, be oriented toward the common good. The relations between the role of the individual and the role of the community in preserving the health or flourishing of the person and the health of the community will be explored further in section I.6. But communal well-being and individual well-being are indeed integrally tied.

The common good, understood as the common end of each member of the community and of the community as a whole along with the means

---

16. Although a person's flourishing is in part constituted by the flourishing of their communities and the common good of those communities, it is also the case that participation in communities will help orient its members toward the common good more generally, to develop the virtue of solidarity. Participation in communities provides a common vision; it often assists in the forming of relationships and the fostering of love and teaches some measure of sacrifice. Participation in communities also helps individuals see the contribution of these communities to others and to life as a whole and helps individuals see the tremendous power and good of people working together, thereby allowing individual persons to see the importance of communities and of the common good in human flourishing.

17. John Paul II (1987, 38). The breadth of this definition of solidarity depends in part on whether the common good is understood as the particular common good of the state rather than the general common good of community flourishing (see footnote 14 above). In this definition of "solidarity," there is moreover some resonance with Aquinas's description of justice as a general virtue ("legal justice") that directs all acts of virtue to the common good (1274/1948, II.II.58.5). The virtue of solidarity arguably extends this further by including not only "the perpetual and constant will to render to each one his right" (1274/1948, II.II.58.1) with respect to the individual and the community but also love (cf. Catholic Church, 2004, 582). One might also construe the difference between general or legal justice and solidarity as the difference between the political common good and the general common good of a flourishing community (see footnote 14 above), although love is required in order to guarantee the political common good (Catholic Church, 2004, 582; see also section III.7h).

to attain it also points toward a more universal common good, that which is found in God.[18] The common good of communities is ultimately the full flourishing of persons as God intended, in community and in love, as part of the attaining of the universal common good of the whole creation.[19] This will be the topic of section I.5.

1.4c. Good community includes flourishing individuals, good relationships, proficient leadership, healthy structures and practices, a welcoming environment and sense of belonging, and a common mission.

There are distinctive features of what is meant by a community that is flourishing *as a community*, or a good or healthy community.[20] The individual members are at the heart of every community. Communal

---

18. The *Compendium of the Social Doctrine of the Church* (Catholic Church, 2004, 170) states that "the common good of society is not an end in itself; it has value only in reference to attaining the ultimate ends of the person and the universal common good of the whole of creation."

19. In Aquinas's *Summa Theologica*, an individual's temporal good is always to be subordinate to the political common good (1274/1948, I.II.90.3, II.II.31.3, 47.10, 68.1, 117.6, 185.2), but the political common good is not only ordered to the temporal good of individuals but also allows for the freedom for each individual to become what God intended. See also Crofts (1973) for an analysis of the central role that the concept of the common good plays in Aquinas's political theory.

20. When one speaks of the "health" of a community, "health" is arguably used metaphorically. Typically it means that a community is whole or intact or is functioning well. Often what is in view is that the community is not in decline or is not likely to end soon or die. One might argue that the notion of the "health of a person" is likewise a metaphorical use of the term "health," that "health" really does principally concern the body and all other uses are metaphorical. This may indeed be the case, and I will not here argue for or against whether the notion of the health of persons is metaphorical or whether the expression "healthy person" in the sentence, "Every day he just sits in his room; he is physically healthy, but he is not a healthy person" can be understood only by way of metaphor. I would maintain, as above, that there is an important distinction to be drawn between the health of the body and the health of the person; and I would maintain moreover that in contemporary discourse around health, much of the confusion, and dispute, concerns not distinguishing between these notions of health of a person and health of a body. Regardless of whether the expression "health of a person" resembles the expression "health of a community" more than it does the expression "health of the body," the distinctions between these two central notions of health are important.

well-being requires the well-being of its members.[21] Although communal well-being extends beyond individual well-being, it is not independent from the well-being of the members of the community. It would be odd to say that a community is flourishing if its individual members were not. Good community is constituted in part by flourishing individuals. The flourishing of a community is made up in part by the well-being of its members.

The importance of good relationships is central to the notion of communal well-being. Relationships in the community should be close. Each person in the community should be respected as a person and trusted. Community well-being requires that people spend time with one another and know one another. A thriving community will be one in which each person contributes to the well-being of others in the community and in which this contribution is experienced and known. When the knowing of one another and that contribution to the other is mutual and extends over long periods of times, it becomes proper to speak of friendship.[22] Good community is constituted in part by good relationships and by friendship.

For a community to flourish and to continue to do so over time, it is also important that there be good leadership. Those in positions of power and authority should care about the well-being of everyone in the community and of the community itself. They should seek the common good and not simply their own private good. The leaders should have the skill and understanding that is needed to lead the community well and should be of sufficient character and consistency that they can be relied upon to do what is right. They should be able to inspire others with their vision for the community's well-being. Good community is constituted in part by proficient leadership.

A well-functioning community will also have healthy practices and structures. There should be structures and practices in place that allow

---

21. Catholic Church (2004, 165); Aquinas (1274/1948, II.II.58.5).

22. Aristotle (4th C BC/1980, Books VIII–IX) distinguishes between what are often referred to as friendships of utility, friendships of pleasure, and friendships of virtue, which aim, respectively, at mutually contributing to one another what is useful, what is pleasurable, and what is good. Complete friendships are such that good people mutually aim at the good of the other. In addition to friendship being a good in its own right, both in *Nicomachean Ethics* (4th C BC/1980, VIII, 1) and *Politics* (4th C BCE/1995, II, 4), Aristotle comments that friendship has an important role in holding together and ensuring unity within the community constituted by the state.

relationships to develop and strengthen, that allow the community to sustain itself, that allow for the appropriate handling of conflicts and disputes, and that allow the community to achieve its primary goals. Good community is constituted in part by healthy practices.[23]

The community should ideally be welcoming and should provide a sense of belonging. There should be a sense that each person is an integral part of the community; there should be a sense of unity. It should be possible for each person to become more integrated into the community over time. The community should be such that each person thinks that it is a good community to be a part of. In most cases, the absence of these things will indicate that something is wrong. This sense of welcome and belonging, of integration and unity, in part contributes to making the community satisfying to be a part of; that is, it should satisfy a desire to be integrated, to be in community.[24] Good community is thus constituted in part by a welcoming environment that creates a sense of belonging and unity.

Finally, a good community should be fulfilling its purpose or function, its own particular common good as a community.[25] A good community will be one that somehow contributes to the lives of its members and thereby also or in other ways helps make the world a better place.

---

23. The *Compendium of the Social Doctrine of the Church* (Catholic Church, 2004, 166) notes that with respect to the state, the demands of the common good as part of the flourishing of a community include a commitment to peace; organized state power; a sound juridical system; protection of the environment; provision of essential services to all, including food, housing, work, education, and access to culture, transportation, basic health care, freedom of communication, and freedom of expression; and the protection of religious freedom.

24. The sense of integration, of unity amid plurality, arguably extends beyond having good relationships, which may concern only two individuals. Community and belonging arguably require more: the relation of each person and of each relationship to the whole. With three or more there emerges, not only notions of relations, but also of harmony, the relations and order amongst the relations themselves. That community is present in the nature of the Trinity as three persons but one God.

25. In *Politics*, Aristotle argued that any partnership or community is established for some purpose or aims at some good or end. This in essence is its mission, whether it is implicit or explicit. In certain cases it may be difficult to precisely articulate what the relevant mission is in a particular community context. In the case of a city-state, Aristotle took that end to be making its citizens good, promoting their flourishing (Aristotle, 4th C BCE/1995, I.1.1252a1–7).

The community's purpose or mission or particular common good would ideally be clear to everyone. A community is thriving as a community if its members are able to do more together than the sum of what each could accomplish individually, and if everyone is needed for the community to fulfill its goals and purposes. Good community is constituted in part by a strong mission or purpose, by a particular sense of its common good.

These various characteristics—flourishing individuals, good relationships, proficient leadership, healthy structures and practices, a welcoming environment and a sense of belonging, and a common mission—are important to various forms of community life, ranging from the family to schools, workplaces, religious communities, neighborhoods, cities, and nations. These things do not exhaust what constitutes a good community, and other necessary elements may depend on the form and goals of community life. A well-functioning nation, for example, needs to sustain various modes of transportation; a well-functioning school needs a curriculum and textbooks or other learning aids. However, each of these elements above is an important part of the life of any community.[26] For a community to flourish, individuals must flourish, but for individuals to flourish—to live in a state in which all aspects of their life are good—communities must also flourish.

---

26. For a community to be flourishing *as a community* it must have good relationships, proficient leadership, healthy practices, unity, and a common mission. The relationships, leadership, practices, and unity are important both because they are constitutive of flourishing as a community, but they are also important as a critical means of attaining the *particular* common good of the community (see footnote 14 above). However, community flourishing, understood as "all aspects of a community's life being good," extends beyond this to include flourishing individuals. Such community flourishing is arguably synonymous with the community's attaining its *general* common good (again, see footnote 14 above). One might thus, in principle, assess community flourishing, or the community's general common good, in terms of (1) flourishing individuals; (2) the various formal facets of a community's flourishing as a community, including its relationships, leadership, practices, and unity; (3) the attaining of its particular common end as a community; and (4) the presence and sustaining of any further means necessary to attain the community's particular common end. See also VanderWeele (2019a) for further description of and a potential assessment concerning community well-being in each of the aforementioned domains: flourishing individuals, good relationships, proficient leadership, healthy structures and practices, satisfying community, and strong mission.

1.4d. Good community requires justice.

For a community to fully flourish, each person within the community must flourish. For each person to flourish, each person should be given what is his or her due or right. This is what is meant by justice.[27] Justice is needed for a community to flourish.[28] Justice facilitates the flourishing of individuals by giving each what is their due. When someone within the community is not given his or her due, the relations between individual persons and between the person and the community are not what they should be. The community is not fully healthy. Good community thus requires justice, with each receiving his or her due.

Understandings of justice have differed across traditions, philosophies, and cultures. What it is precisely that we owe one another—what it is that each is due—is not an entirely straightforward matter.[29] In Christian

---

27. Although Aquinas's most substantial treatment of justice in the *Summa Theologica* frames justice as a virtue (1274/1948, II.II.57–122) that concerns the "habit whereby a man renders to each one his due by a constant and perpetual will" (II.II.58.1), he also refers to justice as a state of affairs (II.II.57.1), a property of laws (I.II.90.2; I.II.95.2), an art whereby it is known what is just (II.II.56.1.ad 1), and that which is administered by a judge (II.II.57.1.ad 1).

28. The general common good of the community, or community flourishing, is arguably a broader and more fundamental notion than justice. Community flourishing or the general common good of a community includes more than justice. That this is so can be seen in part by the fact that the scope of the general common good and of community flourishing, as described in sections I.4b and I.4c above, is considerably broader. It can also be seen in that while justice is of critical importance in the community constituted by a state, justice does not have the same level of centrality in other types of communities, such as the family or religious communities. It is not that justice is not a concern in these other communities, but it plays less of a role than it does in a state. Moreover, even with respect to the state, attaining both the particular and general common good arguably requires not only justice but also love (John Paul II, 1980, 14; Catholic Church, 2004, 580–583). See also sections III.2 and III.7h. Although justice renders to each his or her due on account of the other person's being human and on account of the laws that are in place, the virtue of charity or love renders to each person his or her due on account of an agent's love for God.

29. I will make no attempt here to offer any sort of substantive account of justice. Rather, the focus of the cursory remarks in this section will pertain to the need for justice, understood abstractly as a state in which each receives his or her due so a community and its individual members can be healthy. See sections II.2, II.7c–d, and III.7h for more discussion of the relationship between justice and rights and between

theology, what we are due follows in part from the fact that we are created in the image of God.[30] This endows us with certain rights by virtue of the fact that we are human and are created in God's image.[31] Individuals are not to harm one another and are not to kill one another. We have a right to life. Each person also has a right to be respected, to be treated as a person of worth and dignity. We were also created free and that freedom too should be respected. We should in general be free to share our thoughts and ideas, free to associate with others, and free to seek the transcendent, to practice religion so as to seek God, as God intended. We were also created to be relational, to form friendships, and in some cases to marry and form families, and our freedom to do so and to raise and support those families should also be preserved.[32] The preservation of these human rights is a matter of justice. If these human rights are violated, the health and flourishing of persons will be impeded, the relations of individuals with one another and with the community will not be rightly ordered, and the community will not be fully healthy. Good community requires respect for human rights; good community requires justice.

---

justice and health. See Gilby (1958), Finnis (1998), and Krom (2020) for more substantive accounts of Aquinas on justice.

30. The *Compendium of the Social Doctrine of the Church* (Catholic Church, 2004, 153) grounds rights in the dignity of the human person and in the fact that the human person is created by God.

31. A distinction is often drawn between human and natural rights—that is, rights that follow simply from being human ("human rights," e.g., the right to life) or by the nature of things ("natural rights," e.g., the right of parents to care for their children)—and legal and conferred rights—that is, rights that are granted by authoritative political bodies ("legal rights," e.g., a right to health care) or derive from agreements among parties ("conferred rights," e.g., the right to expect a promise be fulfilled).

32. The *Compendium of the Social Doctrine of the Church* (Catholic Church, 2004, 155; cf. John Paul II, 1991, 47) includes among human rights "the right to life, an integral part of which is the right of the child to develop in the mother's womb from the moment of conception; the right to live in a united family and in a moral environment conducive to the growth of the child's personality; the right to develop one's intelligence and freedom in seeking and knowing the truth; the right to share in the work which makes wise use of the earth's material resources, and to derive from that work the means to support oneself and one's dependents; and the right freely to establish a family, to have and to rear children through the responsible exercise of one's sexuality. In a certain sense, the source and synthesis of these rights is religious freedom, understood as the right to live in the truth of one's faith and in conformity with one's transcendent dignity as a person."

Being both by nature and by God's intent relational and social creatures, we have also organized ourselves into societies and nations to enhance the health of bodies and the health of persons—to promote human flourishing. These nations grant rights, which may be referred to as legal rights, to members or citizens and provide various goods and services and systems of protection, and help ensure that each person is able to enjoy various liberties, all to enable people to flourish.[33] Fulfilling those obligations and creating laws and legal systems to ensure that citizens have these rights is ultimately the responsibility of the state.[34] However, the capacity of a state to protect these rights and liberties, fulfill

---

33. A state can, and arguably should, grant legal rights and goods and services that are within its means to provide and that enable individuals and communities to flourish; that is, that promote the common good. Paul VI (1965, 26) described these rights and goods as "the sum of those conditions of social life which allow social groups and their individual members relatively thorough and ready access to their own fulfillment." Such legal rights and goods and services generally extend beyond what follows from human rights alone. The *Compendium of the Social Doctrine of the Church* (Catholic Church, 2004, 166) teaches that "the demands of the common good . . . concern . . . the provision of essential services to all, some of which are at the same time human rights: food, housing, work, education and access to culture, transportation, basic health care, the freedom of communication and expression, and the protection of religious freedom." A commitment to provide such essential services constitutes important and reasonable legal rights that a state may grant. Within the context of the state, justice, the rendering to each his or her due, might be understood not just as protecting human, natural, and legal rights but also as involving the proper expansion of legal rights, in proportion to the means available, to enable the common good.

34. Aquinas defines law as "an ordinance of reason for the common good, made by him who has care of the community, and promulgated" (1274/1948, I.II.90.4). A law is just when it is made by a competent authority (I.II.90.3), is according to reason (I.II.95.2, I.II.90.1), and is conducive to the common good (I.II.90.2). See also Vermeule (2022, 63) for an account of the justice of laws in terms of a common good framework such that "(1) the public authority acting within its constitutional sphere of competence (2) may act on a reasonable conception of the common good . . . by (3) making reasonable, nonarbitrary determinations about the means to promote its stated public purposes." Vermeule argues that when the determinations of a public authority and its laws conform to these criteria, judges should defer to those laws, but when such determinations do not so conform, judges should invalidate them. Vermeule also makes the case that the US Constitution is best seen as being grounded in, and best interpreted in light of, the classical legal tradition and a common good framework.

obligations, and provide goods and services also ultimately relies on the cooperation of the members or citizens of that state.[35] Rights entail the duty to maintain, respect, and fulfill them. Preserving rights—both the rights we have by nature of being human and the rights the state grants— is a matter of justice. When rights are violated, individuals do not have what is their due. Their flourishing is inhibited; relations between individuals and with the community are not rightly ordered; the community is not healthy.

Justice is thus needed for good community in part both because individuals need this in order to flourish but also because it is part of the common good of the state.[36] The particular common good a state offers is its capacity to help develop, build, and promote "the sum of those conditions of social life which allow social groups and their individual members relatively thorough and ready access to their own fulfillment,"[37] and that involves maintaining justice. Justice is thus important for good community not only because it is important for each individual person but also because it is part of the particular common good of the state. Justice is constitutive of healthy community. Good community requires justice.

---

35. This is so because political leaders are themselves members of the state, and also because the provision of these goods and services and the respecting of human rights and legal rights will depend on the members of the state more generally. The *Compendium of the Social Doctrine of the Church* (Catholic Church, 2004, 167–168) teaches that "the common good therefore involves all members of society . . . according to each one's possibilities, in attaining it and developing it. . . . The responsibility for attaining the common good . . . belongs also to the State, since the common good is the reason that the political authority exists . . . in order that the common good may be attained with the contribution of every citizen." It is the exercise of justice as a virtue (Aquinas, 1274/1948, II.II.57–122), understood as the "habit whereby a man renders to each one his due by a constant and perpetual will" (II.II.58.1), on the part of both the leaders and all the citizens of the state, that ultimately ensures the state of justice, in which each person receives what is his or her due, and that helps bring about the common good.

36. With respect to the flourishing of the state as a community, justice as a virtue and as a state of affairs is constitutive of both proficient leadership and of healthy structures and practices and is central to the state's attaining its particular common good.

37. Paul VI (1965, 26); cf. Catholic Church (2004), 164.

1.4e. Healthy families are needed for the health of bodies, the health of persons, and the health of communities.

Although the state and justice are needed if individuals and communities are to flourish, more than this is required. The human person develops slowly throughout infancy and childhood and thereafter and requires nurturing. The primary context for that nurturing occurs in the family.

The family is the first community most children experience—a community of parents and often of siblings and relatives, a nurturing community of love. Parents nurture and care for their children, both with regard to their bodily needs and with regard to their intellectual, emotional, behavioral, and spiritual development. The stability of the family community established by the wedding vows helps provide children with a secure context in which to grow, to develop, and to be formed and loved.[38] Parents and families share, along with schools, religious communities, and other organizations, the task of forming the character of children and promoting their flourishing.[39] However, the

---

38. Catholic Church (2000, 1643–1658); Catholic Church, (2004, chapter 5); Girgis et al. (2012). The traditional understanding of marriage as a vow of permanent union between a man and a woman has been challenged by the phenomenon of same-sex marriage and was challenged before that by the rise of no-fault divorce and in some cases by the alteration of vows so that lifelong fidelity is not necessarily included. The Catholic Church's understanding of marriage is still one of "a permanent union . . . between one man and one woman" (Catholic Church, 2004, 227), and this is distinguished from de facto unions involving a simple agreement to live together without vows and from same-sex unions (Catholic Church, 2004, 227–228). The former are distinct from marriage because they do not provide the stability needed to best nurture children. The latter are distinct from marriage "by the objective impossibility of making the partnership fruitful through the transmission of life . . . [and] the absence of the conditions for that interpersonal complementarity between male and female" (Catholic Church, 2004, 228). Other Christian groups have modified their understanding of marriage to allow for same-sex unions. Much of the determination comes down to the question of how the relation between procreation and marriage as an institution is understood. See also Girgis et al. (2012) for philosophical, legal, and practical considerations and the appendix of VanderWeele (2023) for some discussion within the context of public health.

39. See Cuñado and de Gracia (2012), Powdthavee et al. (2015), and VanderWeele (2017b) for empirical longitudinal evidence concerning the important role of schools and education in shaping the subsequent physical, mental, social, and financial well-being of children, and see Chen and VanderWeele (2018) for empirical evidence

chief responsibilities in this regard generally fall to parents and to families. Families are thus critical in the formation of children. Because families raise the next generation, they have a critical role in sustaining society, in sustaining other communities, and in promoting human flourishing—the health of persons, the health of bodies, and the health of communities.

Healthy families will seek to enable each person to flourish; they will involve good relationships and systems of trust. A marriage between spouses involves vows to be with and love the other throughout life; it establishes a bond, a communion, a friendship that gives rise to a unity and faithfulness in marriage.[40] Marriage facilitates the flourishing of spouses.[41] Marriage and the development and flourishing of the spouses then enable the flourishing of other members of the family.[42] Healthy families require the wisdom and insight of the parents and other adults to help guide and direct the development of the children and the communal life of the family. Healthy families have practices that nurture each individual and their shared community life together. Healthy families help each child and each member to know that they are loved and included in the rich fabric of family life. Families are often able to welcome others, to provide hospitality,

---

concerning the role of religious communities in shaping the subsequent health and well-being of children.

40. Catholic Church (2004), 215–220; Catholic Church (2000), 1638–1654. See also Abbey and Den Uyl (2001) for a philosophical discussion of marriage as friendship and its relevance in the context of contemporary Western society.

41. Longitudinal studies indicate that marriage is associated with better mental health, physical health, and longevity; higher levels of happiness, personal growth, and meaning; and lower levels of loneliness and financial struggles (Marks and Lambert, 1998; Manzoli et al., 2007; Wood et al., 2007; VanderWeele, 2017b; Chen et al., 2023). Conversely, divorce is associated longitudinally with poorer mental and physical health outcomes; lower levels of happiness, meaning, and positive relations; and greater levels of poverty for both children and mothers (Marks and Lambert, 1998; Wilcox, 2011; VanderWeele, 2017b; Chen et al., 2023).

42. Marriage has profound effects on the lives of children. Children within, rather than outside, marriage are more likely to have better mental and physical health, to be happier in childhood and later in life, less likely to engage in delinquent and criminal behaviors, more likely to have better relationships with their parents, and less likely to later divorce (Amato and Sobolewski, 2001; Wood et al., 2007; Wilcox, 2011; VanderWeele, 2017b).

to show others love, emanating from the deep love the family members have for one another. Families have their own common good—the nurturing and development of children, of spouses, and of all who participate in the life of the family. Families thus are critical not only to preserving bodily health but also to fostering the health of persons.

Bringing new life into the world and nurturing that life is constitutive of human flourishing. In the Genesis creation story, after creating human persons—man and woman—God blesses them and says "be fruitful and multiply, and fill the earth" (Genesis 1:28). Having children and raising children is part of life as intended by God. Jesus himself grew up within the context of a family. God's intent was for children to be raised in the context of family life. Said another way, having children and raising of children is human flourishing.

Moreover, by shaping and forming each successive generation, families play a critical role in sustaining other communities. Were it not for procreation and the nurturing of children, society would cease.[43] The health of persons, shaped by the health of families, in turn shapes the health of other communities and of society as a whole. Families form the basic building block of society. Higher levels of community both depend upon and also should support the life of the family while respecting family rights and responsibilities and also without usurping the role of families.[44] Declines in family life will adversely affect the flourishing of persons and consequently the flourishing of society. The formation of families is both constitutive of and contributes to human flourishing. Healthy families are needed for the health of bodies, the health of persons, and the health of communities.

---

43. See *Compendium of the Social Doctrine of the Church* (Catholic Church, 2004, chapter 5), for further theological reflection on the role of families in shaping and sustaining society.

44. That families' rights and responsibilities should by respected by higher levels of community is an example of what, in Catholic social teaching and elsewhere, is sometimes referred to as the principle of subsidiarity, namely that "it is an injustice . . . to assign to a greater and higher association what lesser and subordinate organizations can do" (Catholic Church, 2004, 186), since the lower levels are the more effective and appropriate levels in which to exercise freedom, initiative, and fulfillment of responsibility.

Propositional Summary 1.4. The complete health of the person includes a flourishing community.

1.4a. The complete wholeness of a person entails the wholeness of his or her community.

1.4b. A community involves a common good, and this implies that the flourishing of one person ultimately depends on the well-being of others in the community.

1.4c. Good community includes flourishing individuals, good relationships, proficient leadership, healthy structures and practices, a welcoming environment and sense of belonging, and a common mission.

1.4d. Good community requires justice.

1.4e. Healthy families are needed for the health of bodies, the health of persons, and the health of communities.

I.5. Health and Spiritual Well-Being

Proposition 1.5. The complete health of the person includes communion with God.

1.5a. The final end of the person is communion with God.

The health or wholeness of the person is a state in which all aspects of life are good, in which a person is fully living life as intended by God. God's final intent for the human person is communion with himself.[1] That communion is to be freely chosen and pursued. Life here is ultimately to be oriented toward that final communion with God. That goal shapes how human pursuits and human function are to be understood in this life.

As discussed in section I.1 above, while human flourishing or the complete health or wholeness of a person might be conceived of as living in a state in which all aspects of a person's life are good, eternal flourishing (or perfect well-being) may be conceived as the attainment of the final goal of the human person, complete communion with God. Spiritual well-being in this life can then be understood as a state in which one's life is oriented toward eternal flourishing or as a state in which all aspects of a person's life are good with respect to his or her final communion with God, and this is the ideal toward which we are to aim. Temporal flourishing is constituted by the aspects of human flourishing that pertain to the goods in this life, including, for example, happiness and life satisfaction, physical and mental health, meaning and purpose, character and virtue, and close social relationships and communal well-being. Human flourishing thus encompasses both spiritual and temporal well-being. From a Christian perspective, spiritual well-being is the component that is most central; it is what brings a person to his or her final communion with God.

---

1. Aquinas (1274/1948, I.II.1–5); Westminster Assembly (1647/2014, Q1); Catholic Church (2000, 1045).

Often the pursuit of such spiritual well-being and temporal flourishing will be consonant with one another. Health of body and mind and a set of supportive relationships will often facilitate spiritual and religious practices that promote spiritual well-being. Likewise, spiritual practices can contribute to temporal flourishing by developing community, facilitating mental health, shaping character, and giving a person a sense of understanding, meaning, purpose, and satisfaction.[2] However, as discussed further in part II, in the fallenness of the world, sometimes these goods and ends come into conflict. In such cases, from the perspective of Christian theology, priority is to be given to spiritual well-being. In St. Paul's first letter to Timothy, he writes, "While physical training is of some value, godliness is valuable in every way, holding promise for both the present life and the life to come" (1 Timothy 4:8). Aquinas, in commenting on Jesus's question, "For what does it profit a man, if he gain the whole world, and suffer the loss of his own soul?" remarks that "the loss of the soul is an inestimable injury."[3] Jesus's beatitudes—"Blessed are the poor in spirit. . . . Blessed are those who mourn. . . . Blessed are those who are persecuted for the sake of righteousness" (Matthew 5:3–12)—likewise illustrate the potential for tension between temporal and spiritual well-being in this life.[4] Health of the body, and even other aspects of the health of the persons, are relative goods. From the standpoint of

---

[2]. Koenig et al. (2023); VanderWeele (2017c); Balboni et al. (2022).

[3]. Aquinas (1270, 16:26).

[4]. Although the Scriptures do not explicitly use the word "flourishing," the notion of "shalom" in the Old Testament, sometimes also translated as "peace," arguably captures a similar conceptual range. The New Testament notion of "blessedness," "happiness" in some translations, perhaps likewise conveys a biblical notion of flourishing, although, as per the beatitudes, with a much stronger emphasis on spiritual well-being and orientation toward eternal flourishing. Some notion of flourishing is likewise arguably in view in Jesus's rendering of his mission with respect to humanity as "I came that they may have life and have it abundantly" (John 10:10) and, perhaps especially when used in the Gospel of St. John, in the notion of "eternal life" as encompassing both the present life and the life to come. As discussed in greater detail in part II, the potential tension in this life between temporal and spiritual well-being is a result of sin, and as per part III of the book, some tasks of redemption are to realign temporal life and affairs toward spiritual well-being and eternal flourishing. See also sections II.6 and III.5 for further discussion of how that tension, and even sometimes the accompanying suffering, can present opportunities for a greater spiritual well-being.

Christian theology, spiritual well-being is the most important aspect of flourishing in this life and provides the path to attain the final goal of the human person, the perfection of flourishing in God. From the perspective of Christian theology, human flourishing must thus always be understood in a two-tiered manner: temporal flourishing in this life and orientation toward and final attainment of a perfect flourishing in God in the life to come.[5]

---

5. In conceiving of flourishing as two-tiered with regard to temporal flourishing in this life and eternal flourishing in the life to come, it becomes easier to situate this proposed Christian conception of flourishing within the traditional philosophical theories of well-being. See also footnotes 13 and 36–40 in section I.1. Four theories of well-being have been put forward and developed in a variety of ways in the contemporary philosophical literature on well-being (Fletcher, 2016): hedonism theories, desire fulfillment theories, objective list theories, and perfectionist theories. Hedonism effectively equates well-being with the greatest balance of pleasure over pain, although how pleasure and pain are understood varies across these theories. Desire fulfillment theories equate well-being with the satisfaction of desires, or, in alternative formulations, with the satisfaction of rationally informed desires (Brandt, 1979; Sidgwick, 1981; Railton, 1986). Objective list theories conceive of well-being as the attaining of some list of items that are viewed as objectively good. Perfectionist theories conceptualize well-being in terms of that which perfects an individual's nature (Hurka, 1993). There are numerous variations on these theories of well-being, including hybrid versions that combine elements of more than one of them (e.g., Lauinger, 2013). Particular specifications of each of these theories might in fact be considered adequate as Christian theories of eternal flourishing. If eternal flourishing is conceived of as final communion with God (for Aquinas, attained by a vision of the divine essence) and this is considered to be (1) the highest happiness or pleasure, infinitely greater than all others; (2) the complete satisfaction of the will and all its desires; (3) ultimately, in the final state, the only relevant objective good; and (4) the perfection of human nature in charity and union with God, then each of the four theories of well-being, thus construed, might effectively serve as an alternative, but adequate, characterization of eternal flourishing. The relation of a Christian understanding of temporal flourishing to the four well-being theories is arguably more complex. One might say a potentially infinite list of objective goods corresponding to "all aspects of a person's life being good" might be viewed as an adequate characterization of temporal flourishing (see also footnotes 36–40 in section I.1). Likewise, a desire fulfillment theory that made reference to fully rationally informed desires, understood as in alignment with God's intent, might likewise be thought to be an adequate characterization of temporal flourishing (see also footnote 13 in section I.1). However, hedonistic theories of well-being do not provide an adequate characterization of a Christian understanding of temporal flourishing because there is more to well-being than the balance of pleasure over pain in this life. Likewise, perfectionist theories of well-being, conceived of as the perfection of human nature according to

1.5b. Communion with God requires approaching God in faith, hope, and love.

Within the Christian tradition, three theological virtues are central in the spiritual life: faith, hope, and love.[6] These will be discussed at greater length in part III. Faith may be conceived of as a trust in God and all that God has revealed, including a conviction that communion with God is the final goal. Hope may be thought of as a pursuit of and orientation to that final goal, guiding all of life but with the realization that only God can ultimately bring this about. Love, or charity, may be seen as a friendship with God.[7]

That communion, viewed as friendship with God, is one that develops over the course of a life.[8] As in any friendship, it develops out of who the persons are, what they do, and the time they spend together.[9] The development of that friendship with God thus involves the transformation of one's character, rightly ordered actions and the carrying out of one's calling, and time with God in prayer and contemplation. These will be the topics of the next three sections.

1.5c. Communion with God requires growth in character and knowledge.

Charity, or friendship with God, ultimately directs all actions toward final communion with God.[10] Friendship with God, or love of God, includes love of neighbors, who are loved for the sake of God (1 John 4:20). Such love includes a desire for their good and actions to bring it about

---

God's intent, are perhaps not entirely adequate accounts of temporal flourishing because although they might capture what is most important with respect to temporal flourishing, such *temporal* flourishing also consists of not only a perfection of one's nature but also various external goods, such as food and shelter or relationships with others. The perfecting of one's nature as a human that was accompanied by imprisonment and severe undernourishment would arguably not constitute full *temporal* flourishing. Thus, while such perfectionist theories perhaps adequately capture what is most important with respect to temporal flourishing and what is to be prioritized, they do not provide a complete account of temporal flourishing.

    6. Aquinas (1274/1948 I.II.62).
    7. Aquinas (1274/1948 II.II.23.1).
    8. Aquinas (1274/1948 II.II.24.4–7).
    9. Aquinas (1274/1948 II.II.27.2).
    10. Aquinas (1274/1948 I.II.65.2–3).

and a desire to help them also attain final communion with God.[11] As Jesus taught, such love is to extend so far so as to also include loving one's enemies (Matthew 5:43–48).[12] That love, that seeking of the good for the other, even for one's enemies, requires a transformation of character.

To love God and neighbors well requires the development of other virtues as well.[13] To love well requires practical wisdom to understand what that good is and how to bring it about, justice to understand right action and rightly adjudicate between competing claims about what each person is due, fortitude to continue to seek good in the face of difficulties, and temperance that regulates desires and actions in the face of lower competing desires. As discussed in section I.1c, these four aspects of character—practical wisdom or prudence, justice, fortitude, and temperance are sometimes referred to in the classical and Christian traditions as the cardinal virtues, the virtues upon which other moral virtues depend. In the Christian tradition, these other virtues are strengthened and transformed by charity, or friendship with God.[14] In loving God, it is the desire for final communion with God that directs all actions and one's very being. As that transformation of character occurs, friendship with God can grow further.

1.5d. Growth in character, faith, hope, and love requires community, service, and the carrying out of one's calling.

Friendship with God is accomplished in part by transformation of character, and that is often brought about by action and service. Character is formed out of habits of mind and action.[15] By repeated action in accord with reason to attain some good oriented toward one's proper end, character is formed and right action thereby also become easier and are empowered. Those actions, if they are actions of love and of service toward neighbors, are also actions of love for God (1 Corinthians 10:31). Those actions of love are a part of friendship with God. They will include helping others attain a wholeness of person—actions that contribute to

---

11. Aquinas (1274/1948 II.II.25.1).
12. Aquinas (1274/1948 II.II.25.8,9).
13. Aquinas (1274/1948 I.II.65.3).
14. Aquinas (1274/1948 II.II.23.4,6–8).
15. Aquinas (1274/1948 I.II.51.2, 1274/1948 I.II.55.1–3).

the happiness, health, meaning, character, or relationships of others or help provide for others the means of achieving these important goods. Such actions of love for God and for one's neighbor will also include actions that help others understand and pursue final communion with God as well.[16]

The proper way to love God and to love one's neighbor will in part depend on one's calling. The Christian notion of a calling or a vocation has both a universal and a particular sense. A calling or vocation might be understood as a singular life mission that generates and orders various further purposes and goals and helps one decide among these when and if they come into conflict. The universal sense of a calling or a vocation is a calling to God, to one's final communion with God. This is a calling that is in some sense shared by all. However, the sense of calling or vocation may also be more particular, shaped by a person's circumstances, who they are as a person and the needs that intersect with that person's life and communities. This will in turn affect the work that a person undertakes and the relationships and communal involvements that he or she pursues. A person's particular calling or vocation is discerned over time and is gradually made manifest in reflection, prayer, and the unfolding of life events and life decisions. A calling or a vocation provides order and focus to the loving actions a person is to carry out.[17] It gives a sense of purpose and meaning to life, its attainment results in happiness, it shapes and forms relationships, and it is often the context for growth in character, both in the discernment of that calling and in working through the challenges that might be encountered in trying to carry out that calling. A sense of a calling or a vocation helps a person flourish and find wholeness. The complete health of the person is aided by an understanding of and the pursuit of their calling.

Both the universal and the particular sense of calling will often also play a central role in the development of the theological virtues of faith, hope, and love. In the pursuit of one's calling, of loving one's neighbor in those particular ways that one's life circumstances and one's being seem to demand, there may be struggles and difficulties along the way. Those difficulties can be seen as opportunities for faith, hope and love: faith that

---

16. Aquinas (1274/1948 II.II.25.1).
17. Aquinas (1274/1948 II.II.26.6–12).

God is working through them to accomplish some good, hope that in the end all will be well and that the present difficulties will be overshadowed by the person's final communion with God; and love, that regardless of the circumstances, one can always try to respond to them by loving God and loving one's neighbor. Even challenging circumstances can be an occasion for a deeper charity, a deeper friendship with God. The carrying out of one's calling in loving actions until one's final communion with God thus helps bring about friendship with God, the wholeness of the person that includes spiritual well-being both for oneself and for others.

1.5e. Communion with God requires and is found in prayer and contemplation.

Communion with God is in some sense attained most directly by prayer and contemplation of God. Prayer is essentially time with and for God.[18] It is bringing oneself, one's requests and petitions, to God; expressing one's gratitude for God's gifts and presence; coming to God in confession with hope of transformation; and adoration or contemplation of God. In prayer, friendship with God is partially brought about and experienced. There is a bringing of one's self and one's life to God in prayer. There is a receiving, in turn, of love from God.

A transformation of character and actions and the pursuit of one's calling in love are important preparations for prayer. But prayer and contemplation require that time be taken to simply be present with God. Time with God is essential for charity, for friendship with God.

We will consider prayer and contemplation at greater length in part III as the attaining and restoration of wholeness and in its relation to the final end of the human person. However, time with the other is central in any friendship. That time may consist of having conversations with the other, of doing things together, or simply being present with and contemplating the other. Prayer may be seen as in some ways analogous to conversation, loving action as analogous to joint activity, and contemplation as simply being present with and beholding the other.

In the Christian tradition, contemplation of God is sometimes conceived of as a passive receiving of a vision of who God is: seeing,

---

18. Philippe (2005).

knowing, experiencing, and participating in God.[19] This may take place in very ordinary cognitive and affective modes or through more exceptional or mystical experiences. Regardless, this experience of contemplation is viewed, in faith, as true experiential knowledge of God. Such contemplation gives a vision of God's goodness; it will often bring joy but may also lead to a reorientation of life resulting from a deeper understanding of God.

Experience or contemplation of God in some sense constitutes the closest we can come to the final end of the human person as full communion with God. It is both partially constitutive of and helps facilitate our final end. It is central to spiritual well-being, to the wholeness of the person. Contemplation, or vision of or experiential knowledge of God, is for the most part viewed as passive, as being a gift of God. It is something that is received. One makes oneself open; one spends time in prayer and in silence. It is God's initiative to bring about that experience of himself.

1.5f. Charity, including the love of God and love of neighbor, is central in attaining communion with God.

Of the three theological virtues, love, or charity, is seen as most central (1 Corinthians 13). Upon the full attainment of one's final communion with God, faith and hope are no longer necessary, as that communion is attained directly.[20] However, charity—one's friendship, one's relationship with God—remains and is what constitutes one's final communion with God.[21]

The centrality of love is present throughout the biblical texts. It is present in the summary of the law as "You shall love the Lord your God with all your heart, and with all your soul, and with all your mind. This is the greatest and first commandment. And a second is like it: You shall love your neighbor as yourself" (Matthew 22:34–40). It is present in the relative ordering of the theological virtues: "And now faith, hope, and love abide, these three; and the greatest of these is love" (1 Corinthians 13:13). It is present in descriptions of the very nature of God: "God is

---

19. See Pieper (1998); Garrigou-Lagrange (1999).
20. Aquinas (1274/1948 I.II.67.3–4).
21. Aquinas (1274/1948 I.II.67.6).

love" (1 John 4). Throughout the Christian tradition, love is preeminent among the theological virtues and indeed among all virtues.[22] The other virtues are necessary, but charity directs them to their final purpose and helps form them.[23]

Charity produces a peace wherein all a person's desires are consonant with one another and with the good, and those desires are attained in God.[24] And charity further produces joy, the experience of that attainment of one's final communion with God.[25]

1.5g. God's initiation and grace are necessary to bring about full communion with him.

If spiritual well-being is understood as friendship with God, such friendship requires a certain mutuality.[26] There must be reciprocation. As discussed above, that reciprocation is found in part in prayer. Much of the preceding discussion, however, has focused upon the actions a person can take to help bring about such spiritual well-being, to develop a friendship with God. However, within the Christian tradition, it is also understood that that development of spiritual well-being, and even its origin, comes out of initiative taken by God.[27] It is God's grace, God's free initiation and sustenance of a person's spiritual life, that brings about a person's response (Ephesians 2:8).[28] As will be discussed in greater detail in part III of the book, there are ways a person can become open to the receiving of God's grace through the Church and through the sacraments, but God's grace and his initiative remain central.

As discussed above, the theological virtues of faith, hope, and love are central in bringing a person to his or her final communion with God. There is within Christianity a tradition that the theological virtues are

---

22. 1 Corinthians 13:13; Aquinas (1274/1948 I.II.62.4, 1274/1948 I.II.66.6, 1274/1948 II.II.23.6).

23. Aquinas (1274/1948 I.II.114.7, 1274/1948 II.II.23.8). Aquinas refers to charity as the "mother of the other virtues" (1274/1948 II.II.23.8.ad 3).

24. Aquinas (1274/1948 II.II.29).

25. Aquinas (1274/1948 II.II.30).

26. Aquinas (1274/1948 II.II.23.1).

27. Aquinas (1274/1948 II.II.24.2).

28. Aquinas (1274/1948 I.II.109.6,9,10; 1274/1948 I.II.112.3).

not acquired by habit but are rather infused by God.[29] This is part of God's grace and God's initiative. God's action through his Spirit in the person's life initiates faith, builds hope, and sustains love. Fellowship with God is above human capacity and must be given by God and God's Spirit.[30] The person's response is important, however. Charity, or friendship with God, can be lost or obscured by actions that are contrary to the love of God or by rejecting God's love.[31] The person's response to God's initiative is free. However, such charity or friendship with God cannot come about except by God's initiative. God's initiative and grace are necessary to begin the spiritual life and are necessary to sustain it and to bring it to completion in full communion with God.[32] Spiritual well-being is facilitated by and can only be brought about by God's action. This is part of the reciprocal nature of friendship, of communion.

From a Christian perspective, this spiritual well-being, this charity or friendship with God, constitutes not the only but the most important aspect of the health of the person. It is what brings about that final and perfect flourishing, that communion with God, that is the final goal of the human person.

> *Propositional Summary 1.5: The complete health of the person includes communion with God.*
> 1.5a. The final end of the person is communion with God.
> 1.5b. Communion with God requires approaching God in faith, hope, and love.
> 1.5c. Communion with God requires growth in character and knowledge.
> 1.5d. Growth in character, faith, hope, and love requires community, service, and the carrying out of one's calling.
> 1.5e. Communion with God requires and is found in prayer and contemplation.
> 1.5f. Charity, including the love of God and love of neighbor, is central in attaining communion with God.
> 1.5g. God's initiation and grace are necessary to bring about full communion with him.

---
29. Aquinas (1274/1948 I.II.62.1, 1274/1948 II.II.24.2).
30. Aquinas (1274/1948 II.II.24.2, 1274/1948 I.II.109.3).
31. Aquinas (1274/1948 II.II.24.10–12).
32. Aquinas (1274/1948 I.II.109.9–10).

I.6. Health and Responsibility

Proposition 1.6. Health is the responsibility of the individual and of the community, but it depends also on circumstances beyond the control of either.

1.6a. The causes of health are diverse.

The things that support and sustain bodily health are diverse. Health is shaped by one's genetic background; by one's upbringing and the resources and experiences therein; by one's health behaviors, including diet, exercise, sleep and rest; by one's access to social and material resources, including access to health care; by maintaining one's mental and psychological well-being; by a safe environment; by one's exposure to pathogens; and by one's actions and behaviors.[1] In this section, we will briefly consider both individual and communal responsibility for sustaining physical health, mental health, and the health of the person.

1.6b. Fundamental approaches in sustaining health include regular use of the systems that maintain health, avoiding abuse of those systems, and seeking repair of those systems when necessary.

Fundamental approaches in sustaining health include the regular use of the systems involved that are to be maintained; avoiding the abuse, misuse, or overexertion of those systems; and the repair of those systems when needed. Regular use ensures that a system is working and is whole; avoiding abuse helps prevent damage to the system; and repair brings a restoration to a state of wholeness. We will consider these practices both as they relate to the health of the body and to the health of the person. From the perspective of Christian theology, God's intent for the body and

---

1. See, for example, Detels et al. (2015) for an overview of the contribution of each these various determinants of health.

for all that one is endowed with as a person is proper stewardship of the body and of all that one has been given. That stewardship consists in part in care, in avoiding abuse, and in healing.

1.6c. Practices to sustain physical health include exercise, good diet, good sanitation, temperance, sleep and rest, and medical care.

The body's various systems and parts will function well when they are used as intended. As discussed in section I.3, health is in some sense the body's natural state. When the body's systems are used without excessive strain this can help sustain their functionality. Much of this happens through the ordinary daily processes of movement, respiration, circulation, and so forth. In contemporary times, regular physical exercise has become an important behavior to offset what has often become a more sedentary pattern of life whereby the body's physical systems do not get the extent of use that might have been the case in past times. Good diet likewise maintains the health of the body, supplying the body with the sustenance it needs and making appropriate use of the digestive system.

However, avoiding abuse of the body's system is also important in sustaining health. Excessive physical strain or stress may compromise the health of the body. Foods and diets not well suited to the body's digestive system can lead to bodily changes that compromise its functionality. Excessive alcohol intake can cause damage to the body's systems. Pollutants, toxins, and chemicals, whether they are in the air or water or are consumed through tobacco or narcotic products or other drugs, can affect the body's respiratory and circulatory systems and other aspects of the body's function. Inadequate rest can also cause damage to the body and to cellular functioning. The sustaining of health is facilitated by avoiding these abuses of the body's physiological systems.

Finally, health is sustained in part by seeking repair when damage occurs. As noted in section I.2, the body carries out some of that repair naturally. Repair is also facilitated by rest and sleep and good nutrition. Advances in medical care have gone a considerable way in allowing for further repair of the body when it has been subjected to extensive forms of damage.

Thus, regular use of the body's systems, avoiding abuse to those systems, and seeking repair of those systems when they are damaged are all important in sustaining health, and more specific practices to sustain physical health include exercise, good diet, good sanitation, temperance, sleep, rest, and seeking medical care when required. Many of these practices involve the formation of habits. Healthy habits bring about and sustain health. In his treatise on habits, Aquinas identifies health itself as a habit.[2] Health results from a pattern of behaviors and activities that promote it. Habits are behaviors that are done with sufficient frequency and are sufficiently integrated into the person's life that they become difficult to change and can then be sustained without need for deliberation. Health as a habit involves both actions to promote health as a pattern and the bodily response and readiness to do what is needed to maintain health. The person forms these habits through repeated action and thus has some responsibility for the development of such habits. Health might thus be seen both as a state and as a habit. Health is something that can be partially lost, but even then, there is often still some possibility of, and the individual has responsibility for, restoring and retaining what health is still possible.

In section I.2, the health of the body was defined as the state where the body's parts and systems are normal and function as normal so as to allow for the full range of activities characteristic of the human body. Health as such was conceived of as a state. Such a state is compatible, in the short term at least, with the absence of practices or health behaviors that sustain health. This is perhaps particularly evident in one's young adulthood when, for many, bodily health, for a time, will often seem very good even when the body is subjected to various abuses with regard to lack of exercise, poor diet, excessive alcohol intake, or smoking. When bodily health is viewed simply as a state, it does not seem to require healthy practices or behaviors. However, when we view bodily health within the broader context of a person's life and longer term flourishing, it becomes clear that maintaining bodily health is important for the health of the person. Healthy habits are long-term investments in bodily health and thus are also relevant for the flourishing of the person throughout life. We might say that healthy habits or practices and maintaining health are part of the physical health *of the person* even though bodily health, as a state, does not necessarily entail that at a given time such practices are present.

---

2. Aquinas (1274/1920, I.II.49–54); cf. Dobson (2014).

The term "physical health" is somewhat ambiguous and may be used in two distinct senses. First, "physical health" may often be used synonymously with "health of the body," defined as the body's parts and systems being intact and functioning as normal to allow for the full range of activities characteristic of the human body. But second, "physical health" might be used to refer to the health or wholeness of the person in all his or her physical aspects. This is perhaps better described as physical well-being.[3] In this definition, physical aspects of the person are in view from the perspective of both a body that is functioning well and in the body's broader role in the person's life.[4] This second and broader sense of physical health in some sense mirrors the broader conceptualization of mental health considered in section 1.2d, the wholeness of the mind, or mental well-being, as it pertains to the flourishing of the person. Practices that maintain health are arguably not a constitutive part of bodily health (that is, physical health in the narrow sense) because the body can be healthy for a time, even if practices are not in place to sustain health. However, health behaviors and practices that sustain health are a constitutive part of physical health in its broader sense; they are important for the longer-term flourishing of the individual; they sustain bodily health, in the narrow sense, over longer periods of time.

---

3. We might thus define physical health (in the broad sense, as pertaining to the person) or physical well-being as a state in which all aspects of a person's physical life are good, or the wholeness of the person in all physical aspects.

4. The distinction between bodily health and physical health or well-being (in its broad sense) is also made more evident when it comes to questions of physical appearance and beauty. A great deal of attention has been paid throughout history to the beauty and the appearance of the body. In some sense, the body can be whole— its systems functioning as they normally do and capable of the full range of activities characteristic of the human body—without the person being considered, by most, to be beautiful. Bodily health can contribute to beauty, but beauty extends beyond mere bodily health. The physical beauty or appearance of a person can contribute to—or sometimes perhaps also impede—a person's flourishing. These are physical aspects of the person and often ones that individuals spend a great deal of time fostering and cultivating, but these physical aspects of the person extend beyond bodily health; physical appearance and beauty concern persons. These aspects of physical appearance might thus not necessarily be considered part of bodily health, but still considered part of physical health, interpreted in its broader sense of physical well-being, which again could be conceived of what concerns the body and is partially constitutive of an individual's flourishing.

1.6d. Mental health is sustained by the stimulation and proper use of the mind, by rest, and by mental health care as necessary.

As with bodily health, mental health, in both its narrower and broader senses pertaining both to the brain and to the person, is sustained by regular practice, by avoiding abuse, and by seeking repair when necessary. The mind is often used in the normal course of life in human interaction, in problem solving, in work, in at least some leisure activities, and in reflection and thought. The extent of the mind's stimulation or use may vary across people or contexts, but for many people, its regular exercise or use is natural within the contexts of everyday life. This helps, in part at least, keep the mind healthy and whole and functioning well, both with respect to the proper functioning of the brain and in the context of a person's life as a whole. Cases of considerable social isolation, such as prisoners in solitary confinement or sometimes among the elderly in later stages of aging, can give rise to contexts in which the regular use of the mind does not necessarily come naturally. In such cases, special effort is sometimes required to bring about regular mental stimulation. Cognitive exercises, music, and other forms of mental stimulation can help prevent further mental decline in elderly people.[5] The principle is that use contributes to good functioning.

Avoiding abuse of and excessive strain of the mind is likewise important for mental health. Abuse of the mind and of the brain may take the form of excessive alcohol intake or the use of drugs or of extreme stress or lack of rest or of extended periods of sadness, fear, anxiety, or anger. These things are all constitutive of poor mental health and render the mind less able to function optimally. Avoiding such abuses is important for preserving mental health.

When mental health does deteriorate, treatment and repair can be sought. As discussed in section I.2, treatment may take the form of cognitive behavioral therapy or various forms of psychotherapy or may involve pharmacological treatment. Such therapies and treatments sometimes can help address more severe forms of depression, anxiety, or anger. Repair of poorer mental health can sometimes be addressed through rest or through one's social relationships.

---

5. See Sajeev et al. (2016) and Baird and Thompson (2018).

Each of these approaches can be important in sustaining mental health in the narrow sense of good functioning of the brain. Each thus also constitutes an important way to sustain mental health in its broader sense, the wholeness of the mind as it pertains to the flourishing of the person. However, once we turn to mental health in this broader sense, maintaining mental health goes beyond regular use and stimulation, avoidance of abuse, and seeking repair of the processes of the brain that sustain the mind. With regard to sustaining mental health in its broader sense as it pertains to human flourishing, the mind must be concerned with more definitive positive content concerning what is good. What is then in view is human flourishing and it makes sense to consider this in the broader context of all of the practices that sustain human flourishing itself.

1.6e. Human flourishing, or the health of the person, is sustained by pursuits and purposes, by commitments to relationships and institutions, by spiritual practices, by rest and balance and leisure, and by addressing the domains of life in which one is flourishing least.

The health of a person, or human flourishing, may be understood as living in a state in which all aspects of a person's life are good. This is an expansive notion of wholeness or health. Sustaining flourishing relates to all aspects of a person's life and activity. In section I.6c and I.6d, we considered various practices that sustain the health of the body and the brain. In section I.5, we considered various spiritual practices to sustain spiritual well-being and how they can also sometimes contribute to temporal flourishing. Here we will focus on various other aspects of temporal flourishing, including happiness, meaning and purpose, character, and relationships.

A number of simple activities have been proposed in the recent positive psychology literature that are intended to improve various aspects of subjective or psychological well-being. They include regular practices of gratitude, doing acts of kindness, and imagining one's best possible self. There is now evidence that these activities do indeed seem to promote some degree of greater happiness and perhaps somewhat better health.[6]

---

6. For reviews of activities and the empirical evidence, see Bolier et al. (2013), Sin and Lyubomirsky (2009), Hendriks et al. (2019), and VanderWeele (2020a).

These activities and practices are valuable in sustaining various aspects of well-being over time. However, they seem less effective at giving one a sense of meaning and purpose or building character or sustaining social relationships.[7]

Commitments to relationships and institutions may be especially important for these other aspects of flourishing. Such engagement may be critical in giving one a sense of purpose, strengthening character, and fostering close social relationships and perhaps may contribute to health and happiness. Engaging in work or pursuing education both provide opportunities for purpose, character, and relationships. Marriage, as discussed in section I.4, forms one of the closest types of relationships and can profoundly shape character, and the formation of a family can constitute one of life's most substantial pursuits, giving rise to a sense of purpose. Religious community can likewise foster relationships, form character, provide a system of meaning, and help shape the pursuit of one's final communion with God. Each of these commitments—to work, to education, to marriage, and to religious community—can be powerful pathways to flourishing.[8]

Often these longer-term commitments or pursuits are required to alter not only health and happiness but also character, meaning, and relationships. In section I.5d, we discussed the notion of calling or vocation from a Christian theological perspective and its role in fostering character, purpose, relationships, and love. More substantial longer-term pursuits can likewise provide opportunities for the formation of character and purpose. When these pursuits are made within the context of a community, that community provides the opportunity for close relationships and those relationships further enhance the sense of meaning and purpose and the opportunities for the formation of character. It is perhaps in part because of the interconnectedness among commitments to work,

---

7. VanderWeele (2020a).

8. Elsewhere, I have reviewed the empirical evidence for work, education, family, and religious community being important pathways to flourishing (VanderWeele, 2017a) and have argued that each of these institutional or relational pathways is common or prevalent and has important effects across various domains of flourishing, including happiness, health, meaning, character, and relationships. Within public health, these two criteria of being relatively prevalent with reasonably large effects are often taken as the two criteria for identifying important factors that shape population health.

education, marriage, and religious community that they can so powerfully foster and sustain flourishing.

Flourishing, conceived of as a state in which all aspects of a person's life are good, includes all domains of human life. The sustaining of flourishing over time can be impeded if some important aspect of life is neglected. The complete neglect of some aspect of flourishing can lead to the deterioration of others over time. Declines in physical health may make it difficult to pursue one's purposes or relationships. A failure of character may lead to wrong action, wrong pursuits, and bad relationships. Deteriorating relationships may lead to unhappiness, poorer health, and a loss of meaning. For flourishing to be sustained, each of the domains of flourishing is important not only in its own right but also because of the effects it may have on other domains of life. Individuals will inevitably flourish in different ways and to different degrees and may sacrifice certain goods or aspects of flourishing in order to attain others. However, some awareness of the domains of life in which one is least flourishing may be helpful in addressing challenges and impediments to flourishing and in ensuring that flourishing does not deteriorate too far in any domain of life. Through awareness and reflection and from trying to understand the whole of one's life, one can try to discern what changes to one's life and activities may be important and how best to redirect one's pursuits.

Rest and reflection are critical in maintaining both physical health and the health of persons. Rest sustains health, provides time for reflection, provides opportunities to discover meaning, allows space for relationships, and can uncover which aspects of character need improvement. Rest and leisure are often foundational in experiencing a profound happiness—a celebration of the goodness of life itself—and in religious and spiritual practices that both constitute and bring about spiritual well-being.[9]

In some sense, the fundamental approaches to sustaining flourishing, or the health of persons, over time concern regular practice, avoiding abuse, and seeking repair. Regular practice with respect to commitments to relationships and institutions may include engagement in work, education, family, and religious community, all of which tend to promote

---

9. Pieper (2009).

flourishing over time. Ensuring awareness of how one is flourishing and how one is not and reflection upon these matters can prevent neglect of certain aspects of life or subjecting one's person and being to abuse. Identifying and seeking to rectify or repair domains of life where flourishing is weakest and having adequate rest both to reflect and to flourish are likewise important in achieving the wholeness of the person that is human flourishing.

1.6f. Habits that sustain the health of the mind and the health of the person will also contribute to the sustaining of bodily health.

In our discussion of the sustaining of bodily health, we considered the practices of exercise, good diet, good sanitation, temperance, sleep and rest, and seeking medical care when needed. However, as was also discussed in section I.3, the health of the mind and spiritual health also affect bodily health. Thus, the practices that sustain other aspects of flourishing—mental, social, and spiritual health—will often also contribute to bodily health. Stimulation and proper use of the mind, rest, and mental health care as needed can all contribute to one's mental health and thereby potentially to bodily health as well. Pursuing various purposes, making commitments to relationships and institutions, ensuring adequate rest and leisure, having a balance among activities, and taking time to reflect will all contribute to various aspects of the flourishing of the person and may thereby also contribute to bodily health as well. Prayer, the love of neighbors, the transformation of character, the pursuit of vocation, participation in religious community, faith, and hope all promote and are constitutive of spiritual well-being and may often contribute to bodily health also. We do not often think of these things as practices for bodily health or as being important health behaviors, but given the integrated nature of the human person, these other aspects of flourishing, or the wholeness or health of persons, will often be important health assets for physical health as well.[10]

---

10. For reviews and meta-analyses of the empirical evidence concerning effects on physical health, see Roest et al. (2010), Martín-María et al. (2017), Hernandez et al. (2018), Trudel-Fitzgerald et al. (2019), and Steptoe (2019) for mental health and psychological well-being; Berkman et al. (2014) and Holt-Lunstad et al. (2015) for social well-being; and Chida et al. (2009), Koenig et al. (2023), VanderWeele (2017c), and Balboni et al. (2022) for spiritual and religious well-being.

1.6g. What we value shapes our capacity to flourish.

Our values, our desires, and our loves all shape our capacity to flourish. This is in part because happiness, as part of flourishing, consists of satisfying the will and its desires. We are made at least partially happy when our desires are satisfied, and our capacity to satisfy those desires depends in part on what it is that we value. Desires that cannot be met will leave us unsatisfied, at least in part. Plato, Aristotle, and other ancient philosophers acknowledged that when one values virtue as constitutive of well-being, then one's well-being could at most only very partially be affected by life circumstances because circumstances generally cannot preclude one's capacity to act rightly and develop one's character.[11] Valuing virtue thus potentially shapes the nature of flourishing and one's capacity for flourishing.[12]

The Christian tradition assigns similar importance to the valuing of virtue and character, although within the Christian faith, the various other virtues are to contribute to and to be informed by what is considered the highest virtue, charity, a friendship with God that includes love of God and love of neighbors. St. Paul wrote, "As God's chosen ones, holy and beloved, clothe yourselves with compassion, kindness, humility, meekness, and patience. . . . Above all, clothe yourselves with love, which binds everything together in perfect harmony" (Colossians 3:12–14) and he instructs us to "seek the things that are above, where Christ is, seated at the right hand of God. Set your minds on the things that are above, not on the things that are on earth, for . . . your life is hidden with Christ in God" (Colossians 3:1–3). The Christian teaching applies the insight that well-being found in virtue is not subject to changes in external circumstances to the theological virtues and to spiritual well-being.[13] If what we are pursuing in this life is charity—love of God and

---

11. Aristotle (4th C BCE/1925, book I); Plato (4th C BCE/2004).

12. There is empirical support for the notion that the valuing of various aspects of flourishing affects subsequent actual flourishing, both with respect to enhancing the domain that valued and to flourishing more generally, with maybe also some indication that with respect to potentially valuing the emotional, physical, purposive, character-related, social, and financial aspects of well-being, the effects on well-being as a whole are perhaps greatest for valuing virtue (Węziak-Bialowolska et al., 2023).

13. Other Scriptural references to the value and comparative robustness to circumstances of the theological virtues of faith, hope, and love include: "In this you rejoice, even if now for a little while you have had to suffer various trials, so that the

love of neighbors—and ultimately God himself, then our well-being will not be subject to changes in circumstances. Jesus taught, "Do not store up for yourselves treasures on earth, where moth and rust consume and where thieves break in and steal, but store up for yourselves treasures in heaven, where neither moth nor rust consumes and where thieves do not break in and steal" (Matthew 6:19–20). Spiritual well-being is not subject to corruption in the same way that external goods are, and spiritual well-being is more valuable than any earthly good.

Our desires arise from the perception of something we consider good, and our loves are shaped by our experience of that good.[14] The experience of something good shapes and strengthens our desire further and thus shapes our actions, our habits, and who we are as persons. What we perceive as good and what we value thus shapes our being. It shapes what satisfies our desires and what makes us happy and it shapes our character and our capacity to attain other goods and the most important goods. In comparing earthly to heavenly goods, Jesus taught that "where your treasure is, there your heart will be also" (Matthew 6:21). It is thus important to our well-being that our values and our loves are properly ordered.[15] If what we love shapes our well-being, then it is important to have our loves rightly aligned. We need to be able to perceive what is of greatest value so that our desires and our loves are shaped accordingly. Jesus continued his teachings with this statement: "The eye is the lamp of the body. So if your eye is healthy, your whole body will be full of light, but if your eye is unhealthy, your whole body will be full of darkness. If, then, the light in you is darkness, how great is the darkness! No one can serve two masters, for a slave will either hate the one and love

---

genuineness of your faith—being more precious than gold that, though perishable, is tested by fire—may be found to result in praise and glory and honor when Jesus Christ is revealed." (1 Peter 1:6–7); "We also boast in our afflictions, knowing that affliction produces endurance, and endurance produces character, and character produces hope, and hope does not put us to shame, because God's love has been poured into our hearts through the Holy Spirit that has been given to us" (Romans 5:3–4); and "If I give away all my possessions and if I hand over my body so that I may boast but do not have love, I gain nothing. . . . And now faith, hope, and love remain, these three, and the greatest of these is love" (1 Corinthians 6:3–13).

14. Aquinas (1274/1920, I.II.26.1–2, I.II.30.1–2, I.II.25.2).

15. See 1274/1920, II.II.26 for Aquinas's discussion of the proper ordering of charity, or love.

the other or be devoted to the one and despise the other" (Matthew 6:22–24). What we perceive, what we choose to focus on, what we think about and expose ourselves to will shape our values, our desires, our loves, our being, and the potential for and the nature of our flourishing.

The Christian understanding is that the greatest good is God himself and that when one has this perspective, one's well-being is more grounded, here and now, and is more oriented toward eternal flourishing.[16] However, the insight is applicable more broadly. It pertains to other aspects of life as well. In our work, in our relationships, and in our rest and leisure, what we perceive and experience as good shapes what we desire, love, and value. What we value shapes the actions we take; it shapes our character and shapes the nature of and our capacity for flourishing. Our values affect our capacity to flourish.

All of us desire the fullest flourishing possible. When we do not experience this, when our desires are for things that ultimately do not satisfy, when our values and loves are not properly aligned, we are left longing, however inarticulately, for more. It is thus that St. Augustine writes, "Thou hast made us for thyself, O Lord, and our heart is restless until it finds its rest in thee."[17]

1.6h. Communities and their representatives also bear responsibility for maintaining health because good social relations, material resources, a safe environment, and communal practices are all needed for health and promote health.

An individual's actions and habits clearly contribute to maintaining health of the body and of the person. However, the community that a person is a part of also plays an important role in sustaining health. For a person to maintain the health of the body, the community's organization

---

16. The experience of genuine, but lesser, goods can thus distract a person from the pursuit of the highest goods. Jesus thus taught, "Truly I tell you, it will be hard for a rich person to enter the kingdom of heaven. Again I tell you, it is easier for a camel to go through the eye of a needle than for someone who is rich to enter the kingdom of God" (Matthew 19:23–24) and warned of the "cares of this age and the lure of wealth" (Matthew 13:22) distracting a person from the pursuit of what is of greatest value and from fruitfulness and true flourishing.

17. Augustine (400/1991, I, 1).

and its practices, policies, and economic structure should be such that each person has the resources to access affordable housing and nutritious food,[18] that members of the community have sufficient time for rest and leisure and to spend time with others,[19] that both working and living environments are relatively free of pollutants and toxic chemicals,[20] and that the community is safe and free from violence and discrimination.[21] Each of these aspects of the life of the community is important in maintaining the bodily health of individuals.[22]

Theologically, as discussed in section I.4b, the idea of the common good includes the concept that the community is partially responsible for maintaining health, where this "common good" may be defined as "the sum of those conditions of social life which allow social groups and their individual members relatively thorough and ready access to their own fulfillment."[23] It is the responsibility of each person and of the community as a whole to contribute to this common good, including the conditions that help bring about the health of the body and the health of the person.[24] In section III.4 we will consider further the distinctive contribution of church communities to healing and to restoring persons to health.

The communities we live in also have a central role in providing the context for the relationships, cohesion, and sense of belonging that are important health assets for bodily health. The community is also important in sustaining health because certain members of the community are entrusted to promote health and public health, including addressing issues such sanitation, clean water, vaccinations, and various aspects of environmental health and safety. These public health issues are important in the promotion of individual health and are best approached at the level of a community. Other individuals in the community, those within medicine, are entrusted with the task of restoring health. This too is

---

18. Leo XIII (1891).
19. John Paul II (1981).
20. Francis (2015).
21. John XXIII (1963). See Massingale (2014) for discussion of Catholic theology concerning racial justice and opportunities for further engagement on issues concerning discrimination.
22. See Berkman et al. (2014) for empirical evidence and discussion concerning many of these various social determinants of health.
23. Paul VI (1965).
24. Catholic Church (2004, 164–170).

important in sustaining the health of individuals. In part III, we will consider this important role further and also explore further ways that the community is important for, contributes to, and bears some responsibility for the health of individuals.

The responsibility of the community for individual health arises from the opportunities a community has to contribute to the good of health. These must be balanced against the opportunities for pursuing other goods, and the right allocation of resources within a community and across individuals is a question of what constitutes a just society.[25] Bodily health is just one of the many important goods that a society can seek to promote with its allocation of resources. Different political and organizational structures will inevitably result in different allocations of resources, and there is not necessarily a correct answer to the extent to which resources are to be devoted to physical health. However, physical health is a good that contributes to the pursuit of many other goods and aspects of flourishing, and as societies advance, they often devote a substantial portion of their resources to promoting and restoring health. While individual responsibility for maintaining health is important, the community can and often does play a critical role in that endeavor.

Another way that different communities contribute to and bear some responsibility for the physical health of individuals is in contributing to their flourishing more broadly. As discussed above, many aspects of human flourishing contribute to bodily health. These other aspects of flourishing are also sought as their own end, and a community has numerous opportunities to promote human flourishing through, for example, education, or family, or religious community and also through work.

1.6i. Facilitating flourishing at work will facilitate flourishing in life.

One of the ways that particular communities contribute to human flourishing is through work. We spend much of our lives working. That work, rightly understood, is constituted by effortful activities to help fulfill the needs, aspirations, desires, and good of human persons. Work contributes to the health of persons. Much work—including work directed at producing food, shelter, medicine, and public health—contributes

---

25. Tasioulas and Vayena (2020); cf. Catholic Church (2004, chapter 4).

specifically to the bodily health of others. However, work also contributes to the health and well-being of the person working. Work provides an opportunity to develop one's abilities and one's character because providing goods and services to others can be sources of meaning and working alongside others can foster relationships. Work contributes to human flourishing.[26]

Work is arguably also constitutive of human flourishing. In the creation stories in Genesis, even before the fall, we read of God placing man in the garden he had created "to till it and keep it" (Genesis 2:15). Work is part of God's intent. That generative creative activity in some sense reflects God's creative activity and the fact that human persons are created in God's image.[27] The health of a person—a life lived in accordance with God's intent—involves some form of work or creative activity. This is constitutive of flourishing.

Through rational human capacities, societies have devised ways to do work more collectively and efficiently through organizations and companies and through the use of technologies and systems of distribution that have the capacity to contribute more than is possible without cooperation. Such organizations can and have facilitated human flourishing—both bodily health and the health of persons—in various ways. Human persons can do more together than they can as individuals. This is manifest in countless ways in workplace settings. Organizations and companies can also help individuals care for one another. There are, however, also dangers that can accompany organizations that efficiently coordinate work and productive activity, including seeing persons as means rather than ends, the potential to exploit people, the glorification of work to the exclusion of other goods in human life, and the concentration of power to few people who then have the capacity to use that power in ways that detract from rather than enhance human flourishing. It is important that the rights of workers and the dignity of workers be respected and that action

---

26. See Hanson (2022a) for an account of the history of the philosophy of work and the role of work in human flourishing. See Catholic Church (2004, chapter 6) for theological teaching concerning the role of work in human well-being. Empirical evidence likewise indicates that work contributes substantially to physical, mental, and social health and well-being (McKee-Ryan et al., 2005; Paul and Moser, 2009; Sayer et al., 2011; VanderWeele, 2017a).

27. Catholic Church (2004, 255, 270, 275).

be taken by the state, by companies, and by the workers themselves to ensure that work is directed toward human flourishing.[28]

Because we spend so much of our life working and because we were in some sense intended by God to work, work is critical to the health of persons and to the health of bodies. What takes place at the workplace will affect life more broadly.[29] Companies and organizations that produce goods and services that genuinely contribute to human well-being have enormous potential to make life better for numerous people and peoples around the world. Moreover, workplaces that help persons find meaning in their work, foster relationships at work, and exercise their creative capacities have tremendous potential to facilitate the well-being of employees, which can in turn affect the well-being of their families and communities.[30] Workplaces also contribute directly to the health and well-being of their employees and their families by providing wages in compensation for the work that is done. Workplaces thus have tremendous potential to contribute to bodily health and to the health of persons, and they ought to be organized to fulfill that potential. Leaders of companies and organizations thus have special responsibility to ensure that they do so—both with regard to the goods and services they provide and with regard to the lives of their employees and their families. Facilitating flourishing at work will facilitate the flourishing in life of persons and of society.

1.6j. The flourishing of a society facilitates the flourishing of the individual.

A well-functioning government and society that has sufficient material resources is critical for helping provide the opportunities and the

---

28. Catholic Church (2004, 301–304).
29. See, for example, Węziak-Bialowolska et al. (2020) and Bowling et al. (2010) for empirical evidence concerning the reciprocal causal relations between flourishing at work and flourishing in life.
30. The job-crafting practices of helping employees find meaning in work, foster better relationships in work, and find more efficient ways of working have considerable potential to promote employee well-being and greater work engagement (Wrzesniewski and Dutton, 2001; Frederick and VanderWeele, 2020). Company-level practices to help employees navigate work-family conflict likewise are critical in enhancing employee well-being (Fox et al., 2021).

material resources necessary to sustain health and the pursuit of other goods. A well-functioning community is also important for sustaining the pathways described above that promote individual flourishing. An efficient and effective government, a well-functioning financial system, the absence of corruption, and civic stability are all important in supporting families, work, education, and religious communities in the promotion of individual flourishing. The community provides not only the context and opportunities for the sustaining of bodily health but also the context and opportunities for flourishing.

As discussed in section I.4, one's community is also constitutive of one's well-being. If the health of a person, or human flourishing, is understood as a state in which all aspects of a person's life are good, then flourishing also entails that the person's community be good. The community supplies the set of relationships, structures and practices, and sense of belonging that make up much of the fabric of an individual's life. For a person to be fully flourishing, his or her community must be flourishing as well.

1.6k. The flourishing of individuals can facilitate the flourishing of society.

A community is made up of its members. The relevant contributions of the members and the whole community thus operate in both directions. The flourishing of a society, its state of government, and its policies, can help enable individuals to flourish. But individual flourishing—individual health, relationships, happiness, purpose, and, perhaps especially, virtue will likely also contribute to the strengthening of the institutions that enable a society to thrive. Indeed, for a society to be just, both the society's leaders and its other members must act justly. Individual flourishing facilitates the flourishing of a society.

1.6l. Although personal and communal responsibility are necessary for maintaining health, there are limits to what can be attained and some experience of ill health is inevitable.

Individual actions and habits contribute to health, and the individual bears considerable responsibility for maintaining their health. However, the community also makes critical contributions to health and bears responsibility for maintaining the health of its members. When individuals and communities are functioning well, they will be supportive of each other in preserving the health of individual and the health of society. However, there are limits to the sustaining of that health. Often disease arises, despite individual and community efforts. Injuries, sometimes permanent, do occur, and the process of aging inevitably results in limits to sustaining health over time.[31] Health inevitably eventually declines. These limitations must be understood and accepted. Some progress can be made in improving health and extending longevity, but there are limits, and it is also important to understand these limits and their causes, so as to understand how best to promote flourishing.

This first part of the book has presented an understanding of human flourishing as wholeness as intended by God. This is a positive vision of what flourishing consists of. But part of this positive vision is human freedom, a freedom that is required for genuine love. With that freedom comes the possibility of its misuse, of choosing not to pursue God's intent, of choosing not to love, of rejecting flourishing as God intended. The dark side of the profound freedom of the human person will be the subject of part II of this book, which will consider the fundamental causes of the ill health of the body and of the person. From a Christian understanding, the fundamental cause is sin, a voluntary departure from wholeness as God intended. The tension between the positive vision in part I and the darker considerations in part II will be addressed more substantially in part III, which considers the restoration and fulfillment of wholeness in light of the brokenness of the human person and the world and the misuse of freedom.

Propositional Summary 1.6: Health is the responsibility of the individual and of the community, but it also depends on circumstances beyond the control of either.
1.6a. The causes of health are diverse.
1.6b. Fundamental approaches in sustaining health include regular use of the systems that maintain health, avoiding abuse of those systems, and seeking repair of those systems when necessary.

---

31. See also Moyse and Hordern (2021) for discussion of some of the existential challenges and difficulties that arise in aging.

1.6c. Practices to sustain physical health include exercise, good diet, good sanitation, temperance, sleep and rest, and medical care.

1.6d Mental health is sustained by the stimulation and proper use of the mind, by rest, and by mental health care as necessary.

1.6e. Human flourishing, or the health of the person, is sustained by pursuits and purposes, by commitments to relationships and institutions, by spiritual practices, by rest and balance and leisure, and by addressing the domains of life in which one is flourishing least.

1.6f. Habits that sustain the health of the mind and of the person contribute to the sustaining of bodily health.

1.6g. What we value shapes our capacity to flourish.

1.6h. Communities and their representatives also bear responsibility for maintaining health because good social relations, material resources, a safe environment, and communal practices are all needed for health and promote health.

1.6i. Facilitating flourishing at work will facilitate flourishing in life.

1.6j. The flourishing of a society facilitates the flourishing of the individual.

1.6k. The flourishing of individuals can facilitate the flourishing of society.

1.6l. Although personal and communal responsibility are necessary for maintaining health, there are limits to what can be attained and some experience of ill health is inevitable.

I.7. The Implications of Health as Wholeness

In this section, we will consider the implications of the notion of health conceived of as wholeness of the body and of the person and the implications of the unity and goodness of the body and the person, of community well-being and spiritual well-being as part of flourishing, and of the responsibility we each have for health as these pertain to the practice of medicine, public health, and public policy.

I.7a. In discussions of health, greater clarity is needed about whether the topic is the health of the body or the health of the person.

As noted at the beginning of part I of this text, the word "health" is often used and understood in diverse ways. I argued above that in fact we have two distinct notions of health: health of the body and health of the person. Both notions of health pertain to wholeness. Bodily health may be understood as wholeness of the body with the body's parts and systems being and functioning as normal so as to allow for the full range of activities characteristic of the human body. The health of the person may be understood as complete human well-being, as having attained a state of physical, mental, social, and spiritual well-being. It would be useful in discussions of health to determine whether the health of the body or the health of the person is what is in view. Many discussions of health seem to locate the concept of health somewhere between these two conceptions of health. Greater clarity could be achieved if it were simply kept in mind that two distinct notions of health are present in our language.

Of course, acknowledging that there are two distinct notions of health does not resolve what aspects of health should be aimed for or promoted in any given context or setting. Different institutions, organizations, and practices may appropriately set as their goals different aspects of health, either of the body or of the person. Much of the dispute over the definition of health may pertain more to what the proper goals of medicine or public health or some specific organizations are. Often, these will often not be entirely straightforward questions. However, to acknowledge both the narrower and the broader conceptions of health that are present in our language can help provide clarity about what is under discussion. Promoting, facilitating, and maintaining both the health of the body and the health of the person are laudable goals. However, different institutions and organizations have different roles in promoting health.

The notion of the health of the person, complete human well-being, is multifaceted and includes physical, mental, social, and spiritual dimensions, and different institutions and organizations will play different roles with regard to promoting the health of the person in each of these dimensions. However, with these distinctions in place, discussion can perhaps more appropriately shift from the definition of health to debates about the proper purview of different institutions and practices with regard to promoting, maintaining, and restoring health. As noted above, determining the appropriate scope is not always straightforward. However, in light of the discussion and distinctions mentioned above, the next several sections present proposals for what might be taken as the proper purview of medicine, psychiatry, public health, and public policy with regard to the health of the body and the health of the person.

1.7b. The purview of medicine includes the health of the body and the aspects of the health of the person that pertain to decisions about the health of the body.

It seems clear that the practice of medicine ought to attend to maintaining and restoring the health of the body. The role of medicine with regard to maintaining and restoring the health of the person is perhaps more complex. On the one hand, many of the decisions concerning the health of the body affect an individual's mental and social life and potentially even their spiritual life. In some instances, promoting physical health will positively contribute to a patient's mental and social well-being. However, in other cases, various goods and ends may come into conflict.[1] Various surgeries may extend years of disease-free survival but also seriously compromise a person's quality of life or their capacity to

---

1. See VanderWeele et al. (2019b) and Section I.7g for examples.

work or their ability to function sexually. In such cases, the goal of bodily health or longevity may come into conflict with other aspects of well-being. Decisions related to promoting various aspects of the health of the body may adversely affect other aspects of the health of the person. Although it seems reasonable that a clinician should take such implications into account in deciding, along with the patient, on the best course of action, it also seems clear that the role of the clinician is not appropriately construed as the maximization of all aspects of a patient's flourishing. The physician is not interchangeable with a marital counselor, priest, or career coach. Different institutions and different caring offices have different roles with regard to addressing different aspects of well-being.

However, given the implications of medical decisions about the health of the body for the health of the person, one way to construe the proper purview of medicine might be as follows: the proper purview of medicine may be taken to be the health of the body and those aspects of the health of the person that are affected by decisions about the health of the body.[2] This in no way makes clinicians responsible for the full flourishing of the person, but it acknowledges that their actions have a role in promoting, restoring, and maintaining such flourishing.[3] Often, promoting bodily health will be consonant with the health or well-being of a person in a broader sense. Resetting and putting a cast on a broken arm in almost all cases will not only foster restored physical well-being but will also eventually facilitate mental and social well-being. However, when surgeries or medications have serious side effects, various ends and goals can come into conflict. In such cases, it is important to consider the well-being of patients and their preferences and goals and the priorities they give to various goals more holistically. This is arguably part of the purview of medicine.

---

2. This proposal was initially put forward in VanderWeele et al. (2019a) and developed further in VanderWeele (2024), along with the proposals in sections I.7c and I.7e below.

3. I do not view the position put forward here that the proper purview of medicine is "the health of the body along with those aspects of the health of the person that are affected by decisions concerning the health of the body" to be in conflict with the position taken by others that the end of medicine is health (Kass, 1975; Curlin and Tollefsen, 2021), with "health" understood as what I refer to as bodily health. That the purview or scope of considerations for medicine extends beyond what might be taken as its proper end, bodily health, follows because of the relation of medicine and the decisions made within medicine to other ends.

The consideration of issues related to the health or well-being of the person in medical decision-making pertains to the role of clinicians as caregivers. Patients desire care for the whole person, and most health care practitioners desire to care for the person, not just the body. Patients will often care about their capacity to carry out different roles in life, often in the workplace or in the family, and the capacity to fulfill such roles pertains more to the health of the person, to well-being.[4] Such care for the person requires that the clinician have a sense of the whole of a person's life. Although specialization and division of labor in medicine has advantages with regard to technical capacity, they also have the potential to threaten the sense of the whole.[5] Attention must be given to a patient's emotional, relational, and potentially spiritual well-being, and such matters cannot be easily addressed or documented in a series of notes or medical records that are readily transferable across countless medical practitioners. Addressing the well-being of the patient even in a limited scope as it pertains to decisions about health of the body will require time and care. It will require training beyond narrow technical confines. It will require an understanding of what is constituted by the health of the person, a genuine concern for the well-being of others, and health care systems and practices that allow clinicians to be attentive to such matters.

1.7c. The purview of psychiatry is wholeness of the mind as it pertains to the proper functioning of the brain and to the aspects of flourishing that the patient and clinician together agree to address through dialogue, and the purview of counseling likewise consists of the aspects of flourishing that the patient and counselor together agree to address through dialogue.

The remarks and proposal above about the purview of medicine as the health of the body and the aspects of the health of the person that are affected by decisions about the health of the body arguably pertain to the practice of medicine outside of psychiatry. The proper purview of psychiatry is broader still.

---

4. Gadamer (1996, chapter 10).
5. Gadamer (1996, chapter 6).

Psychiatry is not infrequently envisioned as broadly addressing mental health and not just the health or wholeness of the brain. When considering "mental health," we must, as discussed in section I.2, confront issues of what is meant by the wholeness of the mind and we are thus led to philosophical questions of the nature of the mind and what constitutes a life well lived with respect to the mind and mental well-being.[6]

Mental health, understood in its broader conception of the wholeness of the mind as it pertains to the entire human person, is not coextensive with but does include a substantial portion of what is meant by flourishing. This might well be viewed by some as being too broad a concern for psychiatry to reasonably deal with. Some may embrace this potentially expansive scope for psychiatry as enhancing mental health in a broader sense; that is, of enhancing numerous aspects of a person's flourishing, but others may consider this beyond the proper purview of psychiatric practice.

If mental health is understood in its narrower sense as wholeness of the mind as it pertains to the proper functioning of the brain, this tightens the conception considerably. If the concept of the absence of wholeness of the mind is restricted to malfunctions of the brain that can be documented in some manner and if there can be sufficient consensus about what constitutes normal mental functioning, then most people might mental health and mental illness, understood in its more narrow sense (see section I.2d), as being within the purview of psychiatry.[7] This reduction does not entirely get around the difficulties of how wholeness of the mind is to be understood or what types of mental functioning are to be considered normal. Thus, normative judgements will still be required. There will be disputed territory, but the same is true with other aspects of health and medicine.

However, some may feel that restricting the purview of psychiatry to addressing mental health in this narrower sense may be too restrictive,

---

6. See Stein (2021).

7. Much of the discussion of the scope of psychiatry concerns expansions of the category of "mental disorder" and expansions in the diagnostic classifications of disorders (e.g., Rose, 2006; Michels and Frances, 2013) rather than questions about whether the purview of psychiatry should be restricted to mental disorders or whether it should be broader.

especially in light of the connections between mental well-being and a person's physical, social, and spiritual life. A person may experience a substantial decline in mental well-being because of the loss of a particular relationship or some other good. They may experience depressive symptoms, but their brain may be functioning properly and the mental experience, although negative, may still be reasonable and normal in light of that loss, as is often the case with bereavement. Is helping a patient through that loss or through a relationship difficulty or through what many may perceive as a relatively normal process of grief really beyond the purview of psychiatry?

An intermediate position might be to take the purview of psychiatry to be promoting, maintaining, and restoring mental health in its narrow sense (lack of wholeness of the mind arising from malfunction of the brain) *along with* those aspects of flourishing or the health of the person that the patient and clinician agree, through dialogue, to pursue together.[8] Such a position would take as the object of psychiatric care the wholeness of the mind that arises from malfunction of the brain and would allow the psychiatrist to restrict his or her attention to this narrower conception of mental health. However, it would also allow, for psychiatrists and patients who desired it, the joint pursuit of other aspects of the patient's flourishing, or mental health in its broader sense. Such a position admittedly introduces potential heterogeneity in scope in the practice of psychiatry. However, it allows a minimum set of goals that psychiatric practice should adhere to while also allowing flexibility regarding its aim or the aims of specific psychiatrists or practices.

Such a perspective would open the possibility for various activities and interventions in the practice of psychiatry intended to promote well-being (sometimes referred to as "positive psychiatry")[9] or foster virtue,[10]

---

8. See McHugh and Slavney (1998) for a perspective on psychiatry that considers not only disease, behavior, and dimensions of personality but also a person's life story.

9. See, for example, Jeste et al. (2015) for discussion of the development of a "positive psychiatry," Wood and Tarrier (2010) for "positive clinical psychology," or Peteet (2018) for discussion of a "fourth wave" of psychotherapies that explicitly promote well-being.

10. See, for example, Woolfolk (2012), Waring (2016), Titus (2017), and Peteet (2022) for further discussion of the role of the virtues within psychiatric practice and psychotherapy and the opportunities and challenges within psychiatry for promoting

rather than more narrowly restricting the focus to addressing mental disorders. For such approaches to be effective it would be important that the psychiatrist and the patient be aligned regarding these broader aims within the clinical relationship. It is not necessarily essential that the psychiatrist and patient fully agree on their understanding of flourishing so long as there is sufficient agreement to pursue particular broader aspects of well-being that the patient values. Moreover, there may, in many cases, be considerable overlap in the patient's and the clinician's understanding of well-being, even if this agreement is not complete. In any case, agreement about joint pursuit of broader aims for the patient's flourishing will often be possible only through dialogue about the life and goals of the patient and both the patient's and the clinician's understanding of well-being.[11] Although clarification about how well-being is to be understood and what aspects of well-being are to be pursued may be viewed as a lofty aspiration, psychiatric practice will often contain an implicit understanding of what goods and ends are being sought.[12] It may often be helpful to clarify this more explicitly in order to facilitate better care and to come to an awareness of both areas of agreement and differences in perspective regarding what the patient and the clinician see as the most important goals to pursue.

Similar considerations pertain to counseling. In clinical psychology or counseling more broadly, the focus will generally be less on the proper functioning of the brain and more on the person's life as a whole, on the person's flourishing. It may be the case that a clinical psychologist or a counselor will not necessarily feel comfortable addressing all aspects of a person's flourishing but may feel comfortable addressing some subset of the aspects of a person's flourishing. Through dialogue, it will often be possible for the counselor and the client to come to an agreement about which aspects of the client's flourishing will be discussed and pursued.

---

virtue as its own end and to facilitate other forms of healing. See Jankowski et al. (2020) and VanderWeele (2022b) for a review of some of the empirical evidence concerning interventions to promote character development and virtue as it pertains to the psychiatric context.

11. See Curlin and Hall (2005) for a proposal to extend such dialogue to broader clinical contexts.

12. See Tjeltveit (2004) and Fowers (2005) for discussion of perspectives on how psychotherapy is inherently value laden and embeds implicit views of what constitutes healthy living.

An understanding of the client's and the counselor's various views and values will be helpful in clarifying the scope of what might be addressed. Consonant values and understandings may help broaden the scope of care, but once again a number of goals, such as improving relationships and growth in character, may be shared even if the counselor and patient come from somewhat different perspectives.

1.7d. Given that flourishing will be understood differently across persons and communities, there ought to be room for tradition-specific practices of medicine, psychiatry, and counseling.

The proposal in the sections above was that the purview of medicine was promoting, maintaining, and restoring the health of the body and those aspects of the health of the person that pertain to decisions about the health of the body and that the purview of psychiatry was promoting, maintaining, and restoring wholeness of the mind as it pertains to the proper functioning of the brain, along with those aspects of flourishing the patient and clinician agree through dialogue to pursue together, with the purview of counseling also including this latter arena.

The proposed purviews of the practice of medicine and psychiatry are thus not all aspects of flourishing but potentially include numerous elements of flourishing as they relate to the decisions and persons involved. However, as was noted in section I.1, how flourishing is understood is likely to vary somewhat across individuals and communities. That this is the case has the potential to introduce conflict in decision-making with respect to the goals (or the relative value placed on those goals) the patient and the clinician may think reasonable to pursue. In numerous cases, such conflict will likely not arise or come into play. These issues will not often arise, for example, in treating a burn or bandaging a wound. However, in other settings, such as how to proceed with an unwanted pregnancy or how to address a patient's or client's fears about being punished by God, the values, beliefs, and differing understandings of what constitutes human well-being may strongly influence decision-making in clinical contexts.

One way to navigate such complexities would be to introduce tradition-specific practices of medicine. Such practices might in principle share a common understanding of the research that grounds evidence-based medicine but acknowledge and take into account a differing set of values in the context of clinical decision-making. To some extent, such tradition-specific practices already exist. Religious hospitals may be somewhat more likely to raise religious and spiritual values in the context of clinical care than similar nonreligious institutions.[13] However, these considerations and differences are perhaps less explicit or intentional than they might be.[14]

The emergence of tradition-specific practices of medicine would likely require a gradual transition from the practices of contemporary medicine in the Western context. In a recent book, Balboni and Balboni[15] analyzed the role of differing religious and cultural values in the context of medicine and presented a potential model and set of principles to help facilitate tradition-specific practices. Their model operates in the context of what they refer to as structural pluralism, the conscious organization of coexistence and tolerance in shared medical structures of different religious and moral systems and world views, one that embraces religious

---

13. More research is needed that compares religiously and nonreligiously affiliated hospitals. Koenig et al. (2023) note, using somewhat older data, higher rates of chaplain-to-patient ratios among religiously affiliated hospitals (cf. VandeCreek and Burton, 2001; Cadge et al. 2008). See Handzo et al. (2017) for somewhat more recent data indicating similar conclusions. However, these papers do not look explicitly at the spiritual care received by patients, which can also be provided by clinicians. There has been considerably more discussion of the restrictions in practices that may be entailed by the ethical and moral norms at religious hospitals and health care systems than there has been concerning the opportunities for the provision of spiritual care and spiritually integrated care that religiously affiliated health systems might facilitate. Such facilitation might take place in part by providing an environment and mission more conducive to the provision of such care and in part because of the greater likelihood of concordance between the religious traditions of a patient and a clinician. The development of more explicitly tradition-specific practices would further facilitate such care and might also in many cases alleviate tensions about practices that are restricted by moral and ethical norms, as patients and clinicians would be more likely to share the same moral framework or there would likely be at least somewhat greater awareness of, and comfort with, those restrictions as being entailed by the particular religious tradition.

14. An alternative to tradition-specific practices might be to retain the current structures of health care for the most part but give patients a greater opportunity to request religious concordance with regard to the clinician assigned to care for them. See Blythe and Curlin (2019) for further discussion of the potential for and challenges with such an approach.

15. Balboni and Balboni (2018, chapter 15).

diversity and freedom. Although they acknowledge the potential challenges, including concerns about proselytization, abuse of authority, and clinicians' discomfort with addressing spiritual needs, they note that under their proposed model, no clinician is required to address matters outside their own set of values and understanding, and they support the current practice of relatively secularized medicine as one of many traditions (and presumably the one that will be dominant for some time to come) in the structural pluralism that they envision.

Movement toward a system that allows for tradition-specific practices would require sensible guiding principles to navigate the challenges that such a pluralistic system might give rise to. Balboni and Balboni thus also put forward a set of principles that they believe would support structural pluralism in practice. They suggest first that each spiritual or cultural tradition be permitted to express itself in its own way of life and understanding without truncation or reduction. They suggest, second, that patients and clinicians have freedom to participate and identify with the spiritual or cultural tradition of their choosing without coercion. Patients are thus free to choose a system that does not in any way entail elements of proselytization. Finally, they propose that each spiritual tradition creates its own visible social structures in medicine that are incrementally developed and publicly accessible through scientific evaluation and understanding. Over time, it might be possible to work toward systems that seek and attain greater patient-clinician spiritual and cultural concordance and to explore the possibilities of allowing for tradition-specific spaces. The structural pluralism they envision could encourage new models of medical education: training for spiritually and culturally sensitive care could be strengthened.

Allowing for such structural pluralism and for tradition-specific practices has a number of potential advantages. Balboni and Balboni propose that only in such a system can there be a more adequate return to care of the person, not just of the body, and that such a system is needed for resisting having the forces of the market, bureaucracy, and technology to determine all forms of care.[16] They argue that clinicians

---

16. In a subsequent chapter, Balboni and Balboni (2018) also address objections that such a system of structural pluralism would undermine the seeming unity of medicine. They argue that three foundational values in almost all religious and cultural traditions can help overcome these obstacles and provide some unity: first,

need to take responsibility for transforming medicine from impersonal to personal, from the care of bodies to the care of persons. Although the model of structural pluralism they propose could go a long way toward allowing the practice of medicine and of psychiatry to promote the health of persons, it would admittedly be a relatively long path from the current practices of Western medicine to the model they envision. Nevertheless, creating more space for such tradition-specific practices, interactions, and clinician-patient relationships could, at least partially, achieve some of the advantages they describe and help allow the practice of medicine to aim at a fuller flourishing.

Such tradition-specific practices are already rather more prominent in the context of counseling. Considerable thought and scholarship has, for example, gone into integrating psychotherapy with particular religious beliefs, including Christianity[17] and other religious traditions,[18] along with addressing psychotherapy in distinctively religiously pluralistic or secular contexts.[19] Large organizations exist that provide directories of, networks for, and conferences pertaining to spiritually integrated counseling.[20] In some ways, the need for tradition-specific approaches is even clearer in the context of psychotherapy and counseling than in medicine, since the aims and ends of such counseling almost always extend beyond the body and pertain to numerous other aspects of flourishing. However, as noted above, many decisions in medicine affect aspects of a person's flourishing in ways that extend beyond the

---

notions of patient-centered care is a part of almost all traditions; second, there will continue to be powerful partnership with science and empirical methods and most traditions support these methods; and third, there is the practice of hospitality, the welcoming and providing for the stranger and of those in need that should be placed back at the center of the practice of medicine.

17. Stevenson et al. (2007); McMinn and Campbell (2007).

18. Rosmarin et al. (2009); Abu Raiya and Pargament (2010).

19. Zinnbauer and Pargament (2000); Morgan and Sandage (2016); Vieten and Lukoff (2022).

20. The American Association of Christian Counselors, for example, has over 50,000 members; convenes several thousand participants at its annual conference; and publishes two journals. Although notably smaller, the International Network of Orthodox Mental Health Professionals aims to bring together Orthodox Jewish professionals and rabbis to address mental health issues on an individual and communal level and has an international presence and an annual conference attended by several hundred participants each year.

body, so tradition-specific practices may often be of benefit in medicine as well. The work that has been done—both in scholarship and in institutions—to establish tradition-specific practices of counseling may be taken as models for or as sources of ideas about what might be possible in medicine.

1.7e. The purview of public health and public policy ought to be the aspects of the health of persons, or human flourishing, around which societal consensus can be attained.

Although it might in principle be possible to achieve some level of agreement about the understanding of flourishing and about the most important values, goods, and ends between a patient and a clinician or potentially even between a patient and an entire practice, these considerations of agreement and consensus become more challenging in the context of public health and public policy. In such contexts, decision-making in a pluralistic society must often take place amid differing and competing visions about what constitutes the good. As such, public health and policy priorities are often reduced to matters of physical or bodily health and economic considerations. This is arguably often done because these are goods about which it seems to be comparatively easier to attain consensus. Physical health is nearly universally valued and is considered important both in its own right but also because it facilitates achieving other goals. Economic considerations likewise constitute important means in the pursuit of numerous, and potentially divergent, goals. However, to reduce public health and policy considerations to bodily health and economic resources is to effectively embrace a highly impoverished view of human well-being. Public health and public policy efforts ought to aspire to something greater. The difficulty is that in a pluralistic context it can seem difficult to navigate competing conceptions of the good.

However, even in pluralistic contexts, there is more potential for achieving broader consensus about well-being than is often acknowledged. The vast majority of people value bodily health and having sufficient financial resources, but they also care about more than physical health and money. Almost everyone desires to be happy; almost everyone wants to have a sense of meaning and purpose in life; almost everyone wants to strive to be a good person; almost everyone wants good relationships. These are other aspects of well-being about which it might be possible to achieve a relatively broad consensus. If this is so, the potential implications for public health and public policy efforts could be far-reaching. Instead of a near-exclusive focus on physical health and economic considerations, it might be proposed that the proper purview of public health and public policy ought to be the flourishing of persons to the extent that consensus can be obtained about which aspects of flourishing constitute the good. In most contexts, this would include happiness and life satisfaction, meaning and purpose, character and virtue, and close social relationships.[21] The specification and expansion of the goals considered in the context of policy do not necessarily lead to straightforward decision-making, as certain policies may enhance the flourishing of some but hinder that of others. However, an expansion of the ends in view would result in a rather broader set of considerations in such decision-making than is the case at present.

Such considerations relate closely to the notion of integral human development in Catholic social teaching—the notion that development ought to focus not just on economic outcomes but on the development of the whole person for all people.[22] In the 1967 encyclical *Populorum progressio*, Pope Paul VI wrote, "The development we speak of here cannot be restricted to economic growth alone. To be authentic, it must be well rounded; it must foster the development of each man and of the whole man."[23] The twofold principle is that development should pertain

---

21. See VanderWeele (2017b) for further development of this argument and for a brief proposed assessment of these various aspects of human flourishing.

22. The origin of the concept is often traced to Pope Paul VI's encyclical *Populorum progressio* (Paul VI, 1967), but clearly it has earlier roots such as Maritain's *Integral Humanism* (1936/1996). Integral human development is the stated subject of Pope Benedict XVI's final encyclical, *Caritas in veritate* (Benedict XVI, 2009), and the notion of integral human development was extended further in Pope Francis's encyclical *Laudato si'* (2015) to an "integral ecology" (cf. Pfeil, 2018). *The Compendium of the Social Doctrine of the Church* (Catholic Church, 2004) begins with a description of how the Church's teaching and social doctrine opens the way for an "integral and solidarity humanism." See also Heinrich et al. (2009) for a USAID-funded guide prepared by Catholic Relief Services to a practical framework for integral human development.

23. Paul VI (1967, 14).

to all people and that it should pertain to the whole of the person.[24] What we should be seeking is ultimately the flourishing of all people.

Given that as individuals we are ultimately aiming at the health of the person, at flourishing, and that we arguably ought to be doing so collectively as a society, a shift of public health and policy efforts to promote well-being, at least insofar as we can obtain general consensus, would seem desirable.[25] Moreover, there is now ample evidence that various aspects of psychological and social well-being affect both physical health and economic outcomes.[26] The ends that are being sought are often consonant with one another. Further attention concerning what efforts might be made at national and international scales to promote well-being, to promote health of the persons, will be given in the implications portion of section III.7. However, the time has come for a broadening of and a change in emphasis in public health and public policy.

---

24. The *Compendium of the Social Doctrine of the Church* puts forward four permanent principles to help direct social action toward promoting an integral humanism (Catholic Church, 2004, 7, 160). These are the principles of the dignity of the human person, the common good, subsidiarity, and solidarity. The specific statements of these principles, inferred from the text, might be summarized as follows: the principle of human dignity as "all people have the same dignity as creatures made in [God's] image and likeness" (144); the principle of the common good as "every aspect of social life must be related [to the common good] if it is to attain its fullest meaning" (164) with the common good understood as "the sum total of social conditions which allow people, either as groups or as individuals, to reach their fulfilment more fully and more easily" (164; see also Section I.4b); the principle of subsidiarity as "it is an injustice . . . to assign to a greater and higher association what lesser and subordinate organizations can do" (186); and the principle of solidarity as "interdependence between individuals and peoples . . . [and] we are all really responsible for all" (193).

25. The seventeen Sustainable Development Goals of the United Nations (Sachs et al., 2021) are an important step in this direction, but nevertheless still focus on material conditions. "Good health and well-being" constitutes only one of the seventeen goals and is focused principally on physical health. Little or no attention is given to matters of happiness, meaning, purpose, or character in the targets and indicators (although the Sustainable Development Index now includes a question on subjective life evaluation using Cantril's ladder; see Sachs et al., 2021). The specific targets of the Sustainable Development Goals concerning communities likewise emphasize principally material conditions. Some of this is perhaps necessitated by the difficulties of measuring more subjective aspects of well-being, which will be discussed in the next section.

26. See, for example, Lyubomirsky et al. (2005), Holt-Lunstad et al. (2015), Martín-María et al. (2017), and Trudel-Fitzgerald et al. (2019).

1.7f. In medical, public health, and public policy contexts, assessments should be made of human well-being and not only of physical health and financial circumstances.

The implications of an expansion of the purview of medicine, public health, and public policy are potentially far reaching and would bring a much wider set of considerations into play in decision-making. However, in order to do so and in order to evaluate the consequences of decisions, considerable progress would have to be made with respect to measurement. To facilitate this, we should measure various aspects of human flourishing beyond bodily health and financial circumstances. At a national level, instead of focusing on GDP and on various assessments of physical health and longevity, evaluation of a society's progress and the indicators used to evaluate that progress should be extended to include measures of happiness and life satisfaction, meaning and purpose, character, and social relationships.[27] The measurement of these other aspects of well-being is in no way straightforward, and disagreements over what precisely to measure are likely to persist long into the future. However, such disagreements are not adequate grounds for their relative neglect in

---

27. See VanderWeele (2017b) for a proposed brief assessment of these various aspects of human flourishing with two questions assessed in each of six domains: happiness and life satisfaction, physical and mental health, meaning and purpose, character and virtue, close social relationships, and financial and material stability. These questions (self-rated on a scale from 0 to 10, with different anchors, or degrees of agreement, specified for each item) are as follows: Q1. Overall, how satisfied are you with life as a whole these days? Q2. In general, how happy or unhappy do you usually feel? Q3. In general, how would you rate your physical health? Q4. How would you rate your overall mental health? Q5. Overall, to what extent do you feel the things you do in your life are worthwhile? Q6. I understand my purpose in life. Q7. I always act to promote good in all circumstances, even in difficult and challenging situations. Q8. I am always able to give up some happiness now for greater happiness later. Q9. I am content with my friendships and relationships. Q10. My relationships are as satisfying as I would want them to be. Q11. How often do you worry about being able to meet normal monthly living expenses? Q12. How often do you worry about safety, food, or housing? Anchors are:

Q1 (0 = Not Satisfied at All, 10 = Completely Satisfied); Q2 (0 = Extreme Unhappy, 10 = Extremely Happy); Q3 and Q4 (0 = Poor, 10 = Excellent); Q5 (0 = Not at All Worthwhile, 10 = Completely Worthwhile); Q6, Q9, and Q10 (0 = Strongly Disagree, 10 = Strongly Agree); Q7 and Q8 (0 = Not True of Me, 10 = Completely True of Me); Q11 and Q12 (0 = Worry All of the Time, 10 = Do Not Ever Worry).

policy and public health discussions. Although there will always be disputes over what to measure, existing measures are often highly correlated.[28] Moreover, even in the realm of physical health, we are faced with a range of disparate indicators ranging from life expectancy to infant mortality rates to obesity prevalence and others, as reflected in the Sustainable Development Goals.[29] The full range of these various indicators gives a more complete picture of the physical health of a country than only a single summary would. The same is true with regard to assessments of happiness and life satisfaction, of meaning and purpose, of character, and of social relationships. That a particular well-being construct is multidimensional does not mean that it should be neglected.

Such is also the case with physical health and with other aspects of well-being. Moreover, just as life expectancy is sometimes given greater prominence as a national indicator of physical health, various more prominent assessments of well-being have emerged.[30] This does not mean that the other assessments of well-being should be neglected.[31]

---

28. See Goodman et al. (2018) for one such empirical comparison indicating strong correlation between conceptually different assessments.

29. Sachs et al. (2021).

30. Measures of life evaluation based on Cantril's ladder (Cantril, 1965) or of life satisfaction have taken on an especially prominent role in cross-country dialogues and comparisons. The United Nations' World Happiness Report, authored by eminent economists (Helliwell et al., 2021), has since 2012 used Cantril's ladder data from the Gallup World Poll to rank countries on self-reported life evaluation each year. Cantril's ladder assesses where an individual would place themselves on a ladder with steps numbered 0 to 10, with 10 representing the "best possible life" and 0 representing the "worst possible life." A number of countries are now also independently collecting data on life satisfaction. Life satisfaction assessments often proceed by asking a question along the lines of "Overall, how satisfied are you with life as a whole these days?" with responses ranging from 0 = Completely Dissatisfied to 10 = Completely Satisfied.

31. Although life evaluation or life satisfaction assessment, as per the previous footnote, may be some of the best possible single-item assessments, they are inadequate for giving a fuller picture of well-being. The World Happiness Report, for example, does not draw attention to the fact that while life evaluations are typically higher in richer developed countries, assessments of meaning and purpose are often higher in poorer developing countries (Diener et al., 2011). In keeping with principles of integral human development, it is not only life evaluation or life satisfaction that should be promoted and assessed but also, as best as possible, all aspects of a person's life. Of course, in assessment settings, it may only be possible or financially feasible to carry out a single-item assessment, and life evaluation or life satisfaction

Rather, the situation with well-being indicators is analogous to the present use of physical health indicators. We need an expansion of well-being assessments in medical, public health, and public policy contexts.

In some ways, the success of GDP as a measure of national progress has arisen from the fact that it constitutes a single number. Well-being of a person in his or her entirety or of a nation of course cannot be reduced to a single number. The summaries are useful and valuable but are not all that there is to life. To resist reducing the human person and human society and human progress to purely material and economic terms, it is important to remember that well-being is multidimensional. Various aspects of well-being should be assessed, evaluated, and discussed and should constitute aims of public health institutions and public policy. It may be important to restrict primary attention to those aspects of well-being about which there is general consensus, but, as argued above, such consensus is much broader than the current restrictions to physical health and economic circumstances would suggest.[32]

---

may be the best single-item assessments in certain contexts. Some assessment is better than none at all (Lee et al., 2021, chapter 19). However, when using single-item assessments, what may be missing by using such a simplistic approach should always be kept in mind. Someone may in principle be satisfied and yet addicted to narcotics or satisfied and yet completely socially isolated by their own choosing. The inadequacy of life satisfaction or life evaluation assessments is also evident in individual decision-making. For example, someone who feels a moral obligation to do what is right might make choices that they know will result in lower self-assessment on the ladder (because of, say, the difficult consequences across numerous domains of one's life that result from that right moral action), yet this would still arguably be the right choice. Said another way, not everyone is a utilitarian seeking to maximize their lifetime average score on Cantril's ladder. Cantil's ladder may be the best single-item global assessment we have, but it does not capture all of the elements of well-being or flourishing, which are inherently multidimensional. See also VanderWeele et al. (2020a) and Lee et al. (2021) for a consensus-based set of recommendations for well-being assessments based on the number of items available and the type of setting in which the assessment is done. As discussed in footnote 27, when ten or twelve items are available, the indicators that make up the flourishing index (VanderWeele, 2017a) provide a crude assessment of flourishing across a reasonably broad set of domains: happiness and life satisfaction, physical and mental health, meaning and purpose, character and virtue, close social relationships, and financial and material stability.

32. And again would arguably include happiness and life satisfaction, physical and mental health, meaning and purpose, character, and close social relationships (VanderWeele, 2017b).

What we measure shapes what we discuss, what we care about, what we know, what we aim for, and the policies we put in place to achieve our goals.[33] It is thus important that we begin to assess the various aspects of well-being more comprehensively. Public health and public policy efforts should not stop at measurement, however, but should take broader assessments of well-being into consideration when evaluating different interventions, actions, and policies. Considerable reflection and effort would still be required to develop a public health of well-being or a public policy of well-being approach, but enough work and reflection has gone into these matters already that we ought to begin to shape public health and policy efforts to promote human well-being more broadly.[34]

1.7g. An exclusive focus on the health of the body leads to poor decision-making.

As discussed throughout part I of this book, ultimately it is the health of persons, including, but not limited to, health of the body, that we should be aiming at in individual decision-making, in public policy, in public health, and even, in certain ways, in medicine. Ultimately, we want to promote full human flourishing. Restricting attention more narrowly to an exclusive focus on the health of the body has the potential to give rise to poor decision-making. This will not always be the case. Sometimes the ends of physical health and other aspects of flourishing will be fully consonant, with the former supporting the latter. But in other cases, the ends of physical health and other aspects of flourishing may diverge and be in tension.

Consider the following examples.[35] Perhaps a man is struggling with treatment decisions over bladder cancer at a relatively advanced stage. He knows that a cystectomy will maximize life expectancy but might considerably hamper his quality of life and happiness. Or perhaps a scientist experiences occasional psychotic symptoms and is told that

---

33. See, for example, Stiglitz et al. (2009) and Hall and Rickard (2013) for further discussion.

34. Diener et al. (2009); Adler and Fleurbaey (2016); Trudel-Fitzgerald et al. (2019); Stiglitz et al. (2019); Plough (2020).

35. These examples are drawn from VanderWeele et al. (2019b), which also provides an introduction to the use of the concept of flourishing in medicine.

antipsychotic medications could suppress these episodes but would potentially impede his capacity for scientific work. Or maybe a young woman tests positive in screening for the BRCA gene and it becomes clear that prophylactic removal of her ovaries could be effective as a cancer prevention intervention but would also make her infertile, potentially threatening her happiness, her capacity to have children, and her social well-being. Or maybe a celebrity chef faces surgery options for tongue cancer such that removal of his tongue would maximize his chances of survival but would impede his speech and effectively end his career. In each of these cases, bodily health, or at least longevity, comes into some conflict with some other aspect of flourishing. Depending on the agent's preferences and situation in life, it may, in some instances, be the best decision to proceed with the medical intervention and to extend life in spite of the loss that may occur to mental or social well-being or capacity to work. However, it is not clear that this will always be so. In some instances, the patient may think that his or her flourishing will be best fostered by sacrificing some degree of physical health or longevity for some other good pertaining to relationships, quality of life, happiness, capacity for work, or meaning and purpose. There can be real trade-offs between various aspects of flourishing across different domains of a person's life. Asking what a patient considers important across the different domains of flourishing would thus be critical in evaluating the appropriate course of action. An exclusive focus on bodily health has the potential to lead to poor decisions that do not respect the values of the patient and what the patient considers most important.

Similar considerations can arise in public health and public policy. The recent COVID-19 pandemic has made clear that often there are real trade-offs between the maximal preservation of physical health versus social well-being or mental health. Of course, physical health considerations and morbidity, mortality, and loss following infection can lead to losses in social well-being or happiness or mental health. However, it is likewise the case that policies that focus exclusively on bodily health and neglect mental, social, and spiritual well-being may lead to higher mortality risk; the loss of a job, social isolation, or depression may bring about poorer physical health.[36] In the realms of

---

36. Roelfs et al. (2011); Holt-Lunstad et al. (2015); VanderWeele (2017b); Wei et al. (2019).

public health and with public policy, there can be real trade-offs across various domains of flourishing. We can and should search for policies that are capable of promoting flourishing across the various domains of life, for which various goods and ends are not in conflict, but such policies are not always possible.[37] Sometimes there are trade-offs.[38] However, to neglect other aspects of flourishing and to focus exclusively on bodily health is both to neglect the other goods and ends that people value in life and the role these other goods and ends have in promoting physical health. Again, exclusive focus on bodily health can lead to poor decisions.

Catholic moral theology has articulated a "principle of totality" that all decisions must prioritize the good of the entire person, taking into account physical, mental, social, and spiritual dimensions.[39] Decisions must be made about the "good of [a person's] being as whole."[40] Decisions should not be made based on bodily health alone. The Second Vatican Council asserted that the "moral aspects of any procedure ... must be determined by objective standards which are based on the nature of the person and the person's acts" and that "human activity must be judged insofar as it refers to the human person integrally and adequately considered."[41] Decisions made by individuals and in the realms of clinical relationships, public health, and public policy should take into account the whole person, all aspects of a person's flourishing.

---

37. I have elsewhere proposed using "outcome-wide" designs (VanderWeele, 2017d; VanderWeele et al., 2020b) to study the effects of an exposure or an intervention on many outcomes simultaneously. Such designs would better allow for the identification of interventions that could improve multiple outcomes simultaneously versus those that may entail trade-offs across outcomes.

38. See VanderWeele (2020b) for one possible approach to making decisions when ends come into conflict that prioritizes life but also takes into account various other aspects of flourishing.

39. The principle of totality is often viewed as having arisen from Aquinas (1274/1920, II.II.65.1). Pope Pius XII (1952) is generally credited with having named the principle (cf. Kelly, 1955; McCormick, 1987). See Schulz (2015) for further discussion and application to the limits of human enhancement.

40. Pius XII (1952).

41. Paul VI (1965). See also McCormick (1987).

1.7h. Psychological theories of well-being are often impoverished by the absence of considerations of bodily health, of virtue, and of communal well-being and thus need to be supplemented with these other aspects of flourishing.

As discussed above, medical and public health decision-making often focuses almost exclusively on bodily health and sometimes on mental health considerations, but often neglects questions of happiness or meaning or relationships without taking a holistic approach to decision-making. In contrast, psychological theories of well-being often incorporate considerations of happiness, meaning and sometimes even relationships, but these psychological approaches almost uniformly neglect bodily health.[42] This is perhaps in part because such theories emerge from psychology and thus focus almost exclusively on the mind. It is perhaps also in part because physical health, taken as an outcome, is sometimes used to attempt to justify the importance of these other aspects of well-being. However, bodily health is also a part of human well-being—of flourishing. A person may flourish in various ways but is arguably not *fully* flourishing if they are bedridden or severely ill. Psychological theories of well-being are often impoverished by not adequately considering physical health.

Many, although not all, theories and assessments of psychological well-being also effectively neglect questions of character and virtue, and yet, as noted in section I.1c, character and virtue are central to philosophical, religious, and cultural traditions worldwide. Although some of the most influential empirical character assessment work has arisen from psychology,[43] it is still the case that many theories and assessments of psychological well-being neglect this central aspect of flourishing.[44] To

---

42. For examples of major assessments or conceptualizations of well-being in the psychology literature that neglect bodily health, see Diener et al. (1985), Ryff (1989), Keyes (2002), Seligman (2011), Huppert and So (2013), and Su et al. (2014), among others. Noting the neglect of bodily health in psychological conceptions of well-being, one group of authors has suggested expanding the acronym of Seligman's popular PERMA model (positive emotion, engagement, relationships, meaning, achievement) to PERMAH in order to include health (Kern et al., 2021).

43. Peterson and Seligman (2004).

44. See, as prominent examples, Diener et al. (1985), Seligman (2011), and Huppert and So (2013). Keyes (2002) and Su et al. (2014) include items concerning the

the extent that such theories and assessments ignore character and virtue, they are impoverished and do not offer adequate conceptual or empirical coverage of some of the most central aspects of human life and constituents of flourishing.

Theories of psychological well-being typically focus on the individual. Thus, while some theories and assessments of psychological well-being include social relationships, most ignore any notion of communal well-being.[45] However, as argued in section I.4, flourishing—understood as living in a state in which all aspects of a person's life are good—includes living in a well-functioning community. Flourishing includes communal well-being. A focus on the individual alone, even if the individual's relationships are taken into account, does not fully capture the range of relevant considerations for social well-being, for flourishing. Psychological theories and assessments of well-being thus need to be supplemented by considerations and assessments of communal well-being.

Thus, while psychological theories and assessments of well-being include many aspects of flourishing that are typically neglected in medicine and public health, including happiness, meaning, and sometimes relationships, these psychological approaches often neglect other important aspects of flourishing such as bodily health,

---

contribution one makes to others that might be seen as related to character or the consequences of character. Ryff (1989) has a domain in her model entitled "personal growth" with indicators related to the desire for growth and self-perceived actual growth. However, given that Ryff's "eudaimonic" conception of well-being is supposedly traced back to Aristotle, the absence of emphasis in the assessment on character is conspicuous, though arguably this is simply indicative of the general neglect character has received in psychological conceptions of well-being.

45. See Su et al. (2014) for an assessment of psychological well-being that includes not only social relationships but also communal aspects of well-being, although most (but not all) of the communal well-being items in the assessment pertain to the relationship between the individual and the community (e.g., "I feel a sense of belonging in my community" or "I pitch in to help when my local community needs something done"), rather than to community well-being as such, although perhaps at least an item or two touch on this as well (e.g., "People in my neighborhood can be trusted"). As a contrast, see VanderWeele (2019b) for items that pertain to the well-being of the community, as assessed by the individual, but pertaining to the entire community's relationships, leadership, practices, belonging, and mission.

character, and communal well-being. It would thus be important and advantageous to supplement psychological theories and assessments of psychological well-being with these other aspects of flourishing, both with respect to research and scholarship in psychology, but also with respect to assessing individual and societal flourishing more generally.

1.7i. Since the health of persons includes their social well-being, social and communal well-being should be assessed, and decisions made in clinical contexts and in public health and public policy should take relational considerations into account.

As noted above, the complete health of the person includes good social relationships and living in a healthy community. A person is fully flourishing only if his or her relationships and community are healthy. Medical, public health, and public policy decision-making should take into account the effects of decisions, policies, and actions on relationships and on the well-being of communities. Doing so well will require an understanding of what constitutes the good with respect to relationships and with respect to communities, but it will also require empirical assessments that can support rigorous study and evaluation.

As discussed in section I.1c, good relationships require that each person understand the other, appreciate the other's being, take time to be with the other, and seek the good of the other. In short, good relationships require love, but they also require history, time, and understanding. The health of persons also includes a healthy community. As discussed in section I.4, the health of a community consists of more than simply its various members doing well. The health of a community requires also some notion of the common good, that each person cares for the well-being of others, that the well-being of others becomes a part of each individual's own well-being. Communal well-being includes "the sum of those conditions of social life which allow social groups and their individual members relatively thorough and ready access to their own fulfillment."[46] Communal well-being includes good relationships,

---

46. Paul VI (1965, 26).

good leadership, healthy structures and practices, a sense of unity and welcome, and a strong shared mission and vision for common life.[47]

For decisions in public health and public policy and in clinical settings to take into account social relationships and communal well-being more fully, these aspects of flourishing ought to be empirically assessed. Various measures of social connection and loneliness and of communal well-being have been developed, and in some policy contexts greater attention is being given to these issues.[48] Although these measures have been employed increasingly in research, they are underutilized in clinical, public health, and public policy contexts. We are often ignorant of how clinical decisions affect relational dynamics and of basic trends with regard to social connectedness at local and national levels. More work needs to be done.

As one example, there has been considerable debate over whether and the extent to which loneliness has increased in the United States over past decades.[49] The fact that we have not carried out data collection to be able to adequately settle this question points to the inadequate attention that measuring and understanding the distribution of and trends in social well-being has received. Although we now have access to some better data for the past decade, that so little is available from the decades prior makes clear the need for better tracking of the various aspects of social well-being.[50] Moreover, we would ideally want to understand the temporal trends and distributions about not just loneliness but also positive social connectedness, belonging, friendship, social support, trust, and communal well-being. Social well-being is an integral part of the health of persons. Social well-being needs to be more frequently assessed and better taken into account in clinical, public health, and public policy decision-making contexts.

---

47. See VanderWeele (2019b) for further discussion and a template of an empirical assessment for community well-being that includes national, city, neighborhood, family, workplace, school, and religious community contexts. See also Phillips and Wong (2017) for further conceptual and empirical discussion of communal well-being.

48. For measures, see, for example, Russell (1996), Berkman et al. (2014), Holt-Lunstad et al. (2015), Campaign to End Loneliness (2015), and VanderWeele (2019b). With regard to policy attention and interventions, see NHS England (2019) and Murthy (2023).

49. McPherson et al. (2006); Fischer (2009).

50. Twenge et al. (2021).

1.7j. Because the health of persons includes their spiritual well-being, attention should be given to tradition-specific understandings and assessments of spiritual well-being in discussions of public health, medicine, and public policy.

As discussed in section I.5, from the perspective of Christian theology, human flourishing includes also spiritual well-being. However, even in pluralistic contexts, spiritual well-being from a societal perspective should arguably be taken into consideration in clinical, public health, and public policy decision-making. This is because much of the world's population considers spirituality or religion an important or very important aspect of life.[51] For many, it is the most important. Even in the context of a pluralistic society it would seem that decisions should at least in part be shaped by what people consider to be most important. If what is considered most important is religious and spiritual well-being, then this too ought to be taken into account.

However, to do this sensibly in a pluralistic society will require attention to the diversity of understandings of what constitutes spiritual well-being. Such understandings vary across religious, spiritual, and cultural traditions. However, in a given tradition, it can make sense to consider and think about the progress that various religious and spiritual communities see themselves as making toward the ends they deem most important.

To more fully take such considerations into account in public health, public policy, and potentially even in decision-making will require empirical assessments of some form. Although various generic spiritual well-being assessments have been available for some time, these are arguably too generic to adequately capture the ends that religious communities deem most important.[52] To adequately assess spiritual well-being would require the development of tradition-specific measures.[53] These could be developed by clergy, laity, theologians, counselors, and spiritual directors in each of the world's major religious traditions. The point of such assessments would not in any way be to compare which communities are

---

51. Diener et al. (2011).
52. Fisher (2010); Paloutzian and Ellison (1982).
53. VanderWeele (2020c); VanderWeele et al. (2021).

doing better or worse. Such comparisons would effectively be meaningless, given the different measures employed. Rather, the idea of tradition-specific measures would be to give religious communities tools for making some assessment, over time and across individuals and local communities, about the progress such communities saw themselves as making toward the ends they deemed most important.

Such measurement would acknowledge the importance of the goals of spiritual well-being to various religious individuals and communities. It would provide a way to assess progress toward these ends or the lack thereof. It could in principle be used to evaluate the effects of various policy or clinical decisions or interventions on the capacity of individuals to engage in spiritual and religious life fully and adequately and to attain the goals they deemed most important. Such assessments could also in principle be used to allow religious communities to evaluate how their community activities have promoted their goals of spiritual well-being.

Tradition-specific assessments of spiritual well-being might also facilitate the capacity for religious communities to bring forward empirically informed cases for promoting the spiritual goals they deem important into policy discussions. Such advocacy would certainly need to acknowledge competing interests and goals of other communities, but that is always necessary in political life in a pluralistic context. However, there seems no good reason in principle to exclude the consideration of such goals, given their importance to so many. The use of such spiritual well-being assessments might thus help religious communities discern how various government policies do, or do not, affect their principal priorities.

Since so many consider spiritual well-being to be an important part of life—a critical part of flourishing, of the health of the person—it would seem reasonable to make use of empirical assessments and research to promote spiritual well-being.[54] Almost certainly much more could be done in this regard than has been carried out to date; and given the centrality of spiritual well-being to human flourishing, to the health of persons, and given the interconnectedness of human life, it would seem good to bring

---

54. From a Christian understanding, such spiritual well-being is the most central aspect of flourishing, and as argued in Section I.5, contributes to purpose of human life, in some sense the fulfillment of flourishing.

considerations of spiritual well-being, at least to some degree, into public policy, public health, and even clinical decision-making contexts.

1.7k. Because the health of the body and the health of the person are ideals, health, in both senses, is a relative concept, and flourishing should be promoted in various ways even in the absence of bodily health.

The health of the body and the health of the person are ideals. Health in a narrow sense of the health of the body may sometimes be approximately attainable. Perhaps especially for those who are young, this sense of the health of the body is not uncommon. However, the body is at all times going through a process of cellular aging, with defects and entropy, even imperceptibly, progressively increasing over time.[55] Even the health of the body is thus, in some sense, a relative concept.

The fact that human flourishing—the health of the person—is an ideal and that flourishing is thus relative, is yet clearer. Flourishing was defined above as living in a state in which all aspects of a person's life are good. In actual lives, things of course go wrong. We encounter problems, difficulties, relational challenges, unhappiness, troubling existential questions, conflicts in the communities we live in, and numerous other undesired phenomena in addition to deterioration in physical health. No one is fully flourishing in this life. Flourishing is an ideal; flourishing in this life is always relative to that ideal.

Flourishing should thus not be understood in a binary manner such that someone is either flourishing or not.[56] Such a view is inadequate both because flourishing is relative and because flourishing is multidimensional. With regard to any aspect of physical, mental, social, or spiritual well-being, one might be doing better or worse. Perfection in this life is not attainable. There is almost always room for improvement, but

---

55. See, for example, DiLoreto and Murphy (2015) for an overview and for some discussion of how such processes are genetically regulated.

56. Empirical research has noted that the "prevalence" of flourishing varies dramatically depending on the assessment and criteria used (Hone et al., 2014), but this result is based on an artificial dichotomization of individuals into those who are and are not flourishing. Such artificial dichotomization ultimately neglects the fact that flourishing is multidimensional and is always relative.

things could almost always also get worse. Moreover, because flourishing is multidimensional, one can be flourishing in certain ways but not others. One might have good relationships but poor physical health. One might have a strong sense of purpose but be suffering from a lack of happiness. One might have overall good mental health but be struggling with various aspects of character.

The multidimensional and relative nature of flourishing is important in the context of thinking about health. A person can flourish in various ways even in the absence of bodily health. It thus becomes appropriate to speak even of flourishing at the end of life, or flourishing while bedridden, or perhaps even, again in a relative sense, flourishing in the midst of imprisonment. These would all constitute flourishing in a qualified sense: some aspect of flourishing—whether it be physical health or freedom—is diminished and yet it is possible in spite of such limitations to find meaning, to develop character, and perhaps to improve relationships, find some measure of happiness, and deepen one's spiritual life. Flourishing to a degree is possible even amid adverse circumstances, even in the midst of the absence of flourishing with regard to certain other aspects of life. Of course, as noted in section I.3, the human person is an integrated whole and what occurs with regard to one aspect of the person will affect other aspects of the person's life. Flourishing amid physical illness may sometimes prove challenging due to the limitations that such illness imposes. Moreover, because of the unity and interconnectedness of the various aspects of a person's life, it is entirely possible that difficulties in one area of life give rise to difficulties in other areas of life. Poor physical health can give rise to poorer mental health or loss of purpose or poorer relationships, and likewise each of these things can adversely affect physical health. But limitations in one area of life can also provide opportunities for greater flourishing in other areas. Although physical limitations create challenges, they can also give rise to a greater investment in one's relationships or life projects. Suffering or lack of happiness or challenges with mental health may lead to greater growth in character, a discovery of new meanings, or a deeper spiritual life. Sometimes lack of flourishing in one area of life can provide motivation, or even time, for deeper engagement in other aspects of life, potentially giving rise to a fuller flourishing.

This insight is likewise shared by disability theories of health.[57] Someone may be flourishing in various ways even if the health of the body is imperfect or is subject to various limitations. Someone may have considerable health as a person even if struggles with limitations about the health of the body are real. This is not to deny the importance of bodily health, but rather to contextualize it. Disability, or poor bodily health, does not make someone any less of a person.[58] Moreover, as noted above, flourishing occurs in a diversity of ways. Flourishing as a person may be greater among many whose bodily function or bodily health is poorer.

Because flourishing is multidimensional in this way, it can and should be promoted, even in the relative absence of bodily health. Flourishing can and should be promoted even in the presence of disability or in the context of aging and even at the end of life. Although flourishing in this life is subject to constraints and limitations and is always imperfect, there are also always ways that it can be improved. There are always ways that relationships can be deepened, that character growth can occur, that new meanings can be found, that some measure of joy can be attained, and that one can turn to God in faith, and hope, and love. The health of the person is not reducible to bodily health. A person can flourish even in the midst of the decline of bodily health.

Of course, limitations, constraints, and imperfections of health in this life—health of the body and health of the person—are often frustrating and involve struggle. Health, as wholeness of the body and wholeness of the person, is not perfectly attainable here and now,

---

57. Amundson (2000); Merriam (2009); Sulmasy (2009); Messer (2013).

58. *The Compendium of the Social Doctrine of the Church* teaches "Persons with disabilities are fully human subjects, with rights and duties: 'in spite of the limitations and sufferings affecting their bodies and faculties, they point up more clearly the dignity and greatness of man.' Since persons with disabilities are subjects with all their rights, they are to be helped to participate in every dimension of family and social life at every level accessible to them and according to their possibilities. . . . Great attention must be paid not only to the physical and psychological work conditions, to a just wage, to the possibility of promotion and the elimination of obstacles, but also to the affective and sexual dimensions of persons with disabilities: 'They too need to love and to be loved . . . according to their capacities and with respect for the moral order, which is the same for the non-handicapped and the handicapped alike'" (Catholic Church, 2004, 148).

even though we might desire it. We are, moreover, faced with the eventual inevitability of death. We seek to maintain and preserve and restore health, but there are limits. We are in search for a greater wholeness, a fuller flourishing, a more complete healing, but, from the perspective of Christian theology that healing cannot come about without addressing sin as the movement away from wholeness as God intends it, and this will be the topic of Part II of this book.

Propositional Summary:

1.7a. In discussions of health, greater clarity is needed about whether the topic is the health of the body or the health of the person.

1.7b. The purview of medicine includes the health of the body and the aspects of the health of the person that pertain to decisions about the health of the body.

1.7c. The purview of psychiatry is wholeness of the mind as it pertains to the proper functioning of the brain and to the aspects of flourishing that the patient and clinician together agree to address through dialogue, and the purview of counseling likewise consists of those aspects of flourishing that the patient and counselor together agree to address through dialogue.

1.7d. Given that flourishing will be understood differently across persons and communities, there ought to be room for tradition-specific practices of medicine, psychiatry, and counseling.

1.7e. The purview of public health and public policy ought to be the aspects of the health of persons, or human flourishing, around which societal consensus can be attained.

1.7f. In medical, public health, and public policy contexts, assessments should be made of human well-being and not only of physical health and financial circumstances.

1.7g. An exclusive focus on the health of the body leads to poor decision-making.

1.7h. Psychological theories of well-being are often impoverished by the absence of considerations of bodily health, virtue, and communal well-being and thus need to be supplemented with these other aspects of flourishing.

1.7i. Since the health of persons includes their social well-being, social and communal well-being should be assessed, and decisions made in clinical contexts and in public health and public policy should take relational considerations into account.

1.7j. Since the health of persons includes their spiritual well-being, attention should be given to tradition-specific understandings and assessments of spiritual well-being in discussions of public health, medicine, and public policy.

1.7k. Because the health of the body and the health of the person are ideals, health, in both senses, is thus a relative concept, and flourishing should be promoted in various ways even in the absence of bodily health.

PART II

ILL HEALTH AND SIN

"Our heart is restless"
(Augustine, 400/1991, book 1, chapter 1)

Propositional Outline of Part II:
The cause of ill health is sin.

2.0. Ill health is the absence of wholeness.
2.1. Ill health often follows from the wrongful action of ourselves or others.
2.2. Wrongful actions can bring about unjust structures that may result in ill health over extended periods of time and even across generations.
2.3. Human nature is distorted by sin, and this fallenness has disrupted relations between human persons and the world, giving rise to further external causes of ill health.
2.4. Sin has brought about and continues to bring about death.
2.5. Ill health cannot be prevented without addressing sin.
2.6. The experience of distress over brokenness, or lack of wholeness, is suffering, whereby the need for healing and restoration is made clear.
2.7. The implications of ill health and sin.

Introduction

Ill Health as the Absence of Wholeness

Proposition 2.0. Ill health is the absence of wholeness.

If health is wholeness as intended by God in creation, ill health is the absence of such wholeness. Ill health of the body may take the form of disease or injury or defect or frailty. Such ill health is contrary to God's initial intent for the body. Part of the body may be injured or not intact. The body's systems may not be functioning as they ought. Due to injury, infirmity, disease, or malfunction, the body may not be capable of the ordinary range of activities that is characteristic of it. Any of these would ordinarily be referred to as ill health.[1]

Ill health or lack of wholeness of the person may be understood as any aspect of one's life that is not good. We would not ordinarily speak of this as "ill health" but rather as lack of complete flourishing. The use of "ill health" in English carries considerable *physical* connotations, perhaps even more substantially than "health." The antonym of "health"

---

1. We might define disease as "a bodily anomaly constituted by a process of a sequence of changes from normal or abnormal structure;" injury as "bodily anomaly resulting from an extrinsic infliction"; defect as a "state of bodily anomaly"; frailty as "a bodily state of weakened or abnormal function accompanied by comparatively normal structure"; illness as "the human experience of disease"; sickness as "the experience of physical symptoms suggestive of, or similar to what is experienced in, disease"; and ill health (of the body) as "lack of wholeness of the body" or as "the presence of disease, injury, defect, or frailty." All illness is sickness, but not all sickness (e.g., motion sickness) is illness, although all sickness is nevertheless a form of ill health. Note that by defining defect as any "state of bodily anomaly," the two definitions of ill health (of the body) above—"lack of wholeness of the body" and "the presence of disease, injury, defect, or frailty"—effectively become equivalent. See Miettinen (2011) for a number of closely related definitions from which these were partially drawn, although note that Miettinen uses "ill health" and "illness" synonymously.

with respect to the person might perhaps be more appropriately, though nevertheless metaphorically, referred to as "brokenness."

In part I, I discussed how, from a theological perspective, health could be viewed as wholeness according to God's intent. God's intent for the body was that the body be whole and well-functioning and allowing for the capacity to love. God's intent for the person was goodness, a complete flourishing, with the final end of the human person being communion with God himself. Any deviation from that intent, that wholeness of the body or that wholeness of the person, is ill health.

The Christian tradition ultimately identifies sin as the source of ill health,[2] sin being understood as deviation from God's intent.[3] As discussed further below, this does not mean that all ill health results from one's own sin or wrongdoing, but rather from some deviation from God's intent. How does such deviation from God's intent arise? How is it that God, who is all powerful, could not accomplish his intent? One of the traditional Christian responses to this question is that this can occur through human freedom. Human freedom is important in allowing for a free response to God in love.[4] That freedom is important for having a full communion with God, a friendship with God. But that freedom also allows for the potential for rejection of God. That freedom allows for the possibility of sin. In his discussion of sin, Aquinas defines a sin with respect to human action as a "voluntary inordinate act"—an act that is free and contrary to reason and to God's ordering of things.[5] God's intent is not for sin; his intent is for freedom, and a person can choose to act contrary to that intent.[6] Understood in these terms, that sin is a cause of ill health

---

2. Aquinas (1274/1920, I.II.85.5).
3. Aquinas (1274/1920, I.II.71.6).
4. Aquinas (1274/1920, I.II.79.1–2).
5. Sin might alternatively, and within the theology of Aquinas, be defined as a "bad human act" (1274/1920, I.II.71.6), a "word, deed or desire contrary to the eternal law" (I.II.71.6,), a "human act contrary to reason" (I.II.71.6), or "a voluntary inordinate act" (I.II.71.6, I.II.72.1). The text here will frequently employ "wrong action," understood as "a bad human act" or an "act contrary to the moral law," to attempt to make as transparent as possible the claim that *a* central cause of ill health is wrong action, and to argue this even for those who may not hold a distinctively Christian understanding. See also Frey (2018).
6. Aquinas speaks of God's will in the absolute sense of the universal cause of all things that is always fulfilled and cannot fail to produce its effect, but in light of human freedom, Aquinas also distinguishes between God's will antecedently and

follows as a logical conclusion. Ill health is deviation from God's intent of wholeness; the only way such a deviation from God's intent can come about is free action contrary to God's intent, and this is sin.

However, that sin is itself, by definition, a deviation from God's intent implies that something is not right with the person, that the person is not whole. Sin constitutes ill health.[7] That *the* cause of ill health is always sin needs argument, but that sin is always ill health follows by definition of the terms as given above. Sin separates us from our own nature as intended by God. It separates us from God by that deviation from his intent, and as will be described in the sections that follow, it does harm to ourselves and others, physically and with respect to other aspects of human flourishing. Sin can provoke further sin and can result in unjust structures that are not conducive to flourishing. Since the flourishing of a community and the flourishing of an individual are tied together, there is a corporate or communal element to sin that gives rise to the fallenness of the present world and that will likewise be considered in the following sections.

Understood from a Christian perspective, sin, wrongdoing, and rejection of God are ultimately the root cause of brokenness, illness, and death. Sin is understood as the cause of ill health at the most fundamental level. Again, that does not imply that every instance of ill health is the consequence of one's own sin.[8] Rather, ill health can come about from the wrongful actions of others, or, for example, from the seeming brokenness of the world through environmental hazard, toxins, accidents or natural disasters that past sin has introduced. However, while certainly

---

consequently, wherein the latter takes into account some other additional consequent circumstances by which it may be changed. In this regard, what God wills antecedently may not take place, even though it is nevertheless the case that that which seems to depart from the divine will in one order returns into it in another order (1274/1920, I.19.6). It is in this sense of God's antecedent will that we may speak of sin and ill health as being departures from God's intent.

7. Aquinas likens sin to a "sickness of the soul" (1274/1920, I.II.88.1, I.II.72.5), which is sometimes classified as "mortal," by comparison with a disease, if it involves an irreparable defect destroying the vital principle. See also Van Nieuwenhove (2005); 1 John 5:16–17.

8. Aquinas (1274/1920, II.II.108.4). This is evident also in the Gospel of St. John, in Jesus's response concerning the question about the man born blind, "Who sinned, this man or his parents, that he was born blind?" to which Jesus's reply was "Neither" (John 9:1–4). Cf. Book of Job.

not every instance of ill health is attributed to a wrongdoing of the person, the deep connection between sin and ill health is portrayed in the biblical texts in various ways.[9] Ill health is pictured as the consequence of sin, sometimes directly by someone's actions harming another. At other times, the relationship is depicted as disordered behaviors and actions bringing about ill health for oneself or through deficiency in character. Sometimes the relationship between sin and ill health is pictured as divine punishment, although even in such cases, as will be described below, such punishment serves in part to bring human persons back to God.[10] Relatedly, the relationship between sin and ill health is sometimes pictured in the biblical text as the general all-pervasive fallenness and brokenness of the created order that is the consequence of sin and the rejection of God. In the sections that follow, we will consider these various aspects of sin and fallenness and how from a Christian perspective the cause of ill health is sin.

Propositional Summary 2.0: Ill health is the absence of wholeness.
2.0a. Ill health is the absence of wholeness.
2.0b. Ill health of the body may arise from disease, injury, or infirmity.
2.0c. Ill health of the person, or brokenness, is constituted by lack of full flourishing.
2.0d. Ill health is lack of wholeness intended by God, and this has come about by free human action contrary to God's intent.

---

9. See Kee (1992), Wilkinson (1998), and Pilch (2000) for more thorough commentary on the biblical texts.
10. Aquinas (1274/1920, I.48.6, I.II.87.2, 7; see also II.II.108); Aquinas (1270, v.4). See also section II.6 and part III of this book.

II.1. Agency, Sin, and Ill Health

Proposition 2.1. Ill health often follows from the wrongful action of ourselves or others.

2.1a. Wrong action toward others can bring about ill health.

Wrong action toward others can bring about ill health. This may take the form of direct violence and injury to another, ranging from a slap or push to more extreme forms of violence such as murder or rape. Wrong action toward others may also take the form of verbal or psychological abuse, ranging from a simple unkind word to a long pattern of verbal disparagement, ridicule, or contempt. Wrong action toward others might take the form of neglect of a child or an elderly family member, resulting in lack of love and attention or a lack of having material needs met. It may take the form of neglect of a social relationship and the resulting psychological anguish. Wrong action may take the form of theft and the deprivation of the resources someone needs to sustain themselves or their family materially. Wrong action may take the form of deceit, misleading someone or depriving them of the truth needed to live well. Wrong action may take the form of infidelity to a spouse and the disintegration of a family. Wrong action may take the form of not showing proper respect for others or wishing evil upon them. The Ten Commandments (Exodus 20:2–17; Deuteronomy 5:6–17) in some sense document the range of wrong human actions.[1] These are offenses against God and will be considered as such further below, but they are also offenses against one's neighbor.[2] They encompass the list of wrongful actions that bring about ill health. Each of these may adversely affect physical health. Each of these may also adversely affect the health of the person, thereby poten-

---

1. See Aquinas (1274/1920, I.II.100.3–8).
2. A sin toward one's neighbor is likewise a sin against God; see Aquinas (1274/1920, I.II.72.4).

tially bringing about further declines in physical health. Wrong action toward others can bring about ill health for others.

2.1b. Wrong action toward others damages social relationships and community and can bring about ill health.

Wrong action damages social relationships and wounds the fabric of the community. Wrong actions toward others can lead to reciprocation of those wrong actions. They can lead to the end of friendship or of family relationships. They can lessen the sense of love and care and respect a person feels. Wrong actions can render it less likely that others will act generously.[3] Wrong actions can lead to mistrust within a community. This can create a deeply weakened sense of belonging or welcome within the community. It can lead to declines in the extent to which others invest in the community.

Good relationships and good community are constitutive of the health of persons, as described in part I of the book. Social relationships and community are also important resources for preserving and maintaining bodily health.[4] Wrong actions that damage relationships and communities will thus bring about ill health of the person and thereby also ill health of the body.

2.1c. Wrong action can bring about ill health for oneself.

Wrong action can also bring about ill health for oneself. This can take the form of misuse of one's body in ways contrary to God's intent, whether it be neglect, abuse, or failing to care for the body. It can take the form of damage to one's relationships and one's community. This can damage one's own bodily health. Moreover, while generous action toward others can promote one's own health and well-being, harmful actions toward others cause harm not only to others but to oneself.[5] Wrong action toward others also constitutes wrong action against oneself in departing from

---

3. For empirical evidence of the contagion effects of generosity, see Fowler and Christakis (2010), Jordan et al. (2013), and Chancellor et al. (2018).

4. See Holt-Lunstad et al. (2015) for summary of some of the empirical evidence; see also Hong et al. (2023).

5. See Okun et al. (2013), Curry et al. (2018), Post (2017), and Kim et al. (2020) for empirical evidence and summaries.

human nature and who we were created to be.[6] One's own wrong actions bring about ill health for oneself, both of the body and of the person.[7]

2.1d. Poor habits or vices can bring about ill health.

Poor habits and neglect of the body can bring about ill health. Habits of adequate rest, good nutrition, temperance, and exercise sustain health. The absence of such habits can bring about ill health.[8] As described in sections I.2 and I.6, the body is a gift from God, and the person has the responsibility to properly care for it. There can sometimes be competing goods and ends, but giving inadequate attention to the body can sometimes constitute wrong action.

Poor habits that incline one toward wrong action can dispose one to act wrongly and thus bring about ill health for oneself, for others, and for one's community. Repeated wrong actions lead to the development of vices or habits that incline one toward wrong action. Such poor habits or vices and wrong acts can be mutually reinforcing and lead to further wrong acts.[9] Such vices are contrary to virtue and thus they are contrary to and work against inclinations to act in accord with reason to obtain the good.[10] The vices that are most likely to lead to further wrong actions or sins have sometimes been referred to as the capital vices, which are often enumerated as pride, gluttony, lust, covetousness, sloth, envy, and anger.[11] Each of these capital vices, if not actively worked against and held in check, can easily give rise to further wrong actions. Such vices constitute ill health of the person, and through the resulting wrong actions, they can lead not only to further ill health of oneself, others, and one's community but also to separation in sin from God.[12]

---

6. Aquinas (1274/1920, I.II.71.1, I.II.72.4).

7. See Jeffrey and Levin (2020) for a recent overview of empirical evidence, from studies with varying degrees of rigor, regarding the relationship between various behaviors and attitudes, related in one way or another, to one of the "seven deadly sins" (or "capital vices"), namely, lust, gluttony, sloth, anger, greed or covetousness, envy, and pride.

8. See Dobson (2004), Aquinas (1274/1920, I.II.49–54).

9. Aquinas (1274/1920, I.II.71.1–2, I.II.75.4).

10. Aquinas (1274/1920, I.II.71.1).

11. Aquinas (1274/1920, I.II.84.3–4).

12. Aquinas (1274/1920, I.II.78.2).

2.1e. Wrong action separates us from God, which constitutes and brings about ill health.

Wrong action, action contrary to God's intent, is sin. Such action disrupts God's intent for the goodness of the person, the well functioning of the body, and the person's pursuit of their final end in God. Sin—wrong action contrary to God's intent—separates us from God. This constitutes ill health of the person; it constitutes a decline in spiritual well-being. If there is a turning away from our final communion with God, that separation can, by our own choice and will, be permanent.[13] This turning away from God and lack of spiritual well-being may further lead to a neglect of and lack of love for others. It may prompt and facilitate additional wrongful actions toward others. Sin gives rise to separation from God, which can give rise to further sin.[14] Sin and the resulting separation from God brings about ill health of the person and ill health of the body.

2.1f. Wrong action impedes us from being who we were intended to be and produces guilt, which constitutes and results in ill health.

Wrongful action and sin will often ordinarily produce guilt, a sense or conviction that one has done wrong. Such guilt is an indication of ill health of the person, that one has acted wrongly and that one is in some way not whole. Left unaddressed, such guilt can also adversely affect bodily health and mental health.[15] However, guilt is also an indication that certain aspects of the person, for example the person's conscience, are functioning rightly—that the person is aware of wrongdoing and that the person feels remorse and wishes things were otherwise. Such guilt can prompt a sense of needing to reform and a sense of needing to address the wrong, to find a restoration to wholeness and health. Guilt

---

13. Aquinas (1274/1920, I.II.87.3, I.II.88.1–2). See also Frey (2018) for an account of Aquinas's understanding of sin as an orientation away from our shared final end in God.

14. Aquinas (1274/1920, I.II.87.2).

15. There is, for example, empirical evidence that lack of self-forgiveness or lack of a sense of divine forgiveness, and presumably thus implied lingering guilt, is associated with subsequently worse mental health and poorer psychosocial well-being (Long, Chen, et al., 2020).

indicates that not all is well with one's life. It constitutes in part a thirst for healing and restoration, and it is to such healing and restoration that we will turn in part III of this book.

> *Propositional Summary 2.1: Ill health often follows from the wrongful action of ourselves or others.*
> 2.1a. Wrong action toward others can bring about ill health.
> 2.1b. Wrong action toward others damages social relationships and community and can bring about ill health.
> 2.1c. Wrong action can bring about ill health for oneself.
> 2.1d. Poor habits can bring about ill health.
> 2.1e. Wrong action separates us from God, which constitutes and further brings about ill health.
> 2.1f. Wrong action impedes us from being who we were intended to be and produces guilt, which constitutes and results in ill health.

II.2. Injustice and Ill Health

Proposition 2.2. Wrongful actions can bring about unjust structures that may result in ill health over extended periods of time and even across generations.

2.2a. Wrongful human action can give rise to unjust structures.

Wrong actions, or sin, actions that are contrary to God's intent, can give rise to ill health of individuals, both ill health of the person and ill health of the body. However, such wrong actions can, as noted above, also adversely affect communities by weakening relationships, trust, goodwill, a sense of belonging, and welcome, and investment in the community. A community is governed by its relationships, its leadership, its structures and practices. In a healthy well-functioning community, these will be good and the community will contribute to the flourishing of its members. When the relationships, leadership, structures and practices of a community are not good, the life of the community can potentially hinder or diminish the flourishing of individuals. At the individual level, this may manifest in poor relationships, a sense of exclusion, lack of resources to sustain bodily health, lack of opportunities to develop as a person and to flourish, restrictions on freedom, or policies that impede or diminish flourishing. When these impediments to flourishing are embedded in the structures of a community—whether they be in leadership, laws, policies, systematic ill treatment—we sometimes speak of unjust structures[1] or unjust laws,[2] such that it is not the case that each person receives what is due to them. These are not simply wrongful actions of one person toward another; they are ways that harm toward others is perpetuated, even in a systematic way, that arises from the structures, laws, policies, and practices themselves.

---

1. See, for example, Vidal (1987) and Finn (2016) for theological analysis of the notion of a "structure of sin."
2. Aquinas (1274/1920, I.II.96.4).

2.2b. Unjust structures and communal relations can actively diminish human flourishing, give rise to lack of opportunities for flourishing, and impede each person from receiving what is his or her due.

Unjust structures can impede the health of persons and the health of the body in a variety of ways. In some cases, they may directly and actively diminish or thwart human flourishing. They may directly cause harm to others. Examples of this would include the Nazi Holocaust, various genocides throughout history, and slave trade practices. Each of these examples also includes individual wrongdoing of one person toward another, but in each of these cases that wrongdoing is encouraged and promoted by the structures, practices, and leadership that are in place. The wrongdoing becomes the norm. Not simply the individual but also the structures themselves are contrary to God's intent. They are sinful.

Unjust structures can also be present if they systematically prevent certain groups from having opportunities to flourish. This may be the case if certain groups are systematically prevented from having access to education or to sufficient material resources to sustain life or to health or to employment or to opportunities to form families, relationships, and community life or to religious freedom.[3] Examples might include Jim Crow laws in the United States prior to the civil rights movement, poorer-quality schools in economically disadvantaged neighborhoods, restrictions on freedom of association, loss of welfare benefits upon marriage, and lack of religious freedom for certain groups.[4] Often structures that prevent groups from having opportunities to develop and flourish go hand in hand with actions that directly cause harm. However, structures

---

3. Restriction on same-sex marriage is considered by some an instance of such systematic impeding of flourishing. It is the Catholic understanding that this matter in fact concerns the *definition* of marriage, of what marriage is, and that although persons attracted to the same sex "are to be fully respected in their human dignity," marriage by its nature is to be understood as "a permanent union . . . between one man and one woman" and thereby "oriented towards procreation" (Catholic Church, 2004, 227–228). See also footnote 38 in section I.4.

4. See Grim and Finke (2011), Chetty, Friedman, and Rockoff (2014), Krieger et al. (2014), and Rand (2015) for discussion of and empirical evidence relating to some of these examples. See also Berkman et al. (2014) for summaries of empirical evidence on how working conditions, social capital, and discrimination can affect physical and mental health.

and policies may be such that groups are prevented from access to opportunities to flourish even in the absence of obvious action to directly cause harm.

When possible, a society should be structured to allow maximal opportunities for individuals to flourish. A society's resources are limited and careful thought is necessary to ensure that each person has the best possible opportunities to develop and flourish.[5] Societies that are struggling may have difficulties providing adequate resources and the fullest set of opportunities for everyone. Different forms of government and economic systems may have various advantages and disadvantages and may result in differing levels of economic inequality. There are no straightforward thresholds that determine when readjusting levels of inequality, or reallocating resources, has gone too far. Moreover, considerations extend beyond economics and pertain to the distribution of numerous aspects of flourishing that include happiness, health, meaning, growth in character, and good relationships. A minimal goal might be seeking to ensure a certain equality of opportunity, wherein opportunity is present within a society to pursue and attain a flourishing life, regardless of someone's initial circumstances.[6] This can potentially be achieved with differing governmental and economic systems and with differing levels of potential economic equality. However, when certain groups are intentionally kept from opportunities to flourish and these impediments do not arise simply from questions of resource allocation, this implies that these structures themselves are unjust and contrary to God's intent. They are sinful. They prevent the flourishing of individuals.

Unjust structures can also be present in dysfunctional laws and legal systems. Injustices may be present if crimes are left unaddressed or if they are handled differently for some groups than for others. Injustice may arise in unjust agreements and contracts if these are not properly overseen and enforced. Injustice may arise if workers are not

---

5. Catholic Church (2004, 173–175).

6. See Chetty, Hendren, et al. (2014b) for some empirical evidence that such opportunity, at least concerning economic attainment, may in fact be declining in the United States.

properly remunerated for their work.⁷ Injustice may arise if certain people are discriminated against on racial grounds, for instance, or are systematically paid less for the same quality work.⁸ Society's structures, laws, and systems of justice should prevent these things from taking place. When they do not, the structures themselves are unjust. The responsibility of ensuring just legal proceedings lies both with communities and with individuals. An unjust legal or criminal system will have trouble processing an excessive number of incidents in which some law or agreement has been broken and the system will be more liable to collapse. For a legal or criminal system to be effective, these incidents need to be the exception, not the rule. There needs to be trust within a community, and grounds for that trust, in order for the community itself and for social or business relations to function well. The community needs to be flourishing to some degree in order to sustain the legal systems that are necessary to protect it. Although in many cases, wrongful legal or criminal decisions will be the result of a wrong action or wrong decisions of one person toward another, when the structures and laws and practices and authorities facilitate and make wrongful decisions the norm, the structures themselves are unjust and contrary to God's intent. They are sinful.

2.2c. Unjust structures are contrary to God's intent and they constitute ill health of communities and contribute to ill health of individuals.

A structure or authority or set of laws that promotes and makes wrongdoing the norm is contrary to God's intent. It is sinful. It embeds sin, that which is contrary to God's intent, in the community's structures and practices. The biblical witness is consistent in saying that God is opposed to injustice.⁹ The prophets of the Old Testament, speaking on

---

7. Leo XIII (1891, 45).

8. John XXIII (1963, 44, 86, 100). See Massingale (2014) for discussion of Catholic theology concerning racial justice and opportunities for further engagement on issues concerning discrimination.

9. See Mafico (1992) and Westfall and Dyer (2016) for fuller expositions and commentary on biblical themes concerning justice; see also Catholic Church (2004, 20–27, 255–266, 323–329, 377–383, 428–432, 451–455, 488–493).

behalf of God, proclaim God as a God of justice (Isaiah 30:18) and as a God who loves justice, who is deeply opposed to injustice and the exploitation of the poor (Jeremiah 21:12; Isaiah 3:14–15). That opposition extends so far that God will not notice religious practices if issues of injustice have not been addressed (Isaiah 58). The Old Testament law likewise made provisions for the poor, established structures to alleviate poverty, and warned against injustice.[10] The New Testament continues this witness to God's opposition to injustice,[11] but, as described further in part III of the book, extends it so that justice is transformed by love. However, love in these cases includes working against structures that perpetuate poverty and inhibit flourishing.[12]

Unjust structures and practices are constitutive of the ill health of a community. Under these circumstances, the community's practices are contrary to God's intent. The community is not healthy. Moreover, unjust practices and structures will lead to declines in relationships and in the lives of individuals. The community's ill health will detract from the health of individuals; it will detract from their flourishing. Sin is the cause of ill health at an individual level. Sin is the cause of ill health at the community level. There is a corporate element to sin; it can become embedded within a community and in its structures and practices, diminishing the health of both the community and individuals.

---

10. Israel's gleaning laws required that part of the harvest be left for those in need, and provision for the poor was thereby made (Leviticus 19:9–10; Deuteronomy 24:19–22). The law also provided for the lending of productive resources and required that this lending be generous, openhanded, without consideration of personal loss (Deuteronomy 15:7–11), and without interest (Exodus 22:25; Leviticus 25:36; etc.). Families were to provide for one another and to buy back property that a poor relative was forced to sell (Leviticus 25:23–34). The law included provisions in which the debts and slavery of fellow Israelites were to be canceled in the seventh year (Deuteronomy 15:1–15) and a year of jubilee in which every fiftieth year, all land reverted to the family that originally owned it (Leviticus 25:10), thus preventing the long-term loss of land and multigenerational cycles of poverty within families. The law also warned against neglecting justice for the alien, the fatherless, and the widow (Deuteronomy 24:17) and called curses upon those who withheld justice (Deuteronomy 27:19).

11. See Matthew 23:23; James 2:1–3, 5:1–6.

12. Catholic Church (2004, 204–208).

2.2d. Although unjust structures may have arisen from actions of individuals in the past, they may persist if left unaddressed and it is the responsibility of a community to alter unjust structures.

Although unjust structures ultimately arise from free actions that are wrong, once they are established, they can sometimes be sustained even without further intentional wrongful action. Once established, a set of unjust laws that does not give each person their due or that fails to respect human dignity and human rights may remain in place until it is reformed. When practices of racial discrimination are embedded in access to institutions, they will remain until the institutions themselves are changed. When it has become the norm that certain minority religious groups or minority racial groups are not allowed to publicly congregate, these practices will not change until there is active effort to alter these norms. Even if a particular individual does not practice personal discrimination, if the structures and practices are still in place, they affect the lives of others. They impede opportunities for humans to flourish or actively diminish them. They can moreover often normalize wrongdoing at the individual level.

Arguably, the possibility that unjust laws, structures, and practices can be sustained without further individual intentional wrongdoing and that they can promote wrongful action and make it the norm distinguishes injustice at the societal level from individual wrongdoing. Although the individual or group that put the unjust laws and practices into place was originally responsible, it eventually becomes the responsibility of the community and the individuals within it to reform the structures, practices, and laws that are unjust. Justice includes both avoiding evil and doing good. Failure to do some good that is due may be referred to as a sin of omission.[13] When laws, and structures, and practices do not give each person their due or fail to respect human dignity and human rights, it is each person's responsibility to alter them if they are within their control. Failure to do so is sin. The structures that persist and perpetuate harm might be referred to as structures of sin.[14] As will be

---
13. See Aquinas (1274/1920, II.II.79).
14. John Paul II (1987, 36); see also Daly (2011) and Rozier (2016) on "structures of virtue and vice."

discussed in part III, part of the process of healing and restoration of individuals and of communities is the ending of injustice in love, a restoration of the structures and practices of communities to God's intent.

> *Propositional Summary 2.2: Wrongful actions can bring about unjust structures that may result in ill health over extended periods of time and even across generations.*
> 2.2a. Wrongful human action can give rise to unjust structures.
> 2.2b. Unjust structures and communal relations can actively diminish human flourishing, give rise to lack of opportunities for flourishing, and impede each person from receiving what is his or her due.
> 2.2c. Unjust structures are contrary to God's intent and they constitute ill health of communities and contribute to ill health of individuals.
> 2.2d. Although unjust structures may have arisen from actions of individuals in the past, they may persist if left unaddressed and it is the responsibility of a community to alter unjust structures.

II.3. Fallenness and Ill Health

Proposition 2.3. Human nature is distorted by sin, and this fallenness of human nature has disrupted relations between human persons and the world, giving rise to external causes of ill health.

2.3a. Because of wrongful human actions, our nature and our relation to the world around us are fallen and are not as they should be.

The Christian theological understanding of sin includes not only individual and communal elements but extends in a corporate sense to human nature and, in way, to all of creation. Just as the sinful actions of individuals can become embedded in social structures in ways that give rise to more systematic and sustained forms of injustice, so also individual wrongdoing has an effect on the human persons' relationship to creation.

 The creation stories present humanity as having responsibility for governing creation. In the creation story in Genesis 1, following the creation of the human person, God says "Have dominion over the fish of the sea and over the birds of the air and over every living thing that moves upon the earth" (Genesis 1:28). In the account of the fall (Genesis 3), the consequences of first act of human disobedience to God appears to extend not only to individuals, leading to a separation from God, but also to other aspects of God's creation. In addition to the expulsion of Adam and Eve from God's presence, God is said to declare, "Cursed is the ground because of you" (Genesis 3). The consequences of sin extend in some way to all of the creation that humans were to govern. The corporate tie between humanity and the creation is presented as so strong that the latter in some sense suffers from the actions of the former. Just as one nation may impose sanctions upon another for the actions of just one of its leaders so that all its members suffer, so also human nature itself and possibly all of creation suffers from the consequences of wrongdoing of the human persons who were to govern it.[1]

This fall is sometimes understood in a historical sense, sometimes in a metaphorical sense, and sometimes in a way that is in some sense historical but extends beyond the present nature of the world as it currently is. Different theological models have been proposed, none of which has gained complete dominance within the Christian tradition.[2]

Regardless of the sense in which the fall is understood, its implications for the health of the body, the health of the person, the health of the community, and the health of humanity's relation with the world are all profound. In the story of the fall in Genesis 3, sin and the fall are pictured as giving rise to estranged and conflictual social relations. To the woman, it is said, "your desire shall be for your husband, and he shall rule over you." Concerning the estranged relationship to work and to the world, the account continues "cursed is the ground . . . in toil you shall eat of it . . . thorns and thistles it shall bring forth for you." Of deterioration and death, it continues with, "you are dust, and to dust you shall return." Ultimately, of estrangement from God, it concludes, "the man and his wife hid themselves from the presence of the Lord God . . . God sent him forth from the Garden . . . He drove out the man."

The fall is pictured as the result of a free decision of man and woman to not conform to God's intent. It is a fall from an original state of goodness that was sustained by God. It was a fall away from and a turning away from God. This fall, brought about by sin, an intentional act contrary to God's intent, had implications for the human body, human relations, relations with God, and in fact all of creation. The Christian tradition has used the term "original sin" both for that original action, sometimes understood historically, that was contrary to God's intent and for the implications of sin, which corrupts human nature in its physical,

---

1. See Aquinas (1274/1920, I.II.81.1); Romans 8:20–22.
2. See, for example, Stump and Meister (2020) for an overview of several alternative understandings; see also Cavanaugh and Smith (2017) and Houck (2020). As described in the sections that follow, Aquinas sees the original disobedience of Adam and Eve as having corrupted human nature by removing God's gift of original justice, which preserved the body and kept the passions under the rule of reason (Aquinas, 1274/1920, I.II.82–83, I.II.85.1, 5–6); the resulting disordered human nature is transmitted across generations (Aquinas, 1274/1920, I.II.81.1–2).

mental, social, and spiritual aspects.[3] In the sections that follow, we will explore these various corporate aspects of sin and the fall.

2.3b. The body ages and deteriorates with time, bringing about ill health and ultimately bodily death.

Much of Christian theology pictures the human body in a state of original goodness and justice prior to the fall, preserved from decay by God.[4] Sin, the deliberate choosing of that which is contrary to God's intent, disrupts that original state of goodness and preservation and the body is subject to deterioration. The body is subject to disease, injury, defect, and infirmity. As the person ages, the body naturally deteriorates. Its systems gradually stop functioning as well as before, giving rise to infirmity of body and of mind. When the systems of the human body finally fail, this results in bodily death.

2.3c. The mental faculties and social interactions of human persons are not what they should be, and this is both constitutive of and brings about ill health.

The fallenness of humanity extends not only to the body but also to the mind and to social relations. Desires are often now in conflict with one another. Desires and emotions can be in conflict with reason and with what is good; they are often now in conflict with God's intent.[5] Desires for physical pleasure can often overpower the seeking of other and more important goods.[6] The desire for our own good often overpowers the seeking of good for others. Human relations are thereby brought into conflict. As noted in the previous section, these conflicts in human relations can then become embedded in a society, in communal structures, perpetuating harm toward others and promoting wrong action and additional sin. All these things contribute to the ill health of the person and can bring about ill health of the body. The

---

    3. Romans 5:12–21; Aquinas (1274/1920, I.II.81–83).
    4. Aquinas (1274/1920, I.II.85.5–6). See also Houck (2020), Stump and Meister (2020), and Cavanaugh and Smith (2017).
    5. Romans 7:7–25; Aquinas (1274/1920, I.II.82.1–3, I.II.83.4, I.II.85.5).
    6. Aquinas (1274/1920, I.II.77.4–5).

human mind, the human body, the human person are no longer what God intended them to be. This is a consequence of the fall, a fall from that original state of goodness that God preserved when human action was rightly oriented toward his intent. That fall, brought about by voluntary action contrary to God's intent, disrupted the human body and the human mind and the relations between them. Human nature is now such that reason, will, and passions are all imperfect and are often in conflict with one another.[7]

2.3d. Because the human person's relation to creation is fallen, natural disasters, accidents, and pollution all bring about ill health.

The relation between the human person and the world is fallen and is not as it should be. This too reflects the fallenness of the human person in sin.[8] The fallenness of our relation to the world and to creation is present in the fact that the world is subject to corruption, pollution, and toxins resulting from human activity. These bring about ill health for humans, for plants, and for animals. We ourselves can, and do, damage the nature of the world around us. This fallenness of humanity's relation with creation, with the world around us, is a consequence of and is reflective of human sin.[9]

This fallenness is also present in our exposure to the effects of natural disasters—earthquakes, hurricanes, floods—that cause damage

---

7. See Larchet (2002, 26–33) for an account, as understood by the Church fathers and more generally, of the disruption original sin brought to the nature of the human person and how the passions are now often in conflict with reason and with one another. This conflict is a part of the origin of ill health.

8. Some theologians understand creation as corrupted by the fall. They see the possibility of natural disasters as ensuing from the fall. Some also see violence and death among animals as a result of the fall (see Stump and Meister, 2020). An alternative view, however, is that the nature of creation was such that creation is more perfect because it has varying degrees of goodness, including the creation of both corruptible and incorruptible things and things that could, or could not, lose their goodness as humans can by acting voluntarily contrary to God's intent (Aquinas, 1274/1920, I.47.2, I.48.2, I.49.2). In this view, nothing is intrinsically fallen or evil in creation in the presence of an earthquake or a hurricane. These dramatic movements of the earth manifest God's creative power. What is evil is their effects on human persons, from which, following the fall, humanity is no longer protected.

9. Francis (2015, 66).

to the land, to human shelter, to the sustaining of adequate food for human life, and to human life itself. Without a proper structuring of our life together, without care for the earth and for one another, we are more exposed to the effects of natural disasters and accidents that can bring about ill health. Thus, not only are we subject to ill health and death due to natural causes in the world, but the damage we cause to the earth often brings about ill health for us. God created us to care for his creation, to "till and keep it" (Genesis 2:15), and when we do not do so properly, we sin. That sin also is a cause of ill health. The fallenness of our relation with the world, introduced by sin, is thus a further cause of ill health.

2.3e. Corresponding to the free decisions of human persons to depart from God's intent are the free decisions of spiritual beings to depart from God's intent, which results in further ill health of persons.

The Christian tradition and the biblical witness have also consistently affirmed the presence of other created, purely spiritual beings—angels—who likewise can freely obey or disobey God. Those that have chosen to disobey God are referred to as fallen angels or devils or demons. They desire to be like God in a way that is not suited to their nature and perhaps desire to have a command over others in a way that is proper to God alone.[10] The story of the fall in Genesis 3 portrays "a serpent" tempting Adam and Eve by their actions to "be like God." Although the devil or fallen angels are not the direct cause of sin, as sin requires the free action of the human person, fallen spiritual beings or devils are thought to be able to indirectly induce someone to sin by persuasion and by presenting attractive objects that may be the occasions for sin, as in the narrative of the fall.[11] The resulting human sin has brought about the corruption of our nature and the distortion of our relations with the rest of creation. Such sin both brings about and constitutes ill health of the body and of the person in the various ways noted in prior sections.

---

10. Aquinas (1274/1920, I.63.3); Catholic Church (2000, 390–395).
11. Aquinas (1274/1920, I.II.80.1–2, cf. I.II.75.3).

2.3f. The trials of life lead to strain and distress, which constitute and result in ill health.

The fallenness of the body and of the mind, of social relations, and of the world around us creates conditions that continually threaten human life. Life becomes subject to stresses and struggles for survival. These further strain human relations and strain the human body and mind. The stresses and struggles that result from the fallenness of the relation between human persons and creation both arise from and contribute to ill health, ill health of the body, and ill health of the person. The fallenness resulting from sin is manifest in the world around us and is ultimately reflective of and the consequence of sin. That sin, and the fall from the original state of goodness as God intended, now pervades all aspects of the life of the human person, human society, and the world humans inhabit. Sin, through the fall, is the cause of ill health not simply as the direct consequence of individual action but also through the present fallenness and brokenness of human nature and of our relationship to creation.

> *Propositional Summary 2.3: Human nature is distorted by sin, and this fallenness of human nature has disrupted relations between human persons and the world, giving rise to external causes of ill health.*
> 2.3a. Because of wrongful human actions, our nature and our relation to the world around us are fallen and are not as they should be.
> 2.3b. The body ages and deteriorates with time, bringing about ill health.
> 2.3c. The mental faculties and social interactions of human persons are not what they should be, and this is both constitutive of and brings about ill health.
> 2.3d. Because the human person's relation to creation is fallen, natural disasters, accidents, and pollution all bring about ill health.
> 2.3e. Corresponding to the free decisions of human persons to depart from God's intent are the free decisions of spiritual beings to depart from God's intent, which results in further ill health of persons.
> 2.3f. The trials of life lead to strain and distress, which constitute and result in ill health.

II.4. Sin and Death

Proposition 2.4. Sin has brought about and continues to bring about death.

2.4a. Death is the consequence of sin.

The biblical account presents death as the consequence of sin. In the creation stories, God says, regarding obeying his command not to eat from the fruit of the tree of the knowledge of good and evil, "for in the day that you eat of it you shall die" (Genesis 2). The act of disobedience to God, acting contrary to God's intent, is sin and the consequence of this is foretold to be death. Following the fall, the original act of disobedience, death again is affirmed as the consequence: "you are dust, and to dust you shall return" (Genesis 3). The consequence of the sin and the fall is the loss of the original state of goodness by which the body and health were preserved. The body is now subject to ill health, and deterioration, and ultimately death.[1]

The New Testament writings affirm also that death is the consequence of sin. In the letter of Saint Paul to the Romans, he writes "For the wages of sin is death" (Romans 6). There it is likewise pictured that, in the original act of disobedience, death was brought to all people: "sin came into the world through one man, and death came through sin, and so death spread to all because all have sinned" (Romans 5). Again, what is pictured is the loss of that original state of goodness wherein life and health and the body were preserved. Although the consequence of sin being death is understood in a variety of ways, all now face death.[2]

---

1. Aquinas (1270, V.5) distinguishes between death being "natural" to human beings in the sense that their bodies are composed of matter that subject to dissolution and death being not "natural" to human beings by reason of their soul, which cannot pass away. Prior to sin, God protected the body from death.

2. Aquinas (1274/1920, I.II.85.5–6); see also Stump and Meister (2020); Cavanaugh and Smith (2017); Houck (2020).

2.4b. Sin causes ill health which eventually results in death.

Sin furthermore continues to lead to death by the effects of sin on ill health. As already described in previous sections, sin in the form of harmful actions to ourselves and others results in ill health. Sin in the form of unjust structures that perpetuate harms or facilitate and promote wrongful actions brings about ill health. Sin in the form of conflictual relationships and communities brings about ill health. Sin, bringing damage to the earth and greater exposure to natural and man-made harms, brings about ill health. Sin, as separation from God, brings about further wrongful actions and sin, resulting in ill health. Sin brings about ill health of the body and of the person, the latter also contributing yet further to the ill health of the body. As the body's systems and functioning continues to deteriorate through injury, disease, and aging, it finally stops functioning altogether, resulting in death. Sin, by bringing about ill health, brings about death.

2.4c. Sin is separation from God and thus also constitutes spiritual death.

In sin, as action contrary to God's intent, there is a loss of spiritual well-being, of communion with God, that likewise follows.[3] Sin, moreover, as an intentional separating of oneself from God's intent, separates a person from God's grace, and yet further sin may result.[4] The complete separation from God resulting from sin is spiritual death.[5]

In the next section, we will consider the impossibility of fully addressing ill health without addressing sin, and the impossibility of fully addressing sin without God's action and grace; and in part III of the book we will consider in greater detail God's action and salvation that overcome sin and death. But without that action, without that grace, without salvation, the human person, through sin, is subject also to spiritual death, a separation from God.

---

3. Aquinas (1274/1920, I.II.88.1–2).
4. Aquinas (1274/1920, II.II.24.10–12, I.II.75.4).
5. Aquinas (1274/1920, I.II.74.4; cf. III.79.6). See also 1 John 5:16–17.

2.4d. Death, as the ending of life, is also a cessation of ill health in this life.

Death is the cessation of life. The body's systems cease functioning entirely. It is the cessation of the health of the body. Death is the conclusion and outworking of ill health. However, as the cessation of life, it is also the cessation of ill health in this life. Death provides a relief from ill health and the suffering that accompanies it.

As discussed in the previous sections, the present world is subject to fallenness and ill health. There is a lack of complete goodness. There is suffering. There is sin, a deviation from God's intent, and, as will be discussed in the section that follows, such sin cannot be entirely addressed without a restoration accomplished by God. Death is, or can be, in some sense a release from that fallenness and sin. It is a cessation of life in this present fallen world. It can, as discussed in part III of the book, bring about new life, an everlasting life with God, but only with God's work and salvation and a receiving of this gift. However, in the context of that salvation, death can be a transformation and a new beginning. Avoiding death as long as possible is not the proper aim or end of this life, which is instead the formation and development of spiritual life, of charity, of friendship and communion with God. Even the approaching of death can provide the context for such growth and transformation.

However, while death is the ending of ill health in this life and can constitute a release from the suffering of ill health, death is never to be intentionally sought for its own sake. As discussed in section I.4, life, as created by God, is good; it is a gift; it is not to be intentionally destroyed. Moreover, the experience of ill health and its associated suffering can sometimes be a means of transformation, of a growth in character, a finding of new meaning, or a deepening of relationships, and a turning more fully to God. Ill-health and suffering can be the source of a renewed flourishing, a renewed and changed health of the person. We will consider suffering as a source of growth and renewal in section II.6 below. However, this possibility of transformation allows one to find meaning even in ill health and suffering as death approaches. Death is never to be the ultimate intended outcome. Death is ultimately contrary to God's intent. Death is the consequence of sin.

Propositional Summary 2.4 Sin has brought about and continues to bring about death.

2.4a. Death is the consequence of sin.

2.4b. Sin causes ill health which eventually results in death.

2.4c. Sin is separation from God and thus also constitutes spiritual death.

2.4d. Death, as the ending of life, is also a cessation of ill health in this life.

II.5. Incapacity and Sin

Proposition 2.5. Ill health cannot be prevented without addressing sin.

2.5a. Ill health cannot be prevented without addressing sin because sin brings about harmful actions for ourselves and others, unjust structures that perpetuate ill health, poor social relations, and poorly functioning communities.

Ill health cannot be dealt with and health cannot be maintained or restored unless sin is addressed. This is evident in a number of ways. As long as people do actions that harm themselves and others, there will be ill health. As long as there are unjust structures that perpetuate harms and facilitate wrongdoing, there will be ill health. As long as relationships are conflictual, there will be ill health. There will be ill health of persons and ill health of bodies. All of these things—harmful action towards others, unjust structures, and bad relationships—are constitutive of sin; they constitute departures from God's intent. And each of these things brings about ill health. People have freely chosen and continue to freely choose action contrary to God's intent. This is sin and it causes ill health. Ill health cannot be addressed without addressing sin, which is its cause.

2.5b. Ill health cannot be prevented without addressing sin because sin, as separation from God, is constitutive of ill health.

Because sin constitutes a departure from God's intent, it is constitutive of lack of spiritual well-being, of a separation from God. This constitutes ill health of the person because full flourishing of the person includes communion with God. Sin, defined as free action that is contrary to God's intent, separates us from God. Such separation can bring about additional wrongdoing and additional ill health of the person and of the body. Until this lack of spiritual well-being, this lack of wholeness in communion with God, is addressed, until sin is dealt with, the lack of wholeness of the person in separation from God will persist. We cannot maintain the health of persons without addressing sin because sin, as separation from God, is constitutive of ill health.

2.5c. Without God, we cannot address sin as a cause of ill health, and we are incapable of fully preserving or restoring the body, the mind, our relationships, and the world around us to be what God intended them to be.

The human person and even the human community is limited in its capacity to fully address sin as a cause of ill health. We are unable to completely prevent human wrongdoing or prevent people from harming one another. We are unable to prevent conflictual social and communal relations. Despite what are sometimes important and valiant efforts, we seem to be unable to completely rid our communities and governments of injustice. We are unable to preserve and restore the environment and all of creation to a state of goodness. We are unable to eliminate sin.[1]

We are thus unable also to bring about a full restoration of health, since we cannot fully eliminate sin and its consequences. We are limited in our ability to keep the body from aging and deteriorating. We are limited in our ability to promote good health behaviors. We are limited in our ability to bring about mental well-being, to eliminate depression, fear, and anger. We are limited in our ability to preserve and restore relationships. We are limited in our ability to sustain healthy and just communities. We are unable to prevent natural disasters. We seem limited in our ability to avoid pollution and toxins. We can work toward addressing ill health and its causes, but we are unable to do so entirely. We are unable to eliminate ill health because we are unable to eliminate sin.

As described in greater detail in part III of this book, although we are limited in our capacity to bring about full restoration of health, there is much that can be done, and much that can be restored. Through healing and restoration, community and love, medicine and public health, forgiveness and salvation, and other means there can be partial restoration

---

1. Aquinas (1274/1920, I.II.109.2–4, 7–8); see also Romans 7:14–25, 8:3–4.

to health in this life. By our own efforts, however, we cannot fully prevent ill health or fully restore the health of persons. We cannot eliminate ill health. We cannot eliminate sin. For complete restoration and fulfillment of health and wholeness, we need the action of God. For complete restoration to health, we need the fullness of God's salvation.

Propositional Summary 2.5: Ill health cannot be prevented without addressing sin.
2.5a. Ill health cannot be prevented without addressing sin because sin brings about harmful actions for ourselves and others, unjust structures that perpetuate ill health, poor social relations, and poorly functioning communities.
2.5b. Ill health cannot be prevented without addressing sin because sin, as separation from God, is constitutive of ill health.
2.5c. Without God, we cannot address sin as a cause of ill health, and we are incapable of fully preserving or restoring the body, the mind, our relationships, and the world around us to be what God intended them to be.

II.6. Ill Health and Suffering

Proposition 2.6. The experience of distress over brokenness, or lack of wholeness, is suffering, whereby the need for healing and restoration is made clear.

2.6a. Suffering is the anguished experience of a negative physical or mental state of considerable duration or intensity.

In the wake of sin and the presence of ill health and the brokenness of the world, we suffer. We experience pain. We experience sadness, fear, and anger. We experience anguish arising from both the body and the mind. When these negative undesired physical or mental states are experienced for considerable time or with particular intensity, they constitute suffering. These states are often severe enough to disrupt one's major purposes, to threaten one's sense of personhood and relationships and identity, and they sometimes seem to pervade all aspects of one's life. That intense undesired physical or mental experience often seems beyond one's capacity to control or to end, sometimes leading to a sense of deterioration of the person. Suffering sometimes can make the prospect of continuing to exist in one's present state seem unbearable.[1]

In suffering, there is the absence or loss of something that was good: the health of the body, a goal or a purpose, an important relationship, a sense of identity and understanding, a cherished possession, or a sense of peace or security.[2] With the loss of a substantial good we respond negatively to the loss physiologically and psychologically in ways that give rise to anguish and distress. That experience of anguish and distress over the loss or absence of some good is suffering.

---

1. For more on the concept of suffering, see Cassell (1982), Brady (2018), VanderWeele (2019b), and Duffee (2023).
2. The loss or absence of some good effectively constitutes the objective side of suffering; John Paul II (1984).

2.6b. Our experience of suffering reflects the brokenness of the world and of the human person.

In his apostolic letter *Salvifici doloris*, John Paul II addresses the question of the meaning of suffering.[3] Suffering is the subjective dimension of the experience of some evil or loss. It follows from an experience of brokenness, of evil, of the loss of some good. Ill health of the body is one source of suffering, but suffering extends beyond this. The human person suffers whenever he or she experiences any kind of evil; suffering involves a certain pain of the soul. Any ill health or brokenness of the person will entail some degree of suffering; suffering indicates a certain lack of wholeness. Suffering brings us to ask the question "Why?" We ask this question both about the cause of suffering and about its purpose and meaning. This often is a question of one's own suffering and also a question about why there is suffering at all. Suffering results from evil, from the loss of some good, from sin; though again, as noted above, not every instance of suffering results from one's own sin.

The meaning of suffering is the realization that some good has been lost or is absent and that effort must be made to rebuild or regain or adjust to that loss. In short, suffering points to the need for healing and restoration. That restoration, as will be discussed in further detail in part III, comes about through Jesus Christ's sharing in our sufferings in his life, in his defeat of suffering and death on the cross, in our joining with Jesus in compassionate suffering and love for others, in work to alleviate suffering, and in awaiting a final salvation, restoration, and resurrection from God. But suffering reflects the brokenness of the world around us and the brokenness of the human person.

2.6c. Ill health of the body can bring about suffering.

Ill health of the body can bring about suffering. An injury will typically give rise to pain, which will often constitute a form of bodily suffering. Severe injuries can often compromise the functioning of the body, giving rise to further suffering. Disease likewise can cause pain and can impede the functioning of the body, resulting in both physical and mental anguish that is suffering. Disease can furthermore give rise to processes

---

3. John Paul II (1984).

leading to death, the fear of which is often a source of intense suffering. The process of aging, the wearing and deterioration of the body's systems, and the resulting infirmity can all be sources of suffering. Ill health of the body through injury, disease, and infirmity and by foreshadowing death can often be the cause of suffering.

2.6d. Ill health of the person can bring about suffering.

Ill health of the person can also bring about suffering. Poor mental health in the form of severe depression or anxiety or intense anger will often constitute suffering. A severe failure of life to conform to what one had hoped accompanied by an intense dissatisfaction can be a form of suffering. Failure to achieve or accomplish or be what one had hoped can result in mental anguish that constitutes suffering. A sense of meaninglessness can constitute an intense form of suffering. Failures of character, not acting in way one would have hoped to act, bringing harm to others, and the resulting altered self-perception can give rise to guilt and mental anguish and suffering. The loss of an important relationship through death of a loved one or the disintegration of relationships or communities often gives rise to intense suffering. A sense of separation from or abandonment by God, a lack of spiritual well-being, will often include intense suffering and can exacerbate other forms of suffering.[4] In all of these ways, ill health of the person, a lack of flourishing, will often give rise to suffering.

2.6e. Suffering can lead to a transformation in understanding, life orientation, relationships, and character and can thereby bring about a renewed health of the person.

Although ill health of the body or of the person will often bring about suffering, it is also the case that suffering can sometimes bring about growth and transformation in one's understanding or one's orientation to life and in one's character. When suffering is responded to appropriately,

---

[4]. The book of Job presents a paradigmatic, profound, and probing example of such spiritual suffering accompanied by, and in part caused by, many of these other forms of and causes of suffering; see St. John of the Cross (1585/1959).

that growth and transformation may eventually lead to a renewed or even greater flourishing.

The Christian tradition consistently teaches that suffering can produce transformation. Often that transformation is pictured principally as spiritual in nature, but there is strong witness also to the possibility that suffering can produce growth in character. St. Paul writes in his Epistle to the Romans that we "boast in our sufferings, knowing that suffering produces endurance, and endurance produces character" (Romans 5:3–5). Endurance through suffering can bring about a certain perseverance, a greater capacity not to be pulled down by the circumstances of life, a stronger fortitude and greater ability to continue to pursue what is good and right even in the face of difficulties (James 1).

Suffering and the loss of some good can lead to periods of reflection on the loss, on one's life and its circumstances, on how one might regain the good or otherwise cope with or adjust to the loss, and on what is ultimately of greatest importance.[5] Suffering can lead to a reevaluation of life and a refocus on things that matter most. Suffering can bring about a greater attention to the highest and most important goods. It can lead to a greater practical wisdom in terms of discerning the proper end of one's pursuits and actions and the best means to attain that end. Suffering can lead to a reorientation of one's life and pursuits.

Suffering can also lead to a greater empathy toward others and a greater capacity to love. In suffering, one can become more aware of the suffering of others. One can better understand the experience of those who are suffering; one can better understand and respond to their needs; one can better enter into and share their suffering. This greater empathy and greater capacity to respond to others increases one's capacity to love, to truly seek the good of others.[6]

Suffering can sometimes lead to a deepening of relationships and of community. As we turn to others to find comfort in our own suffering and as we reach out to others to assist them in their suffering,

---

5. There is a large empirical literature on coping and religious coping and the effects of such coping (see Pargament et al., 2000, 2011). This work has some conceptual overlap with responses to suffering and growth through suffering, although the latter category is broader.

6. See Brady (2018) for further philosophical discussion of the role of suffering in bringing about virtues such as fortitude, compassion, and wisdom.

relationships and community can be strengthened. Developing a greater capacity to love in our experience of suffering, reflecting on the most important and highest goods, and perhaps becoming reoriented toward the relationships we have and to the good of others and those around us can likewise enhance relationships and community. Suffering can have profound effects in bringing about an enriched relational and communal life. It may not always do so. Suffering can also pull apart relationships and communities. However, when suffering empowers a growth in character, a deepening of love, and a turning to one another, it has the capacity to enhance relationships.

Suffering can thus bring about a transformation in character, in one's capacity to love, in one's relationships and community, in one's understanding of and capacity to seek what is good, and in one's perseverance in obtaining that good.[7] Suffering can redirect the pursuits of one's life. Through that transformation of character and that reorientation of life, it is possible to find meaning even in the midst of suffering through appreciating the effects one's suffering has had on one's own character and direction in life. A transformation of character, a realignment of one's purposes, an enriched sense of meaning, and a deepening of relationships are all constitutive of a greater flourishing. Suffering inevitably entails some loss, but when it is possible to respond to that suffering as a potential means of growth, a renewed flourishing and health of the person is also possible, at least sometimes.

2.6f. God allows suffering to help bring about the free conversion of the will to God's intent and thereby a fuller spiritual well-being.

The existence of evil and of suffering is sometimes thought to be the most substantial challenge to the Christian understanding of God.[8] How

---

7. See, for example, John Paul II (1984), Larchet (2002), and Van Zeller (2015) for more extensive theological accounts of growth amid suffering. In the empirical and psychological literature, such growth and transformation is sometimes described as "post-traumatic growth." There is some evidence that various forms of suffering may lead to greater appreciation for life and changed priorities, closer relationships, recognition of new opportunities in life, greater personal strength, and spiritual development (Tedeschi and Calhoun, 2004; Ramos and Leal, 2013).

8. See, for example, Swinburne (1998), Adams (2000), Larrimore (2000), Van Inwagen (2008), Stump (2010), and Meister and Dew (2017) for a variety of

could it be that an all-powerful, all-knowing, and all-loving God would allow evil and suffering in the world? There is, both experientially and intellectually, a certain mystery to the presence of suffering and to the extent of that suffering.

One of the traditional Christian responses to this question and this challenge—sometimes referred to as the problem of suffering or the problem of evil—is to point to God's intent for the human person to freely respond to him in love. A loving response to God requires that that response be free. Freedom entails the capacity to reject God, and that rejection of God, and acting contrary to God's intent for oneself and toward others and the world, is sin.[9] That sin, that rejection of God's love, is the cause of separation from God, of ill health, of evil, and of suffering.[10]

However, even with this understanding, there is a mystery regarding the extent of the suffering. Although the meaning of suffering may be found in its pointing to the loss of some important good and thus the facilitating of reflection and action oriented toward the restoration of good, often the extent and anguish of suffering seems to far surpass the meaning that can be found in it. We are left with questions about why the extent and severity of suffering is so great. How could a loving God allow a mother, in desperation, without food, to experience her infant dying of starvation? Why is it that suffering is so great?

There are no easy answers to these questions. A mystery remains with regard to the extent and severity of suffering. Although the Christian

---

contemporary theological and philosophical approaches to the problems of evil and suffering.

9. Aquinas insists that God is not the cause of sin (Aquinas (1274/1948, I.II.79.1, 2, see also I.19.9). He is the cause of free will (I.83.1.ad 3) and the capacity to act (I.II.79.2), and he wills that the human person have free will (I.19.4, I.83.1.ad 3; see also I.19.8), but sin is departure, by free will, from the order of God (I.II.79.1,2). God is thus not the cause of sin (I.II.19.1) and never wills sin (I.19.10.ad 2).

10. Aquinas insists that God does not create evil (1274/1948, I.48.2), only its possibility. However, God permits evil to exist because many good things would not be possible if God did not permit evil (I.48.2). God does not will evil except to allow for its possibility in the attaining of certain other goods (I.19.9). God never wills sin (I.19.9, I.19.10.ad 2) but allows sin because of the good of free will (I.48.6; see also I.19.6). God wills justice, which in the presence of sin entails punishment (I.19.9, I.48.6, I.49.2), but this punishment can effectively act as medicine to heal the sinner, prevent further sin, and facilitate a restoration of the soul to God (I.48.6, I.II.87.2, 7).

tradition does point toward the capacity of suffering to bring about transformation of character and the finding of new meaning, there is a greater emphasis on the capacity of suffering to bring about a fuller and deeper conversion to God, a more profound spiritual transformation.

Suffering will often lead to a turning to God in prayer for help or as a source of support or strength. Suffering can lead one to a more profound appreciation of the limitations of the goods in this life and a seeking of that higher, more permanent and final good in God. Suffering as a result of the loss of goods in this life can lead to a greater detachment from earthly goods and ends. It can lead to a more profound focus on one's ultimate end in God and an alignment of one's life and pursuits with that end. It can give rise to a sense of hope wherein one's principal desire and aim is for one's final communion with God with a confidence that God will indeed accomplish this. In his Epistle to the Romans, when St. Paul writes of suffering producing character, those lines conclude with "we . . . boast in our sufferings, knowing that suffering produces endurance, and endurance produces character, and character produces hope, and hope does not disappoint us, because God's love has been poured into our hearts" (Romans 5:3–5). The result of character produced by suffering is hope, to be fulfilled by the experience of God's love.

The Christian understanding of the role of suffering is to allow for a turning back to God, a recognition of the good that was lost through sin and action contrary to God's intent. Sin brings about ill health and suffering, but mysteriously, God uses the suffering that we have effectively brought upon ourselves to redirect us back to himself.[11] Suffering, as the consequence of sin and wrongdoing, is used to heal the sin and wrongdoing that brought it about.[12] Suffering can be seen as an invitation to turn

---

11. Hebrews 12:5–11.

12. Aquinas divides the evils that ensue from voluntary action into moral evils (faults) and penalties (pains) (see 1274/1948, I.48.5–6). Moral evils have more of the nature of evil, understood as the privation of the good, because the evil of pain is the removal of some good, whereas the evil of fault is opposed to God, to the fulfillment of the divine will, and to divine love. God allows pain to prevent fault in ourselves (I.48.6; see also II.II.108.3.ad 2) or in others (I.II.87.2; see also Aquinas, 1270, V.4) or as medicine to restore the soul to God (I.II.87.7, II.II.108.4), although medicine never removes a greater good in order to promote a lesser one (II.II.108.4). In his commentary on Paul's Epistle to the Romans, Aquinas twice (Aquinas, 1272b, 8:28, 11:11), in

back to God. We will explore in part III of this book how and in what ways, from a Christian perspective, that occurs and how each instance of suffering can be seen as an opportunity for a reaffirmation of faith, a strengthening of hope, and a deepening of charity, of love for and friendship with God. The role of suffering is as an invitation to recommit the will to God, to heal the rupture from God brought about by the free decision to act contrary to God's intent. Suffering can help bring this about.[13] Suffering can be the occasion for sacrifice in the giving up of some good to attain a higher good in God.[14] That that end in God in love is seen as the very highest good relativizes all other goods and relativizes even the experience of suffering.[15] Some mystery will remain about the extent and severity of suffering. That mystery is perhaps deepened in God's response to sin and suffering: God became man in the person of Jesus Christ and fully entered into that suffering and took it upon himself.

The goal of the reconversion of the will back to God is such an important, and at times elusive, goal that for some it may require a sustained pursuit of God even amid the apparent experience of God's absence. Within the Christian tradition, there is the notion of the "dark night of the soul," an experience wherein God seems entirely absent, when the consolations brought about by spiritual life appear to be no more, when all experience of the love of God and even love for God seem removed, when the mind is filled with doubts and the heart is drawn to other goods or things contrary to God's will.[16] Such experiences of the dark night of the soul may be brief or may last for very extended periods. Much of the Christian tradition on such experiences is that God allows this experience of his absence to be felt in order to allow the person to more fully commit to the pursuit of God in faith, hope, and love even when there appear to be no outward signs or any inward affections that might incline one to do so. This submission of the will to God, even when circumstances and feelings

---

reference to Augustine, affirms that God "would not permit any evil to occur except for some good, which he draws out of the evil"; cf. Van Nieuwenhove (2005).

13. See Stump (1996) for discussion of Aquinas's commentary on Job concerning the role of suffering in bringing one to one's final end in God.

14. See Scheler (1992) for further exposition of the meaning of suffering being found in sacrifice.

15. See Romans 8:18; 2 Corinthian 4:17–5:4

16. St. John of the Cross (16th C/1959).

would incline one otherwise, strengthens one's commitment and builds one's faith, one's hope, and ultimately one's love for God in ever deeper ways. The conversion of the will to God is of such importance that God allows himself to be felt entirely absent to eventually bring about a greater friendship with him, a deeper spiritual life.

2.6g. The impossibility of our fully alleviating suffering and ill health points to the need for final restoration by God.

Finding meaning in suffering—in the transformation of character, in the conversion of the will to God, in a deepening of faith and hope and love—can provide partial relief from suffering. We can see the good that comes from suffering. There is a certain joy that can come even in the midst of suffering when we see the transformation and the good that can come about. However, this does not eliminate suffering. The losses of good in our lives are real losses; they are real evils. The ill health of the body and the ill health of the person are contrary to God's original and ultimate intent; they are to be mourned. In the absence of these goods, we suffer, and we are to mourn with and suffer with those who have likewise experienced losses and who are suffering.[17]

We can and should seek to mitigate suffering—suffering always indicates the loss or absence of some perceived good—but there are limits to what we can achieve. We can seek to address its causes: injury, infirmity, or disease; meaninglessness, broken relationships, and broken communities; wrong actions, unjust structures, and harm both to and from the environment. We can seek also to alleviate suffering and ill health when it is present. We can provide care for those in need; we can use the arts of medicine to heal a person following disease; we can offer love and support in the wake of broken relationships. These efforts are all important and good, and should be carried out. We should seek to mitigate suffering and to prevent the loss of what is good to the extent possible. However, there are limits to what we can expect to accomplish. We cannot fully address and eliminate sin by our own efforts. We cannot alter human nature or fully eliminate human wrongdoing. There are

---

17. That roughly a third of the Psalms are constituted by psalms of lament points toward the important role of lament and mourning in human experience.

limits, it seems, in our capacity to eliminate unjust structures. We cannot fully undo the damage done to creation. It is important that we do what we can to reduce, as best as possible, sin and injustice and suffering in each of these ways. But it is important also to understand our limitations in this regard. We will never, on our own, be entirely successful. We will not be able to create a utopia. There will continue to be suffering. There will continue to be sin. However, that very impossibility of fully eliminating suffering, along with our continued yearning to do so, points to our need for help. Our limitations point to the need for God's action to restore us and to eliminate suffering and sin and death. It is to that need, and to God's response, that we will turn in part III of this book.

> *Propositional Summary 2.6: The experience of distress over brokenness, or lack of wholeness, is suffering, whereby the need for healing and restoration is made clear.*
> 2.6a. Suffering is the anguished experience of a negative physical or mental state of considerable duration or intensity.
> 2.6b. Our experience of suffering reflects the brokenness of the world and of the human person.
> 2.6c. Ill health of the body can bring about suffering.
> 2.6d. Ill health of the person can bring about suffering.
> 2.6e. Suffering can lead to a transformation in understanding, life orientation, relationships, and character and can thereby bring about a renewed health of the person.
> 2.6f. God allows suffering to help bring about the free conversion of the will to God's intent and thereby a fuller spiritual well-being.
> 2.6g. The impossibility of our fully alleviating suffering and ill health points to the need for final restoration by God.

II.7. The Implications of Ill Health and Sin

Numerous implications arguably follow from an understanding of sin as the cause of ill-cause.

2.7a. Human wrongdoing should not be neglected as a cause of ill health.

The fundamental thesis of part II of this book is that the cause of ill health is sin or wrongdoing. If health is wholeness as intended by God, then a turning away from God's intent, which is sin, results in ill health. As discussed in the various sections above, such turning away from God's intent may be manifest in a variety of ways, including actions that result in harm to oneself, harmful actions toward others, harm to the community or environment, more systematic injustices that can persist over time and even over generations, and the fallen or broken nature of our world and of human life. These things result in ill health. A clear implication of this is that if we are to understand the causes of health and ill health and to try to address the causes of ill health, then we cannot neglect human wrongdoing as a cause of ill health. Ultimately, it is the cause of ill health.

In the contemporary West, and often within public health and medicine, it has become commonplace to not comment on individual wrongdoing as a cause of ill health. There are sometimes legitimate concerns that this might constitute blaming the victim.[1] As discussed in the sections above, the link between human wrongdoing and health is not one of perfect correspondence. It is often the case that it is someone other than the wrongdoer who suffers from the wrongdoer's actions. Our wrongful actions—whether this be violence, harsh words, discrimination, lying, or slander—often harm both the physical and mental health of others as well as other aspects of their well-being.

---

1. See, for example, Sloan (2011) for arguments that discussion of virtue and vice and their relation to health within the context of medicine is problematic.

However, one's own actions can also affect one's own health, both the health of the body and the health of the person. With regard to the health of the body, this can sometimes be manifest in behaviors with results that range from drunkenness to heart disease to acquiring sexually transmitted infections. With regard to the health of the person, any wrong action ultimately causes some harm to one's habits and character and may also adversely affect one's mental health, happiness, sense of meaning and self-understanding; one's relationships; and one's spiritual life.[2] Clearly we bear some responsibility for our own health.

Given the role of human wrongdoing in giving rise to ill health, wrongdoing should not be neglected or denied as a category in discussions of the causes of ill health. To do so is to be blind to one of the forces that ultimately shape health and well-being. Ill health cannot be adequately addressed without addressing human wrongdoing.

2.7b. Character ought to be emphasized as an important factor in maintaining health.

Given the centrality of human wrongdoing as a cause of ill health, it follows that an emphasis on character and on the development of virtue is critical for maintaining and preserving health. Good character involves habits that contribute to the good of oneself and others. Good character involves habits of avoiding human wrongdoing. As such, good character is critical in the avoidance of human wrongdoing that harms the health of oneself and of others. This is clear both conceptually and, as discussed in section I.3e, from the empirical data.[3]

---

2. Beyond violence and abuse, there are perhaps other examples in which wrongdoing is considered problematic within public health, as with discussions of racism as a public health issue (Devakumar et al., 2020), in which it is not only the effects and consequences of action that are considered problematic but the action is as well. Pornography as a public health issue (Rothman, 2021) is also sometimes portrayed as problematic but with less consensus within the public health community as to whether it is only the potential consequences that are problematic, though clearly considered wrong within the Christian tradition (Catholic Church, 2000, 2354). Concerning public policy and wrongdoing, see also George (1995) for discussion of how moral laws can play a role in preserving the moral life in society, since the moral choices people make not only form their own characters but also influence the moral lives of others.

3. See section I.3e and Wade et al. (2014), Chen, Harris, et al. (2019), Long, Kim, et al. (2020), Emmons and McCullough (2003), Davis et al. (2016), Seligman

To link wrongdoing and ill health, or to link character and virtue with good health, need not, however, entail "blaming the victim." Although such concerns should be taken seriously, they are also arguably pressed too far.[4] One can acknowledge that character or the virtues play a role in preserving and restoring health without ascribing every decline in health to a failure in virtue. One can look for opportunities to grow in character without always attributing lack of health to matters of character. Likewise, a caregiver can also look for opportunities to encourage a person or a patient to grow in character without necessarily subjecting them to guilt over past failures. However, given the causal, albeit imperfect, link between wrong actions and harm and ill health and between character and good health, matters of character should be given attention. To neglect these matters entirely is to ignore some of the forces that shape health—health of the body and health of the person—and is to ultimately neglect more holistic care that might be provided.[5]

Character and virtue are also important because they can enhance the well-being of others and of the community. If a virtue is understood as a habit in accord with reason to attain the good for oneself and others, then it follows by definition that virtue, properly understood, will contribute to the good of others. The virtue of justice is sometimes conceived

---

et al. (2005), Schutte and Malouff (2019), Węziak-Białowolska et al. (2021), and VanderWeele (2022a, 2022b).

4. The concern about attributing every mental health deficit to failure in virtue is a real one and ought to be guarded against. The Christian tradition, which places strong emphasis on character, makes these caveats clear. The story of Job in the Old Testament presents an example in which calamity and extreme psychological distress arise through a series of horrific undesired circumstances, not through failure of virtue, even though Job's friends are inclined to attribute it to such failure. New Testament teachings frequently present suffering as an opportunity for growth in character and comment that suffering in fact often arises from goodness or righteousness, but also noting the potential for wrong action to bring suffering (Simundson, 1992). Even Jesus, whom the New Testament portrays as the perfect model of virtue, is described as experiencing intense mental distress, even sweating blood, prior to his approaching death. The spiritual tradition of the "dark night of the soul" connotes a period of intense mental and spiritual distress that ultimately leads to the person's spiritual growth (St. John of the Cross, 1585/1959; May, 2009). Virtue may increase one's capacity to find peace amid difficulties, but it is no guarantee that suffering will be avoided. Indeed, it is possible that virtue may give rise to suffering.

5. See Waring (2016), Peteet (2022), VanderWeele (2022b), and section I.7c for further discussion.

of as "a steady and enduring will to render to each his or her due [or right]"⁶; the virtue of generosity as the habit of "giving good things to others freely and abundantly"⁷; the virtue of mercy or compassion as the habit of "heartfelt sympathy for another's distress, impelling us to [help] him if we can."⁸ Each of these virtues concerns bringing about good for others. Good character contributes to the good of others. There is, moreover, experimental evidence that the recipient of an action of goodwill is more likely to go on to act similarly and that the contagion effects of such beneficent action may extend so far that a positive interaction between two persons can propagate through a social network and ultimately affect the interaction of two other persons who do not know either person in the original pair.⁹ Good character thus has the potential to promote good generous actions among others.

Good character is also critical to maintaining health because the actions and decisions of leaders can powerfully shape the health of communities and even of nations.¹⁰ Leaders need the virtues of practical wisdom and justice to govern wisely and to rightly preserve and promote the health of all, both the health of the body and the health of persons. They often need the virtues of fortitude and temperance to endure the challenges, stresses, and conflicts that good leadership can entail. The character of a community's or country's leaders can profoundly affect the health of others.

Because the character of each person in, and the leaders of, a community are centrally linked to health, the issue of character should be considered of central importance in maintaining health, in discussions about what shapes health, and in promoting the health of populations.

2.7c. Injustices, the social nature of wrongdoing, and unjust structures from past wrongdoing need to be addressed in order to maintain health.

Matters of justice and injustice have been rightly emphasized within public health and public policy.¹¹ In order to maintain health—both

---

6. Justinian (533/1985).
7. Allen (2018).
8. Aquinas (1274/1920, II.II.30.1); see also Augustine (426/1998, book IX, chapter 5).
9. Fowler and Christakis (2010).
10. See Dayrit and Ambegaokar (2015) for further discussion.
11. Kass (2001); Daniels (2008); Hunt et al. (2015).

health of the body and the health of the person—it is critical that each person receives what is his or her due. It is important that a community's resources are distributed such that each person has the opportunity to flourish. It is important that when society's resources and capabilities allow, each person has access to basic health care both to preserve bodily health as its own end and to enable individuals to pursue other goods and ends, to pursue the health or flourishing of persons. Maintaining justice is also important for the health or wholeness of communities. A community is not healthy unless there is justice, unless each person receives his or her due.

Unjust actions that deprive someone of what is their due thus constitute a threat to health—both to bodily health and to the health of persons. As noted in the sections above, such injustices may be constituted by laws or systems that discriminate against certain groups of people, that fail to distribute resources when available to provide for the basic needs of each person, that fail to enforce laws, or that unnecessarily restrict human freedoms. Injustices may also be present even if the laws themselves are not unjust if there is systematic collective discrimination against certain groups of people. Injustices may also be present with regard to unequal access to and inadequate distribution of resources that have arisen from unjust actions and laws and structures of the past. All of these injustices adversely affect health.

Efforts need to be made to develop just laws and structures; to reform unjust laws and structures; to address issues of discrimination, both past and present; and to provide for the needs of all and to give all the opportunity to flourish. Addressing inequalities in access to good education and to health care that have arisen as a result of past discrimination and legacies of slavery and discrimination are critical for providing for the needs of all and giving everyone an opportunity to flourish. Likewise, addressing persisting interpersonal discrimination is important for moving toward a more just society.[12] Emphasis on the equal value

---

12. Although interpersonal discrimination is arguably less prominent in the United States today than it was sixty years ago, it still clearly persists. More empirical work on effective methods of helping to address these issues would be valuable. Although programs to train people to recognize implicit bias are well intentioned, their effectiveness is less substantial than might be hoped, perhaps especially among those for whom biases are greatest (Paluck et al., 2021; Chang et al., 2019; Dobbin

and dignity of every human life can help support efforts to address issues of discrimination and to better ensure that a society is oriented toward maintaining justice. For a just society, efforts also should be made to preserve individual rights, for example, of association, of speech, and of religion. Such rights are central in maintaining the health of persons and of communities, in the pursuit of truth, and in helping people achieve their final and most important ends. Individual liberties sometimes must be suspended for the sake of the common good, but laws and structures should be put in place to minimize the need and occasions for such suspensions.[13]

Injustices of all forms in the present and unjust structures created by past wrongs harm bodily health, the health of persons, and the health of communities. Efforts to maintain and restore justice are critical to maintaining health.

2.7d. Respect for life and the averting of abortion and euthanasia is critical to maintaining health.

The notion of health presupposes life. Life is a gift from God. The deprivation of life is the loss of this gift. The action of a person, as an

---

and Kalev, 2016). More effective strategies might include adopting some of those of the civil rights movement, such as regularly emphasizing the equal value and dignity of all people and promoting love among all people. There is also evidence that interracial mentoring programs may be more effective in altering attitudes (Dobbin and Kalev, 2016), once again involving an emphasis on the good of the person. See also section III.7g.

13. Conflicts can arise between individual liberties and the common good. In Aquinas's understanding of a justly ordered society, the state has the authority to limit individual liberties for the sake of the common good (Aquinas (1274/1920, I. II.90.4, 96.1, 96.4, 97.4). Doing this in a way that improves rather than detracts from overall well-being requires practical wisdom on the part of the community's or nation's leaders. These conflicts and tensions were present throughout the recent COVID-19 pandemic. Arguably, liberties should be suspended when the harm caused by such suspension is outweighed by the contribution to the common good. Reluctance to suspend individual liberties should be proportionate to the burden imposed and to the extent of the good being threatened by the suspension of individual liberties. In the case of the COVID-19 pandemic, the use of masks, while uncomfortable, constitutes a relatively minor inconvenience. The suspension of religious services, in contrast, while perhaps prudent for a time when uncertainties were greatest, constituted a much greater threat to individual and communal well-being.

individual, of intentionally taking the life of another is a violation of God's gift of life, a termination of health, a termination of wholeness.[14] Health and wholeness cannot be preserved without life.

Abortion involves the destruction of developing human life. It is the termination of life, of wholeness; it is the cessation of health; it is a refusal to accept the gift of a new life. Averting abortion is essential for maintaining and preserving life and health. Abortion typically arises as a result of an unwanted life. Such new life is sometimes unwanted or unwelcome because of competing desires or needs for other things that seem threatened by welcoming that new life into the world. The reasons for this lack of welcome, for the desire or felt need to end the developing human life, are diverse, ranging from financial hardship to the absence of a committed marital partnership to concerns about restrictions on freedom.[15] Laws restricting abortion may help bring about reduced numbers of abortions but do not in general address the underlying causes for the desire not to welcome life. Without addressing those underlying causes, many will seek abortion even if it is contrary to the law. To preserve life and foster health, it is necessary to work toward a "culture of life," a culture that respects and welcomes new life, and to address the causes that give rise to the desire or felt need not to welcome new life.[16]

Abortion and the accompanying desire not to welcome life are signs of the lack of health in relationships and in community. The

---

14. Aquinas argues that it is always wrong for a private individual to intentionally take the life of another (1274/1920, II.II.64.3) and that this constitutes murder. However, he also argues that it is lawful for a public authority, in certain cases, to put a criminal to death for the sake of the common good (II.II.64.2,3, 65.1), but in his understanding even in these cases there is strict restriction to those that "inflict an irreparable harm . . . as contain some horrible deformity" (II.II.66.6.ad 2) and "which conduce to the grave undoing of others" (II.II.103.ad 2). See also Koritansky (2012) and footnote 8 in section I.3 concerning current teachings of the Catholic Church on capital punishment. Although cases of capital punishment do not constitute murder, they are nevertheless always best avoided. Likewise, when the death of the other person is not intended but is a consequence of action nonetheless, this does not in general constitute murder (Aquinas, 1274/1920, II.II.64.7–8). However, it is always wrong and a grave sin when a private individual intentionally takes the life of another.

15. See Kirkman et al. (2009) for a review of the empirical literature on reasons women give for abortion.

16. John Paul II (1995).

desire for abortion often arises in the context of the absence of a committed marital relationship, or sexual relations oriented more toward physical pleasure and the satisfaction of powerful urges instead of being ordered toward the good of each person and the openness to new life. The lack of respect for life, for wholeness, for health that is manifest in abortion cannot be addressed without restoring and reinforcing the institution of marriage and addressing the proper orientation of sexual relations.[17]

Concerns about adequate financial resources to care for a child are also often present with regard to desire or felt need for abortion. Although this may in part arise from the absence of a committed marital relationship, it also relates to the distribution of societal resources. Systems and structures of promotion and pay, of welfare, and of child support play a critical role in whether a mother or family feels that resources are sufficient to welcome another child, and a just and flourishing society will be one in which resources are such that the welcoming of new life is facilitated. Concerns about freedom likewise come into play and are real. However, to not welcome life on those grounds and to seek to terminate it is a failure to understand life as the highest value here and now and a failure to understand the great wrong that is committed in the taking of the life of another.

There will inevitably be cases in which a mother genuinely cannot care for a new child. In such instances, an approach that welcomes life and that does not violate the gift of life is to pursue adoption, to find a home for the child in which the child can be welcomed and cared for. To terminate the pregnancy and put an end to the developing life harms the fabric of a culture of life and wholeness, often adversely affecting the mental health of the mother, and ultimately constitutes an action contrary

---

17. Catholic teaching on contraception (Paul VI, 1968) also effectively presupposes sexual intercourse within the context of committed marital relations. Sexual intercourse is to be ordered toward the unity of spouses and the formation of new life. It is in the context of a committed marriage that there can in principle always be openness to new life. Family and societal resources are, of course, also important considerations, and thus sex must take place in a responsible manner that takes into account the whole of the family's context. However, the relation between marriage and contraceptive use or lack thereof is arguably bidirectional. See, for example, Regnerus (2017) for arguments and evidence about how contraception has played a role in declining rates of marriage.

to God's intent for life and wholeness.[18] We should ideally aim for a society in which each family can welcome new life. When that is not possible, adoption, rather than termination, provides the right way forward to health and wholeness.

Concern for life and respect for life and for wholeness is also needed at the end of life. As death approaches, as the body deteriorates, as ill health sets in, there can be a temptation to end life prematurely. But this does not respect life as God's gift. Euthanasia, like abortion, is a violation of the gift of life and of wholeness. A decline in physical health inevitably occurs that can be painful and can result in considerable suffering. But to end life prematurely on these grounds constitutes a devaluing of life and a devaluing of the nonmaterial dimensions of human wellbeing, of meaning and relationships and character, that can often develop and be enhanced even in the midst of or because of challenges and suffering.[19] Euthanasia is a sign of an unwillingness to see the potentially redemptive value in suffering and a sign of the reduction of the human person to material dimensions. As with abortion, so with euthanasia, efforts should be made to understand the causes for the desire or felt

---

18. Mental health difficulties are notably more prevalent among those who have had an abortion than within the general population (see National Collaborating Centre for Mental Health at the Royal College of Psychiatrists, 2011). Some of these studies restrict the comparison to women with unwanted pregnancies, comparing those who had had an abortion with those who had not. Some studies and a meta-analysis indicate that women who chose to have an abortion subsequently had higher rates of depression than those who did not, but not all studies indicate this and the matter is disputed (Coleman, 2011; Steinberg et al., 2012) and may well vary by context. However, in some sense, the debate is only tangentially relevant. Both groups of women have considerably higher rates of depression than the general population. Both need help—both in navigating the difficult set of circumstances and with respect to mental health (VanderWeele, 2023b). For both, the issue stems from an *unwanted* pregnancy and the circumstances that make that pregnancy unwanted. Moving toward a culture of life requires not only helping women in the circumstances they find themselves in and helping them choose not to terminate the pregnancy, but also addressing issues concerning relationships and resources so that life is always welcomed and so that when pregnancies occur, they are not unwanted.

19. Earlier versions of the Hippocratic oath effectively entailed vows not to carry out euthanasia or an abortion, though these clauses have now been removed from modern versions (Scheinman et al., 2018).

need to terminate life.[20] Effort should be made to address physical pain, existential suffering, and potential despair.[21] Efforts should also be made to help a person prepare for death.[22] Addressing the underlying causes of the desire to end life instead of terminating life has the potential both to respect the value of life and to bring some degree of transformation to the one suffering, to help restore or preserve a greater wholeness of the person.

Lack of respect for life is a sign of the ill health of persons and of society. In order to promote health, we need to create a culture of life, a culture that values life and welcomes life, and a just society that facilitates such welcome. Life is a precondition for health, for wholeness. Respect for life, and the averting of abortion and euthanasia, are critical to maintaining health.

2.7e. Care for the environment is critical to maintaining health.

Care for the environment is likewise critical for maintaining health. We are dependent upon the world in which we live, as the place where we dwell, as our source of food and sustenance, as that which God has entrusted us to care for. Care for the environment is needed for human life to flourish. This includes preserving natural beauty and the beauty and diversity of plant and animal life that we find in our world. Care for the environment involves making use of it in ways that are sustainable so that the earth can continue to be a source of food and of sustenance. Care of the environment involves trying to avoid human-induced changes to ecosystems that make the earth less hospitable to life.

Consequently, efforts should be made to preserve and foster natural beauty. Efforts should likewise be made to the extent possible to preserve the diversity of plant and animal life, to protect species that are

---

20. In many cases, these reasons concern difficult existential questions rather than issues of physical pain (Emanuel, 2017) which can now often be addressed.

21. Palliative pain treatment that is proportionate to what is needed to treat symptoms and results in death that is foreseen but not intended is different from intentionally killing the patient (Keenan, 1993). However, see Curlin (2018) for discussion of ethical complexities concerning palliative sedation with respect to its cutting off one existentially from human experience.

22. See, for example, Dugdale (2017, 2021) for discussion of the ethics and practical considerations in "dying well."

endangered. Efforts should be made to confront and counter potential human-caused changes to the climate that threaten human life and plant and animal diversity. Efforts should be made to consume the earth's resources in ways that are consistent with sustaining human life over time.

As human life flourishes and continues to expand, the challenges of caring for the environment become more complex. More and more needs to be done to think through how to inhabit and make use of the earth in sustainable ways. These complexities require our very best scientific knowledge, governance, and international cooperation. We must develop and use technologies in ways that both make use of and preserve the environment as we navigate these complexities and tensions.[23] From the perspective of Christian theology, those complexities and tensions are both reflective of and a result of our fallenness. They require our efforts to mitigate the effects of that fallenness and of further human wrongdoing that can harm both the environment and other people. Unfortunately, there are often real trade-offs involved in the care of the environment between various aspects of human flourishing both at present and with respect to future generations.

Decisions about care for the environment must take into account human needs and questions of human flourishing in all places and at all times. The care of the environment is a duty that is required as a part of the common good and as action that promotes the common good.[24] This is both a shared political responsibility and an individual responsibility. It is a political responsibility because this cannot be adequately achieved without joint collective action. But it is also an individual responsibility because each person's choices matter. Pope John Paul II's *Centesimus annus* (John Paul II, 1991) taught that "serious ecological problems call for an effective change of mentality leading to the adoption of new lifestyles, 'in which the quest for truth, beauty, goodness and communion with others for the sake of the common good are the factors that determine consumer choices, savings and investments.'"[25] Given that the earth is in some sense the shared heritage of the whole human community across generations, both individual efforts and

---

23. See Catholic Church (2004, chapter 10) for further discussion of navigating these challenges from the perspective of Christian theology and ethics.
24. Catholic Church (2004, 466).
25. John Paul II (1991, 36); Catholic Church (2004, 486).

efforts to coordinate such care across countries and across generations are essential.[26]

To not care for the environment is ultimately also to neglect the health of persons. The state of the environment clearly affects physical health.[27] However, the need for the earth to sustain life, not only for the present time but for future generations as well, is such that neglect of the care of the environment is an abandonment of our role in and responsibility for human life and the flourishing of future generations.[28] Care for the environment is critical in efforts to preserve and maintain bodily health and the health of persons in both the present and the future.

2.7f. The notion that we will ultimately overcome ill health and death in this life is a fiction that we need to resist.

Because of the impossibility in this life of completely averting human wrongdoing, because injustices often persist, because of the fallenness and brokenness of our nature and of our world, it will not be possible in this life to completely overcome ill health. All eventually do die. This does not mean that we should not do what we can to address the causes of ill health. Indeed, our efforts to combat ill health and its causes, to rectify evil and human wrongdoing, to establish justice and to work to maintain, preserve, and restore health are critical to human well-being. However, we should also be realistic about what can, and cannot, be accomplished.

The notion that we will, in this life, ultimately overcome ill health and death is a fiction that needs to be resisted. To not do so is to pursue an impossibility, thereby potentially squandering valuable resources that could be used more effectively in maintaining health and in addressing some of the causes of ill health that are potentially within our control. Use of resources in often futile attempts to extend life is in tension with the idea that it is especially the poor and those in adverse conditions that, out of mercy and justice, should be the particular focus of efforts to

---

26. Catholic Church (2004, 467). See Francis (2015) for further theological reflection on the challenges and responsibilities of caring for the earth as our common home.
27. Woodward and Macmillan (2015); von Schirnding (2015).
28. Francis (2015, 159–162).

improve well-being.[29] To invest in extending life more and more, at greater and greater cost, often in neglect of considering what constitutes the health or wholeness of the person, can hinder individual and societal flourishing. It may also constitute a failure of attending to the actual needs of the person approaching death and a failure to help them adequately prepare for death.[30] Ending life prematurely is wrong but attempting to extend it indefinitely can be a foolish and futile pursuit.[31] Allowing someone to die and accepting the inevitability of death is not the same as intentionally ending the life of another.[32]

The desire to completely overcome ill health and death perhaps arises in part from the fact that ill health and death are indeed great evils. It perhaps also arises in part from a desire to achieve some sense of emancipation, or salvation, through the use of science and technology.[33] Death in some sense marks the limits of our scientific and technological ability.[34] These are limits that we are often fearful of today. Many prior cultures gave a prominent role to death in their cultural life; we often try

---

29. Catholic social teaching refers to this principle as the "preferential option for the poor" (Catholic Church, 2004, 182–184).

30. Balboni and Balboni (2018); Dugdale (2017, 2021).

31. Basil of Caesarea (St. Basil the Great, 1962) in his Long Rules, Q. 55., comments, "Whatever requires an undue amount of thought or trouble or involves a large expenditure of effort and causes our whole life to revolve, as it were, around solicitude for the flesh must be avoided by Christians. Consequently, we must take great care to employ this medical art, if it should be necessary, not as making it wholly accountable for our state of health or illness, but as redounding to the glory of God and as a parallel to the care given the soul. In the event that medicine should fail to help, we should not place all hope for the relief of our distress in this art, but we should rest assured that He will not allow us to be tried above that which we are able to bear."

32. Treatments to attempt to sustain life may be disproportionate in being excessively burdensome or effectively useless. The relevant distinction is that it is the *treatment*, rather than the person's *life*, that is judged to be burdensome or useless. As a gift from God, life is never useless. Withholding excessively burdensome or effectively useless treatment is not the same as intentionally killing the patient. See May (2008, chapter 7, section 4) for further discussion; see also Pius XII (1957).

33. See Balboni and Balboni (2018) for discussion of how medicine and its accompanying technologies and institutions in some sense provides an implicit "theology of immanence" suggestive of some form of salvation or liberation from suffering and death.

34. See Gadamer (1996, chapter 4) for an analysis of our experience of death and its relation to our understanding of health.

to hide it. However, even today, religious practices preserve and enact ceremonies concerning life and death, and often even the most secularized members of society participate in these rituals. There is a real need to acknowledge and confront the reality of ill health and death and to prepare for it.

From the perspective of Christian theology, because of the brokenness of the world, understood as arising from and reflective of, sin, the health of the body and of the person will always be imperfect and we will always eventually confront death. We can go some way in addressing the causes of ill health, and indeed we should do so, but we should also understand our limitations. We are best off acknowledging this, understanding the meaning and root causes of ill health and death, responding to these, and ultimately preparing for death. We can appropriately respond to the reality of ill health and death only by adequately acknowledging them as realities. To respond appropriately, we need to resist the notion that we can, in the present life, overcome ill health and death.

2.7g. Medicine, public health, and public policy should be attentive to questions of suffering and not just to mental disorders and physical diseases.

Acknowledging that ill health and death are realities that cannot be overcome in this life allows us to be more attentive to what our response to those intractable realities should be. Such acknowledgment can shift the perspective from a focus on technical problems to be overcome to the more fundamental matters of human experience in facing the realities of ill health and death. It can facilitate a greater care for the person, and not just of the body. It can facilitate a greater attentiveness to suffering.

Suffering is constituted by the undesired nature of the experience of ill health, of a negative physical or mental state, often of considerable duration or intensity. Suffering concerns the person. Suffering reflects the meanings and implications for a person's life as a whole related to being in a state of ill health or confronting death. Although medicine and public health and public policy have made important and impressive progress in preserving and maintaining health and developing institutions of medicine to try to restore health, less emphasis has been given to the human experience of ill health, to suffering. And yet for many patients, it is not just their bodily state that is of concern or that needs attention but also their experience of ill health and its meaning and its implications for the whole of a person's life and their personhood.[35]

Greater attention should be given in medicine, public health, and public policy to assessing suffering and understanding its determinants, to asking patients about their suffering, to finding ways to alleviate suffering when possible, and to finding meaning and transformation within suffering both generally, and also especially when its alleviation is not possible. The role of the institutions of medicine and public health include the health of bodies but, as argued in section I.7, also extends in various ways to the health of persons. It is not possible to care adequately for the health of persons without attending to their suffering. Attending to suffering acknowledges the limits of our medical knowledge and technology in human experience, our limits in fully addressing ill health, in fully addressing its causes, and in postponing and preventing death. Attending to suffering can empower a person to better understand the meaning of their suffering, of ill health, of its causes, and of death, along with the need for a more complete restoration.

2.7h. Medicine, public health, and public policy should be attentive to and address the phenomenon of moral injury.

Wrong action can harm oneself and others. Such harms may be physical, mental, social, or spiritual. Moral injury is one form of harm that may be brought about that is not often addressed in medicine, public health, and public policy. The possibility of moral injury is inherent in wrongdoing. The violation of deep moral beliefs or values by one's own action or that of another can have profound consequences for someone in terms of guilt, shame, a sense of betrayal, or a threatening of one's moral understanding and framework. When such moral emotions cause persistent

---

35. See Cassell (1982, 1991) for an account of how attending to suffering within medicine may help medicine better achieve its ends in the care of persons. See VanderWeele (2019b) for a description of the potential that empirical assessments of suffering might have in the context of patient care and for research directions that might be made possible by more systematic collection of data on suffering in clinical, community, and even national contexts.

distress over time, it may become proper to speak of moral injury.[36] Such injury is a phenomenon related to the health of a person; it is a moral phenomenon that will in general have psychological, social, and spiritual aspects and can have physical consequences. As moral agents, our own wrong actions and those of others can cause not only direct harm to the body and to mental health, narrowly understood, but also to our sense of values, our sense of right and wrong and of good and evil. The health of the person requires that we be attentive to the moral aspects of life and their consequences and to injury that can occur when our moral understanding is deeply violated or threatened by something that has occurred. Such injuries can occur when persons commit acts they thought themselves incapable of or when witnessing such acts carried out by others or by being a victim of such an act. The phenomenon of moral injury is best documented and studied in the context of military personnel and veterans but can occur in civilian life and has received some study among health care providers, professionals, and parents involved with child protection services, police officers, educators, and refugees.[37]

The phenomenon of moral injury has long been discussed and documented in religious and spiritual writings and in literature, but it has not been studied in the fields of science and psychology until recently.[38] Evidence has begun to accumulate that the phenomenon can be distinguished from post-traumatic stress disorder (PTSD).[39] This can also be seen conceptually: moral injury must always concern some action and

---

36. More formally, we might define moral injury as persistent distress that arises because personal experience disrupts or threatens one's sense of the goodness of oneself, of others, of institutions, or of what are understood to be higher powers or one's beliefs or intuitions about right and wrong, or good and evil. Analogously, a potentially morally traumatic experience might be defined as personal experience that disrupts or threatens one's sense of the goodness of oneself, of others, of institutions or of what are understood to be higher powers or one's beliefs or intuitions about right and wrong, or good and evil. Such an event may or may not result in distress that is persistent. However, when such a potentially morally traumatic experience gives rise to persistent distress because of its moral nature, it becomes proper to speak of "moral injury."

37. Koenig and Al Zaben (2021). See Giffin et al. (2019) for additional references and an integrative review.

38. Litz and Kerig (2019). Griffin et al. (2019) argue that the scientific study of moral injury began with the work of Litz et al. (2009).

39. Bryan et al. (2018); Litz and Kerig (2019); Griffin et al. (2019).

event concerning moral action or worth, whereas PTSD may or may not. Conversely, PTSD, at least in its current clinical understanding, must involve a persistent re-experiencing, whereas moral injury may or may not. The possibilities for treatment are likely also different. For example, it is, not clear that prolonged exposure therapy, which is common in treatment for PTSD, will be especially helpful for treating moral injury if questions of guilt or shame or betrayal are not also addressed.[40] Alternative treatments such as adaptive disclosure therapy[41] or approaches that incorporate aspects of spirituality or forgiveness[42] that more directly address moral concerns may be more effective for moral injury than, for instance, in cases of PTSD resulting from what might be devastating occurrences but ones that are less connected with moral transgressions in human action.

As our understanding of moral injury and treatment options expands, it is important that we be attentive to these considerations in medical, public health, and public policy contexts. We are moral agents. We can and do wrong one another. Such wrongs can be deeply unsettling. It is important that we address the guilt and shame, the betrayal and threats to our moral understanding, intuitions, and values associated with such wrongs. To not do so is to neglect the health of the person. In the next part of the book, distinctively Christian approaches to addressing wrongdoing, moral injury, and sin will be developed in further detail, but some of the insights there are applicable more generally in pluralistic contexts. In caring for persons, we need to care for and be attentive to their moral nature. We need to be attentive to matters of moral injury.

Propositional Summary:
2.7a. Human wrongdoing should not be neglected as a cause of ill health.
2.7b. Character ought to be emphasized as an important factor in maintaining health.
2.7c. Injustices, the social nature of wrongdoing, and unjust structures from past wrongdoing need to be addressed in order to maintain health.

---
40. Griffin et al. (2019).
41. Litz et al. (2016).
42. Koenig and Al Zaben (2021).

The Implications of Ill Health and Sin 189

2.7d. Respect for life and the averting of abortion and euthanasia is critical to maintaining health.
2.7e. Care for the environment is critical to maintaining health.
2.7f. The notion that we will ultimately overcome ill health and death in this life is a fiction that we should resist.
2.7g. Medicine, public health, and public policy should be attentive to questions of suffering and not just to mental disorders and physical diseases.
2.7h. Medicine, public health, and public policy should be attentive to and address the phenomenon of moral injury.

PART III

HEALING AND SALVATION

". . . until it finds its rest in thee"
(Augustine, 400/1991, book 1, chapter 1)

Propositional Outline of Part III:
The restoration and fulfillment of health is salvation.

3.0. Healing is the restoration of wholeness.
3.1. Healing of the person cannot fully come about without a healing from sin.
3.2. The principal ways that a restoration and fulfillment of wholeness are brought about are love of God and love of one's neighbor.
3.3. God has brought healing and salvation through Jesus Christ.
3.4. The Church and its members are both agents and recipients of healing, and that healing comes about through communal life, forgiveness, prayer, fasting, the sacraments, growth in character, and the care of others, including the work of medicine.
3.5. There are limits to healing in this life, but healing in relation to God can come about in the midst of and sometimes even through ill health.
3.6. The fulfillment of wholeness, a communion with God and a completion of God's intent, comes only in the resurrection in the life to come and will be accomplished by God.
3.7. The implications of healing and salvation.

Introduction

Healing as the Restoration of Wholeness

Proposition 3.0. Healing is the restoration of wholeness.

Healing is the restoration of wholeness. In our lives, we are confronted with ill health, with a lack of wholeness, and are in need of healing, of a restoration to health. The ill health that we experience may arise from disease, infirmity, or bodily malfunction or it may concern other aspects of the person more broadly, their mental health, their relationships, their character. There is a restlessness that is often experienced, a suffering, a realization that all is not well that is accompanied by a desire to be restored or healed.

As was the case with both health and ill health, so also with healing: we might distinguish between broader and narrower senses in which the word "healing" might be used. We may refer to bodily healing, the restoration of wholeness to the body so that the body's parts and systems are functioning as they normally do so as to allow for the full range of activities characteristic of the human body. We can also refer to the healing of persons, the restoration of wholeness to the entire life of a person, a facilitating of their flourishing.

Like "health," the English word "heal" derives etymologically from the Old English *hælan* ("cure; save; make whole, sound and well") from the Proto-Germanic *"hailjan"* (literally "to make whole"), which derives from the Proto-Indo-European *"kailo-"* ("whole"). Healing is a restoration to wholeness.

In the biblical texts, there is a close connection between health and wholeness and between healing and a restoration to wholeness.[1] The

---

1. See Kee (1992) and Wilkinson (1998) for further discussion of the Greek and Hebrew words related to healing and for further biblical commentary.

Hebrew word "*rapha*," which is often translated as "heal," connotes a restoring to normal. Healing is the restoration to what something is supposed to normally be. The Hebrew word perhaps closest to "health" is "*marpe*," although it is used relatively infrequently. Instead, the Hebrew word "shalom," often translated as "peace," is frequently used with respect to healing and wholeness. That word conveys a sense of general well-being, or right relation to self, others, and God—essentially a wholeness of the person.

Three Greek words are predominantly used in the New Testament for "heal": "*therapevo*," "*iaomai*," and "*sozo*." The word "*therapevo*" is associated with care or attention, the word "*iaomai*" is associated with cure or restoration, and the word "*sozo*" more literally means "save." The Greek word for "to be in health," "*hygiano*," is somewhat similar to the concept of health in English, "to be whole, sound and well." Both the Hebrew and Greek concepts of health and healing thus relate closely to well-being generally or wholeness and to its restoration. As will be discussed further below, healing in the biblical accounts often concerned the whole person and included both physical and spiritual healing.

In this fallen world, the experience of ill health is common and inevitable. However, there are often possibilities for a restoration to health. In many cases, the body has a remarkable capacity to heal itself, to recover from wounds, to restore an equilibrium. Human agency can also facilitate health. The practice of medicine, ranging from pharmacological treatment to surgical procedures, can often bring bodily healing in cases in which the body would not recover on its own. A change in behaviors related to rest, sleep, nutrition, or exercise can sometimes facilitate better health and a recovery from ill health over time.

Similarly, in cases of the brokenness of a person, or lack of flourishing of the person, healing and restoration are sometimes possible. The passage of time or the discovery of new possibilities can sometimes bring healing from sadness over some loss. Broken relationships can sometimes be restored through practices of forgiveness, by the passage of time, or by investing in those relationships in new ways. Deficiencies in character can sometimes be improved by diligent effort, by guidance from others, by moral exemplars, or by a renewed commitment to seeking what is good. Ill health of the body and brokenness of the person can sometimes be addressed. Healing and restoration are sometimes possible.

This healing and restoration is intended by God. God's intent for the human body is that it be whole and well-functioning and capable of giving and receiving love. God's intent for the human person is one of flourishing and ultimately of communion with him. God's intent for human life is health and wholeness of the body and of the person. That the present experience of human life is so often that of ill health is contrary to God's intent.[2] This experience of ill health has come about only because God has given the gift of human freedom, which has been used to bring about a state contrary to God's intent. In the present state of human ill health, God's intent is one of healing and restoration. God's intent is that human freedom be used in conjunction with God's action and healing to bring about a restoration to health and a transformed life for the human person. The restoration to health is a restoration to complete physical, mental, social, and spiritual wholeness and well-being. It is a restoration to full human flourishing. Moreover, God's intent now and in the life to come is not only a restoration, but also a fulfillment of health and wholeness, a bringing about of something new, transformed, and even greater than what was manifest in the original state. God's grace perfects our nature.[3]

Propositional Summary 3.0: Healing is the restoration of wholeness.
3.0a. Healing is the restoration of wholeness.
3.0b. Healing may pertain to the body or, more broadly, to the person.
3.0c. Numerous aspects of ill health can be addressed so that health is restored.
3.0d. God's intent is for health and thus for healing, a restoration to health.
3.0e. Healing of the person is constituted by a restoration to physical, mental, social, and spiritual well-being.
3.0f. God's intent now and in the life to come is the fulfillment of wholeness.

---

2. As per the introduction to part II, speaking of ill health as contrary to God's intent is in respect to God's will considered antecedently (Aquinas, 1274/1920, I.19.6), prior to human action and sin. God wills that human persons be free, but he does not will sin, although he permits it (I.II.79.2, I.48.6, I.19.10.ad 2) because of human freedom. Sin constitutes and brings about ill health, although, as discussed in section II.6, the suffering of ill health may ultimately bring us back to God.

3. Aquinas (1274/1920, I.1.8.ad 2, I.II.109.3, I.II.110, I.II.113, I.II.114.2).

III.1. Healing of Persons and Healing from Sin

Proposition 3.1. Healing of the person cannot fully come about without a healing from sin.

3.1a. Complete healing of the person may seem like an ideal that is not possible to achieve.

Healing of the person is constituted by a restoration to wholeness of all aspects of the person's life. Such healing includes a full restoration to physical, mental, social, and spiritual wholeness. The healing of the person is a restoration to full flourishing. The complete healing of a person—a restoration to the full health of the person—is thus a lofty ideal. It may appear difficult, or impossible, to achieve. This ideal is impeded in countless ways by the brokenness and fallenness of the world and of our own lives. It is impeded by the reality of sin.

3.1b. Restoration to wholeness cannot be achieved without addressing sin and the effects of sin.

As detailed in part II, sin is the cause of ill health. Ill health cannot be addressed, and there can be no complete restoration to health, without addressing sin. Wrong actions often harm ourselves and others and can bring about unjust structures that perpetuate ill health of the body and of the person over time. Wrong actions disrupt our relationships and our communities. Wrong actions disrupt our peace with ourselves. Wrong actions disrupt our peace with God.

Sin has thus affected and continues to affect our daily lives and interactions, along with our health, the health of our bodies, and our health as persons. Sin has disrupted and impedes our flourishing. Sin has ultimately also disrupted our relationship to the world around us and has brought about a world that is fallen and broken. Sin has brought about corruption of the body and of the soul, and disorder in our relationship with creation, further perpetuating ill health.[1]

Although the consequences of sin for ill health can sometimes be addressed by the arts of medicine, by therapies, by public health measures, by cooperation and hard work, and by various other efforts, so long as sin is present, there will be ill health. A complete restoration to health will not be possible by our own efforts.

3.1c. Complete health of the person requires communion with God and thus healing in relation to God so that sin no longer separates a person from God.

More fundamentally, sin separates us from God and from our final communion with God. Complete wholeness of the person is constituted by communion with God, and sin impedes that communion.[2] Sin is voluntary action contrary to God's intent that keeps us from union with God. A complete restoration to wholeness, including spiritual wholeness found in God, cannot be accomplished without addressing sin. There can be no attainment of life as God intended without the healing of the soul, without a healing of that which relates to God within the human person. We need God's help to address sin and to bring about restoration to wholeness as God intended.[3] This help and this restoration, which God accomplishes, is understood as salvation.

3.1d. Salvation is the deliverance from sin and its consequences and thereby a complete restoration and fulfillment of wholeness as God intended.

Salvation is the deliverance from sin and its consequences.[4] If sin is the cause of ill health, then restoration to complete health of the person cannot be accomplished without the removal of sin and without the removal of the consequences of sin, for both the body and the soul. It is this

---

1. Aquinas (1274/1920, I.II.82, 85–86).
2. Aquinas (1274/1920, I.II.88.1–2); Aquinas (1270, V.1).
3. Aquinas (1274/1920, I.II.109).
4. Aquinas (1274/1920, I.II.113); see also van Nieuwenhove (2005).

removal of sin and its consequences that is understood as salvation. That deliverance from sin and its consequences is the healing that is needed for the restoration of the whole person. The healing of the person cannot fully come about without such salvation and deliverance from sin.

For these reasons, healing is often also tied to salvation in the biblical accounts. The prophetic books speak of the "healing" of apostasy and faithlessness.[5] What is healed or restored is the lack of right relation to God, of that within the human person and human community that relates to God. Healing and restoration or salvation are thus often spoken of in parallel in the prophetic books.[6] Likewise, in the healing accounts of the gospels, in several instances where Jesus uses the words "your faith has healed you," it is the Greek word *sozo* that is used, and the more direct translation would thus be "your faith has saved you."[7]

Although it was faith that gave rise to physical healing in the miracle accounts, that faith was also constitutive of a restored relationship to God, which itself was salvation and which was mirrored by the physical healing. Jesus's care for the physical ailments of those he healed highlights the importance of the body, but the healings themselves often symbolically pointed toward or were accompanied by speech concerning spiritual healing and salvation. The New Testament epistles also suggest a link between salvation and healing: faith leads to conversion and the transformation of character by following the example of Jesus, by the work of the Spirit, and by Jesus giving himself for us.[8] Full restoration of the health of the person requires a healing of the soul. Full restoration and fulfillment of health requires salvation.

Propositional Summary 3.1: Healing of the person cannot fully come about without a healing from sin.
    3.1a. Complete healing of the person may seem like an ideal that is not possible to achieve.
    3.1b. Restoration to wholeness cannot be achieved without addressing sin and the effects of sin.

---

5. Hosea 14:4; Jeremiah 3:22.
6. Psalm 103:3; Jeremiah 17:14; Isaiah 6:9–10, 53:4–5.
7. Matthew 9:22; Mark 5:34, 10:52; Luke 17:19, 18:42.
8. Hebrews 12:1–13; 1 Thessalonians 5:19–24; 1 Peter 2:24–25.

3.1c. Complete health of the person requires communion with God and thus healing in relation to God so that sin no longer separates a person from God.
3.1d. Salvation is the deliverance from sin and its consequences and thereby a complete restoration and fulfillment of wholeness as God intended.

III.2. Healing and Love

Proposition 3.2. The principal ways that a restoration and fulfillment of wholeness are brought about are love of God and love of one's neighbor.

3.2a. Love of God is the foundation for healing.

As discussed also in part I, within Christian theology, love is central to wholeness as God intended. God is described as love (1 John 4:8). When Jesus was asked what the greatest commandment is, he responded, "You shall love the Lord your God with all your heart, and with all your soul, and with all your mind. This is the greatest and first commandment. And a second is like it: You shall love your neighbor as yourself" (Matthew 22:34–40). Love is described as the highest virtue without which nothing is ultimately gained (1 Corinthians 13). Love is central to Christian theology. Love is central in the restoration to wholeness.

The salvation brought about by Jesus Christ, the restoration to wholeness, is, as described in the next section, grounded in, constituted by, and an act of, God's love for us: "But God proves his love for us in that while we still were sinners Christ died for us" (Romans 5:8). Our healing is grounded in God's love. Healing, salvation, is brought about by God's work already accomplished in the life, death, and resurrection of Jesus Christ. That work is an act of love.

However, the healing we need continues into the present. As described in section III.4, God's love is made manifest also here and now through God's Spirit and through the Church. And as described in section III.6, God's love will find its fulfillment, and a full healing—a complete restoration to health, a full communion with God—will come about in the resurrection in the life to come. God's love is manifest and operative in the past in the work of Jesus Christ. In the present, it is manifest by the Spirit and in the life of the Church. In the future, it will be brought to fulfillment in the restoration of all things.

However, our healing and our salvation also require a transformation of the person's will to be oriented toward God, to experience God's love, and to live life as God intended. The principal means by which this healing and wholeness is brought about is through our growing in love: love for God and love for one's neighbor. Freedom from sin, from willful deviation from what God intended, involves a freedom to love God and to love our neighbor. The love we are to have for others and for God is the love that God intended. That love is constitutive of healing and brings healing to oneself and to others. Even our love for our neighbors is ultimately also grounded in God's love because the dignity and worth of the human person arises from God's love in the action of creation and from God's love of each person. Our love for our neighbors is also ultimately grounded in our love for God because it is in loving God that we are empowered to love our neighbors. And that love for God and the ensuing love for our neighbors arises from God's love for us—the love God has shown to us in Jesus Christ; God's love for us as he brings about our transformation, salvation, and restoration to wholeness; and in our experience here and now of God's love. The love of God is the foundation for our restoration to wholeness.

3.2b. Loving one's neighbor brings healing to others.

Jesus commanded, "You shall love your neighbor as yourself" (Matthew 22:39). We are to love our neighbors—those around us, who are likewise created in the image of God—in the same manner as we love ourselves[1]: We should seek good for our neighbor by providing for his or her material and spiritual needs. We should wish our neighbor well for our neighbor's sake. We should also seek the highest happiness for our neighbor, a full restoration to wholeness for our neighbor, including ultimately also a healing of the soul, a healing from sin, to attain that final end of communion with God.

Interpersonal love involves both a unitive dimension and a contributory dimension. Love's unitive dimension seeks to be with and in some sense to be one with the other person. Love's contributory dimension

---

1. See Aquinas (1274/1920, II.II.44.7).

seeks to provide what is good for the beloved.[2] We might say that love involves both seeking the good that is constituted by the other and seeking the good for the other. That love for another person, both in its unitive and contributory aspects, can bring healing to the beloved. Both in promoting the other's good and in being with the other person, the beloved's experience of that love can bring about their healing. In being loved, one knows that one is valued and cared for. The goodness of one's very being is affirmed.[3]

Seeking the good for others may of course be constituted by providing for their material needs. But it may extend beyond this to include the flourishing of the beloved more broadly, seeking to enable some measure of happiness, of meaning, of a sense of relational connectedness, and possibly of growth in character. Parts of the Christian tradition distinguish between corporal alms—acts of mercy and love constituted by the provision or meeting of material needs that contribute to another's good—and spiritual alms—acts of mercy that contribute to another's spiritual good. Corporal alms were sometimes enumerated as feeding the hungry, giving drink to the thirsty, clothing the naked, sheltering the homeless, visiting the sick, ransoming the captive, and burying the dead. Spiritual alms are sometimes defined as instructing the ignorant, counseling the doubtful, comforting the sorrowful, reproving the sinner, forgiving injuries, bearing with those who trouble us, and praying for all.[4] All of these can

---

2. Although the uses of the word "love" are unquestionably diverse, almost all involve either a unitive or a contributory component or both. It is often presumed that "real" or "authentic" interpersonal love will involve both unitive and contributory elements, and often if one or the other of these aspects of love is absent in interpersonal love, something is thought to be not entirely right. However, for the use of "love" more generally in ordinary language, either unitive or contributory forms of love typically suffice for us to be willing to employ the term "love." One might thus take as an analytical definition of "love," when used in expressions of the form "he/she loves" the denoting of "a disposition toward either desiring a perceived good or desiring union with it, either as an end itself or with it being a source of delight in itself, or desiring good for a particular object for its own sake" (see VanderWeele, 2023c). The first of these might be referred to as unitive love and the second as contributory love. In interpersonal relationships, we generally expect or hope for both to be present.

3. Pieper (1974).

4. Aquinas (1274/1920, II.II.32.2). See also Matthew 25:31–46; 1 Thessalonians 5:12–18; Galatians 6:1–6.

contribute to the good of the other. All of these meet some sort of material or spiritual need for the other. Acts of goodwill can extend beyond these and beyond a clear evident material lack on the part of another. When actions are taken to help improve relationships, to help others attain a sense of meaning, to bring others happiness, these too contribute to the good of others. Loving one's neighbor can thus contribute both to the health of the body and to the health of the person.

In most cases, seeking to help others flourish, seeking their well-being will make it more likely for the other person's well-being to be enhanced.[5] Moreover, desiring to be with the other person and spending time with the other person is what allows relationships themselves to form, develop, and deepen. There is a joy that comes in loving and a joy that comes in relationships that are loving. There is a sharing of life, a deepening understanding of the other person. We delight in the other person and enjoy their presence. Loving relationships affirm to the other the goodness of their being. The unitive aspect of love involves a recognition

---

5. Rigorous empirical research on love and various aspects of human flourishing is unfortunately somewhat limited. This is arguably in part because the topic is understudied (especially given its importance), and in part because adequate measures have yet to be developed and much empirical research on love focuses only on romantic love. Moreover, understandings of love in the empirical literature are diverse and often deviate substantially from the notion of love found in the Christian tradition. The empirical evidence that love promotes human flourishing must thus mostly be established by more indirect means. There is a moderate body of evidence around parental love or warmth and the subsequent health and well-being of the beloved child (Huppert et al., 2010; Chen, Kuzansky, et al., 2019). Evidence suggests that love from one's parent is one of the most important—if not the most important—factor in shaping numerous outcomes later in life (Chen, Haines, et al., 2019). Likewise, as discussed in section III.4d, there is considerable evidence that forgiveness results in better mental health and well-being and possible physical health outcomes as well (Wade et al. 2014; Toussaint et al., 2015; Chen, Harris, et al., 2019; Long, Worthington, et al., 2020; Ho et al., 2024). Forgiveness—understood as the replacing of ill will toward the offender with goodwill—might itself be understood as a form of love. There is also evidence from randomized trials that interventions to promote compassion and loving-kindness can improve various aspects of well-being (Jazaieri et al., 2014; Galante et al., 2014; Kirby et al., 2017). There is additional evidence that marriage is associated with better health and well-being (Manzoli et al., 2007; Wood et al., 2007; Chen et al., 2023). This evidence is perhaps the most indirect, as love will often be powerfully present within marriage, but the extent to which this is so may vary considerably, and marriage itself shapes life and one's circumstances in ways beyond the presence, and extent, of love.

of, and a delighting in, the goodness of the other person. Contributory love involves the recognition of some good that is absent in the life of another and that might be bestowed. Both unitive and contributory love concern goodness, and both affirm the goodness of the other's being.

Loving others and seeking the good for others not only contributes to their own good but also tends to prompt and promote similar acts of kindness and love in others. There can be a powerful contagion of love and of loving action that can extend not just between two individuals but can spread through an entire community and beyond.[6]

Love ultimately extends beyond beneficent or prosocial acts. Love is the consistent desire to both be with and contribute to the good of the other. Love recognizes, is drawn by, and affirms the goodness of being of the other. Love persists in good action even amid challenges and difficulties.[7] Love arising from the recognition of the goodness, dignity, and worth of the other allows us to contribute to the needs of the other while preserving their dignity and their self-respect, since recognizing the inherent worth of the other and thereby desiring to be present or united with the other affirms to the other their value and worth.[8]

Jesus makes the command to love one's neighbor more radical by teaching that we are to love one another as Jesus loved us: "I give you a new commandment, that you love one another. Just as I have loved you, you also should love one another. By this everyone will know that you are my disciples, if you have love for one another" (John 13:34–35). Jesus's followers are to love as Jesus loved. Jesus provided the perfect example of a life lived in love, one that involved giving his life for the sake of others.[9] Jesus's love is the love we are called to imitate. That love

---

6. Fowler and Christakis (2010) present experimental evidence that the recipient of an action of goodwill is more likely to go on to act similarly, such that the contagion effects of altruistic action may extend so far that a positive interaction between two persons can propagate through a social network and ultimately affect the interaction of two other persons, neither of whom know either person in the original pair.

7. See 1 Corinthians 13:4–8.

8. See Weil (1951).

9. Aquinas speaks of an "order of charity" (1274/1920, II.II.26) in which things are loved: God, oneself, one's neighbor, and one's body. We are to love our neighbor more than our own body because our neighbor participates in divine happiness more directly than our body does, which is more by way of overflow (II.II.26.5). In this way, our own bodily health must sometimes be set aside or

brought powerful healing to those Jesus encountered in his earthly life and work and brought salvation and healing to all humankind in his death and resurrection. God in Jesus showed his love to us, and we are likewise to give our lives in love for others. To do so is to help bring healing and wholeness to our neighbors, to all those around us.

3.2c. Loving one's neighbor brings healing to oneself.

The love of one's neighbor also brings healing to the one who loves. Loving others can bring physical, mental, social, and spiritual wholeness by promoting our relationships, character, meaning, happiness, and possibly also our physical health.[10] Loving others is what God intends. The love of one's neighbor thus helps restore a person to God's intention. That seeking of the good of the other and seeking to be with the other is an affirmation of the goodness of being of the other and an affirmation of the goodness of creation and of the Creator. It is in love and from love that God created all that is, and in loving others, we reflect God's being and it is more manifest that we are made in God's image (Genesis 1).[11] When we love, we are restored to be who and what God intended. It is thus that Jesus's teaching on the greatest command concludes with "on these two commandments hang all the law and the prophets" (Matthew 22:40) and that St. Paul likewise teaches that "the one who loves another has fulfilled the law . . . The commandments . . . are summed up in this word, 'Love your neighbor as yourself.'" (Romans 13:8–10). In loving, we are better brought to be who God intended us to be; we are brought to wholeness.

3.2d. Loving God is integral to a full restoration to wholeness.

Jesus's command, however, was not only to love one's neighbor, but also to love God. Indeed, this was pointed to as the "greatest and first commandment." If God is the highest good, then our love for God ought to surpass

---

sacrificed for the sake of our neighbor—for the spiritual health, or health of the person, of our neighbor.

10. See also footnote 5 above.

11. Aquinas (1274/1920, II.II.30.4). God's love itself gives all of creation its being and goodness (1274/1920, I.20.2).

our love for all other things and ought to guide and relativize all of our other loves. Love for God is integral to a full restoration to wholeness because it is constituted by a right orientation to our final and highest end in God. Our desires are rightly ordered when we love God above all else. Our desires are reoriented to what God intended. In the words of St. Augustine: "Thou hast made us for thyself, O Lord, and our heart is restless until it finds its rest in thee."[12] By loving God above all else, we seek to live as God intended. This is restoration to wholeness. By loving God, we desire union with him, as God intended. By loving God, we experience joy.[13]

Aquinas speaks of the will being transformed by charity—by love of God, by friendship with God—so as to be able to receive God.[14] If final eternal flourishing is constituted by some form of union with God, a vision of God, a being with God, then love for God is both the appropriate response to a proper understanding of God and the chief means to that final end—the fulfillment of wholeness that God intended for us.

3.2e. Loving God empowers one to love one's neighbor.

Love for God also empowers one to love one's neighbor. This may arise in part because it is clear that God has commanded us to love our neighbors and love for God will entail wanting to obey God and please God.[15]

---

12. Augustine (400/1991, book 1, chapter 1).
13. Aquinas (1274/1920, II.II.28.1).
14. Aquinas (1274/1920, I.II.62.3).
15. If love is understood as the disposition to desire or will to be united with or contribute to the good of the beloved (see footnote 2 above), then it may seem problematic that love is commanded. However, one possible cause of unitive love is simply the apprehension that something constitutes a good for oneself and thus is in some sense desirable. Such an apprehension is not sufficient for love because it may be dominated by other desires or one may become distracted, but such an apprehension can, sometimes at least, be a cause of love. In the case of love of God, in its unitive sense, the command to love might be understood to be fulfillable because it is a command to understand God as the greatest good and therefore something to be desired (see Aquinas, 1274/1920, II.II.44.1,4). Moreover, if it is thought that it follows from God being the highest good that each should contribute to his good by seeking to carry out on earth what God wills, then contributory love for God could likewise be commanded. God as the object of love thus resolves the tension in having a command to love and arguably also does so with love for neighbors. As framed above, love of God, in its contributory sense, would be the disposition toward desiring to

However, that love for God will empower one to love one's neighbor insofar as it is seen that all people—and indeed, all of creation—was created good by God, that God wills that goodness to be manifest, and that God wills a restoration of all people and all of creation to his intent.[16] Understanding the goodness of the human person, as created by God and as loved by God, may lead to a fundamental realization of the value of that person, a realization that as a person created good by God, it is worthwhile to come to know them, understand them, and love them. It is worthwhile to contribute to their good and to enjoy the good of who they are. They too have been created in the image of God; they too have a fundamental dignity and worth, established by God himself; they too are loved by God. Love "makes one see in one's neighbor another self."[17]

In loving God, one comes to desire what God wills and thus one comes to will that one's neighbors also be made whole, that they too come to know and love God and to share in everlasting happiness with God. Recognition of the dignity and worth of one's neighbor, God's love for one's neighbor, and a shared destiny with one's neighbor may help create a naturalness and fervor in our love for our neighbor that we might ordinarily only find in our close relationships and friendships.[18]

---

contribute good to God, where that good is understood as bringing about the good on earth that God desires. However, that good that God desires includes good for one's neighbor for the neighbor's sake. Thus, a disposition toward desiring to contribute to good for God entails a disposition toward desiring good for one's neighbor for the neighbor's sake. Thus, contributory love for one's neighbor follows from and is derivative of one's love for God (II.II.25.1, II.II.44.2). In Aquinas's understanding, love of God and love of one's neighbor constitute a single precept, with the latter effectively being encompassed by the former but with the latter being explicitly articulated to make that entailment clear (II.II.44.2). Within this understanding, it becomes comprehensible how love of one's neighbor, conceived of principally as a disposition toward desiring the good of one's neighbor, could be commanded because it follows from love of God. Although love of one's neighbor is arguably to be understood principally as love in its contributory sense, there is also a unitive sense of love for one's neighbor or even one's enemy, insofar as there ought to be a desire for final union with neighbor, in union with God, in the life to come (see Stump, 2006; Aquinas, 1274/1920, II.II.25.1, II.II.25.8). The command to love can thus be given a coherent rendering even under the proposed definitions (see VanderWeele, 2023c).

16. Aquinas (1274/1920, I.20.1–2, II.II.25.1).
17. Catholic Church (2004, 582).
18. See Hanson (2022b) for an interpretation of Jesus's teaching on giving a banquet for the poor (Luke 14:12–14) that pushes in this direction. See also Kierkegaard (1847/1995).

Although such love for all we encounter may seem inaccessible, the lives of many saints are testimony to the possibility of love and friendship with God empowering a deep love for all people one encounters. Loving God empowers our love for our neighbors. The connection between love for God and love for our neighbor—by way of command and by way of the very nature of love—is so deep that, in the first Epistle of St. John we read, "We love because he first loved us. Those who say, 'I love God,' and hate their brothers or sisters, are liars; for those who do not love a brother or sister whom they have seen, cannot love God whom they have not seen" (1 John 4:19–20). Love for God entails and empowers our love for our neighbor.

3.2f. Communities are brought to wholeness by love.

Love needs to be promoted within communities and for the good of communities. Love of others contributes to the good of others, allows for the enjoyment of the good of others, and affirms to the other their own goodness as created by God. When this takes place, not just between two people but between many, community life is allowed to emerge in a fuller richness and is sustained, thereby creating trust, belonging, welcome, mutual support, and care—it becomes a flourishing community. When that love is grounded in the love of God in Jesus Christ through the Spirit, the community that arises is the Church, a community of love that brings healing and restoration to wholeness. This community of love that is the Church is the subject of section III.4.

Consideration of love within community is relevant for other and related forms of community, from families to schools to workplaces to neighborhoods and nations. Love of one another is fundamentally what will allow relationships to develop and community life to flourish. Love may arise naturally in seeing the value of others and coming to desire good for them and to be with them. But love can also be fostered; and if communities are to more fully flourish, love needs to be fostered. There needs to be an understanding of the value of each person, and efforts should be made to facilitate such an understanding. Each person should view every other person as having fundamental value and dignity, as someone it is worthwhile to contribute to, as someone it is good to be with, and, moreover, from the standpoint of the Christian faith, as someone who is loved and created by God.

A return—again and again—to the fundamental value and dignity of the human person and of the importance of love will be needed to facilitate love within communities. In his encyclical *Spe Salvi*, Pope Benedict XVI discusses the human condition, human society, and the economic forces that can sometimes make true flourishing difficult, and comments that we need to create an economy of good and an economy of human love.[19] If love were to be more actively promoted, there would indeed be greater health, greater flourishing, and greater healing. Love brings healing by restoring and strengthening relationships, by providing for the needs of others, and by attaining those purposes for which God created each person. Pope Paul VI thus spoke of creating a "civilization of love."[20]

The *Compendium of the Social Doctrine of the Church* proposes that "in order to make society more human, more worthy of the human person, love in social life—political, economic and cultural—must be given renewed value, becoming the constant and highest norm for all activity. . . . Love must thus enliven every sector of human life and extend to the international order. Only a humanity in which there reigns the 'civilization of love' will be able to enjoy authentic and lasting peace. . . . Charity is the greatest social commandment. It respects others and their rights. It requires the practice of justice, and it alone makes us capable of it. Charity inspires a life of self-giving." Moreover, "it is in relation to God that [love] finds its full effectiveness."[21]

The community provides the forum wherein such love is present and has the opportunity to flourish and to provide healing. That love is needed for a restoration to wholeness of individual persons and the flourishing of communities. And that love is empowered by love for God.

---

19. Benedict XVI (2007, 40).

20. The phrase was introduced in 1970 in Pope Paul VI's Regina Coeli address for Pentecost Sunday (Bulzacchelli, 2012) and was further developed in the theology of Pope John Paul II (Catholic Church, 2004, 580–583; John Paul II, 1991; cf. Osewska and Simonič, 2019).

21. Catholic Church (2004, 582–583).

3.2g. Love of enemies is a pathway to wholeness for all people and communities.

Although all people are created and loved by God and are worthy of being loved, sin disrupts human relationships. The harms that one has experienced from others can make it difficult to love. When such harmful actions are persistent, it may become proper to refer to that other person as one's enemy—someone who consistently desires harm for oneself.

Part of the radical nature of the Christian teaching on love is that love of one's neighbor—a love commanded by God—includes all people. It thus includes one's enemies, those who might desire that harm come to us, those who are opposed to us, those who do not love us. Jesus's teaching on the matter was both radical and direct, "Love your enemies and pray for those who persecute you" (Matthew 5:43). If all people have value and worth and are created by God and loved by God and have their end in God, then all people—including one's enemies—are also to be loved as part of love of one's neighbor.[22] That they perpetuate harm and that there is sin is simply an indication that they have deviated from God's intent, that they too are in need of restoration to wholeness, that they are in need of healing, that they are in need of love. With a love of neighbor grounded in love of God, the sin of and harm from one's enemies are not reasons not to love but rather can be the very grounds that call forth love. That love is an imitation and reflection of God's love for us. St. Paul writes, "God proves his love for us in that while we still were sinners Christ died for us" (Romans 5:8).

That love of one's enemy has the potential to end cycles of hatred. A response of love toward those who wish one harm can sometimes help bring about conversion, healing, peace, or reconciliation.[23] It is not guaranteed to do so because the other person is free, but it might invite such a response. St. Paul writes, "Bless those who persecute you; bless and do not curse them. . . . Do not repay anyone evil for evil, but take thought for what is noble in the sight of all. . . . Never avenge yourselves. . . . 'If your enemies are hungry, feed them; if they are thirsty,

---

22. Aquinas (1274/1920, II.II.23.1.ad 2, II.II.25.8–9, II.II.27.7).
23. Brooks (2019).

give them something to drink.' . . . Do not be overcome by evil, but overcome evil with good." (Romans 12:14–21). The response to one's enemies is to care for them, to love them. Such a response is counterintuitive and paradoxical. It may confuse and confound those who wish one harm. That response of love may even infuriate and provoke them further, but it may bring peace and repentance. It may overcome evil with good.

Such an approach does not ignore the wrong but rather sees it as the grounds for the other's need for healing, for love. Such an approach also does not ignore the harm. When we are harmed, we are often rightly angry, but that anger, when directed properly, is to be used to address the harm and to right the wrong or injustice that was done. Doing so may even involve rebuke or punishment of the wrongdoer, but it should not involve hatred or desiring to harm them simply so that perpetrator might suffer. Rather, the purpose should be to correct or prevent further wrongdoing or to restore justice within the community.[24]

However, when a person has experienced harm, feelings of anger and even hatred may persist. To restore love following some wrongdoing, forgiveness is needed, the replacing of ill will toward the offender with goodwill. This is part of love for one's enemy. Forgiveness, as

---

24. Love does not necessarily preclude punishment. In Aquinas, punishment is understood as a relative harm imposed on the offender, but absolutely speaking, it is a good (1274/1920, II.II.108.1, II.II.19.1). Punishment rightly carried out ultimately aims at some good. Punishment may be understood as a good action to the extent that the offender is receiving what is his or her due, having exceeded what is proper in excessively following his or her own will. It is thus an upholding of justice (II.II.108.4). The good of punishment may be the restraint or reformation of the offender or deterrence of the offender or others or a restoration of justice and a making manifest of evil as evil and good as good (II.II.108.3). Love aims at the good of the offender. Restraint, reformation, and deterrence of the offender all directly aim at the good of the offender. Deterrence of others and the restoration of justice can still be understood as indirectly aiming at the good of the offender because the offender is a member of the community and thus shares in its common good. Punishment may thus, once again, impose a relative harm on the one who is guilty of wrongdoing, but the action of punishment is itself good (see Koritansky, 2012). Punishment in this life mirrors God's punishment for our sins, which likewise aims at the good, our reformation, our turning from sin, and our salvation (see Aquinas, 1265/2014, III.146.1–2). Love thus does not contradict punishment and the seeking of the good of the other, but it does put bounds on what might constitute reasonable punishment.

discussed in section III.4, is an important pathway toward healing, toward restoration of wholeness, toward love.

Love for one's enemies is a pathway toward the end of enmities, toward reconciliation, toward peace and wholeness of all people, toward the healing of communities. Just as acts of love can prompt similar actions in others, so also acts of hatred can prompt hatred in others in return. Something must break the cycle of hatred and acts of hatred. What is required is love.

Love of one's enemy is a radical approach with the intent of breaking cycles of hatred. If it were practiced universally, enmities would cease. Because human persons are free and because that freedom is used to sin, to act in ways contrary to God's intent, there will never be complete cessation of enmities in this life and so there is need to love one's enemies, to counter the cycles of hatred that persist whenever possible. The Christian belief is that God in Jesus Christ both initiated and exemplified love of enemy by giving his life for us, by loving while being persecuted, by loving us in spite of our turning from God, by doing away with our sin upon the cross. "God proves his love for us in that while we still were sinners Christ died for us" (Romans 5:8). We are to follow Jesus in this calling of love—love of God, love of neighbor, love of enemy. Doing so can bring wholeness to communities and to all people.

3.2h. Charity—the virtue of friendship with God, including love of one's neighbor—is brought about by God's grace.

The calling to love—to love God, to love one's neighbor, to love one's enemy—is a high and difficult one. It is not one that comes to us naturally in our broken state.[25] At first encounter, some may even be repelled by the notion of love for one's enemy. It can seem to have the potential to allow for continued harm and offense. In purely temporal terms, it did not seem to lead to a good outcome in Jesus's life. But that is true only from a temporal perspective. From the perspective of the Christian faith, as discussed in the next section, Jesus's life, death, and resurrection and Jesus's love for his enemies accomplished salvation and opened the path

---

25. Aquinas (1274/1920, I.II.109.3).

to healing and wholeness for all people. It created the potential for the end of all hatred and enmity through love.

However, this understanding of the events of Jesus's life and death requires the eyes of faith. It requires a belief in God and a belief that the meaning of Jesus's life, death, and resurrection as put forward by the Christian faith is correct. This perspective and this understanding require faith. This perspective also requires a hope that final wholeness will be found in God in the life to come, a hope that, despite all circumstances, God can and will restore all things. Seeing love—love for God, love for one's neighbor, love for one's enemy—as the proper pathway to healing requires faith and hope. But with that faith and with that hope come charity—a friendship with God.[26] That charity, that friendship with God, that love of God and neighbor, brings healing. It reorients us properly to our final end, it brings healing to others, and it brings healing to ourselves. It makes us who God intended us to be; it transforms our will so that we may both seek and ultimately find joy in God as our last end.[27]

That friendship with God requires God's initiation; it requires God's grace.[28] Faith is brought about by God's revealing his love in Jesus Christ, by God's revelation in history and in the Scriptures, by God's guiding the Church, by the Church's proclamation, by the Spirit's prompting us to believe, by our receiving this as good news. All this is ultimately accomplished by God's grace. Faith comes about as a gift of grace, a gift that must also be freely accepted. Our hope that communion with God is our final end and that God will provide the means to that end likewise arises from our faith and trust in God. And as we see and understand our final end in God, we come to more and more love God as we ought.[29] However, because God—the object of our faith, hope, and love—is so far above our understanding, we ultimately need God himself to initiate and empower our faith, hope, and love.[30] But by that grace, God perfects and fulfills our nature as established in creation and we

---

26. Aquinas (1274/1920, I.II.62.4, I.II.65.5).
27. Aquinas (1274/1920, I.II.62.3, II.II.28.1).
28. Aquinas (1274/1920, I.II.109).
29. Aquinas (1274/1920, I.II.62.4).
30. Aquinas (1274/1920, I.II.62.1, II.II.23.2, II.II.24.2).

more fully experience love of God.[31] It is by God's grace that we are saved, that we are healed, that we come to love, that we are restored to wholeness, and that the wholeness of the human person finds its fulfillment. God has acted in history and has acted in the life, death, and resurrection of Jesus Christ to accomplish this. And it is to God's action in Jesus Christ and by the Spirit to enable us to love God, to love our neighbor, and to overcome sin, that we now turn.

> *Propositional Summary 3.2: The principal ways that a restoration and fulfillment to wholeness are brought about are love of God and love of one's neighbor.*
> 3.2a. Love of God is the foundation for healing.
> 3.2b. Loving one's neighbor brings healing to others.
> 3.2c. Loving one's neighbor brings healing to oneself.
> 3.2d. Loving God is integral to a full restoration to wholeness.
> 3.2e. Loving God empowers one to love one's neighbor.
> 3.2f. Communities are brought to wholeness by love.
> 3.2g. Love of enemies is a pathway to wholeness for all people and communities.
> 3.2h. Charity—the virtue of friendship with God, including love of one's neighbor—is brought about by God's grace.

---

31. Aquinas (1274/1920, I.I.8.ad 2, I.II.109.3, I.II.114.2).

III.3. Healing and Jesus Christ

Proposition 3.3. God has brought healing and salvation through Jesus Christ.

3.3a. God is the principal agent of healing.

Although some degree of healing can be accomplished by our own efforts—by rest, the practice of medicine, the restoration of relationships, and seeking to love—there are limits to what we can accomplish. Disease and injury will often be present. With aging, there inevitably eventually comes infirmity, ill health, frailty, and finally death. Although our efforts at healing and restoration are important, ultimately, from the perspective of Christian theology, only God can provide a fuller healing. God is the principal agent of healing.

Healing in the Bible is often seen as the work of God and of those whom God empowers. In many of the biblical stories, God healed after intercessory prayer was made by another.[1] The prophetic books speak of God's renewal, restoration, and healing of the entire people of Israel.[2] Many of the gospel accounts are occupied with accounts of Jesus's healing by God's power.[3] In response to John the Baptist's question about

---

1. As examples, Abimelech by the prayers of Abraham (Genesis 20:17), Miriam by the prayers of Moses (Numbers 12:13–15), the widow's son by the prayers of Elijah (1 Kings 17:17–24).

2. E.g., Jeremiah 33:1–11; Hosea 14:1–7.

3. See Pilch (2000). Healings occupy a substantial portion of Jesus's ministry. Jesus is reported to have healed a leper (Matthew 8:2), the centurion's servant (Matthew 8:5), Peter's mother-in-law (Matthew 8:14), two men possessed by demons (Matthew 8:28), a man sick with palsy (Matthew 9:2), Jairus's daughter (Matthew 9:18), a woman with an issue of blood (Matthew 9:20), two blind men (Matthew 9:27), a mute demoniac (Matthew 9:32), a man with a withered hand (Matthew 12:9), a blind and dumb demoniac (Matthew 12:22), the Syrophoenician's daughter (Matthew 15:22), a child with an evil spirit (Matthew 17:14), blind Bartimaeus (Matthew 20:30), a man with an unclean spirit (Mark 1:23), a man both deaf and mute (Mark 7:32), a

Jesus's identity, Jesus presented himself as a healer who enabled the blind to see, the lame to walk, the lepers to be cleansed, the deaf to hear, and the dead to be raised.[4] The gospels present Jesus's death on the cross and his resurrection as somehow accomplishing the healing and salvation of the world with God as the agent.[5] The Spirit of God is also spoken of as accomplishing transformation of a person's character, bringing about a restoration to wholeness.[6] God is the one who heals.

From a theological perspective, our efforts to heal are in made collaboration with God's action as healer. God created those things that constitute our medicines and remedies and God equipped the human person with the powers of reason that have led to the development and practice of medicine and of public health prevention and promotion efforts.[7] God is the creator of the human body, which has the capacity for healing and restoration.[8] Even the agency of the human person and thereby all efforts to bring about healing and restoration is a gift God has bestowed. Thus, from the perspective of Christian theology, even in our own efforts at healing, God is still in some sense the principal agent. That is because only God can fully address the problem of sin as the cause of ill health.

3.3b. Sin cannot be fully dealt with through human efforts.

Sin is the cause of ill health. Sin impedes wholeness as God intended. Sin prevents communion with God. Thus, there cannot be full healing, a full restoration to health, without addressing sin. However, our efforts to address sin often fail or, at best, are only partially successful. We often are unable to alter the actions of others; we often have only limited self-mastery, a limited capacity to fully govern ourselves. Unjust structures

---

blind man (Mark 8:22), the widow's son (Luke 7:11), Mary Magdalene (Luke 8:2), a woman bound by Satan (Luke 13:10), a man with dropsy (Luke 14:1), ten lepers (Luke 17:11), Malchus's ear (Luke 22:49), a nobleman's son (John 4:46), a man born blind (John 9:1), Lazarus (John 11:1), and multitudes (Matthew 8:16; Matthew 15:30).

4. Matthew 11:1–6.
5. Matthew 20:28; Colossians 2:12–14; 1 Peter 2:24–25.
6. Romans 5:5; 8:2–11; Galatians 5:16–25. See also Aquinas (1274/1920, I.II.68,70).
7. See also Larchet (2002, 114–116) for further development of this position and its exposition among Church fathers such as St. Basil, Origen, and Theodet of Cyrus.
8. Aquinas (1265/2014, 3.157, 4.72); Aquinas (1274/1920, I.117.1).

that perpetuate harm and sin are often difficult to fully root out and eliminate. We need assistance in our efforts to address sin. We need help from God. We need God's salvation.

Moreover, in any relationship or friendship, an action on the part of one person that constitutes an offense to the other will damage that relationship. Forgiveness can potentially take place whereby the offense no longer impedes goodwill toward the other and no longer separates the two in relationship. However, the offense must be addressed, forgiveness must be granted, and reconciliation must be pursued if the relationship is to be restored. The same things are true in our relationship with God. As voluntary action contrary to God's intent, sin constitutes an offense against God. It disrupts communion with God. For restoration of the relationship with God to take place, forgiveness of those offenses, forgiveness of sin, is needed.[9] This must be action on the part of God. Only God can forgive sins and accomplish the restoration of the relationship with him. The human person cannot attain a restored relationship with God simply by his or her own efforts.[10] Sin cannot be fully dealt with through human effort alone. God's action, God's restoration, God's salvation is necessary.

3.3c. God has dealt with the problem of sin in the person of Jesus Christ.

The Christian doctrine of the atonement is that in the life, death, and resurrection of Jesus Christ, God brought salvation to humanity and to the world. God brought deliverance from sin and its consequences and provided reconciliation between God and human persons. The Christian belief is that in order to do this, God became human in the person of Jesus Christ and entered human history to accomplish this restoration. The mode by which Jesus Christ's life, death, and resurrection provided deliverance from sin and its consequences is presented in different ways in Christian theology, and different aspects of Jesus's life, death, and resurrection are presented as relating differently to the restoration of the human person to God's intent.

---

9. Aquinas (1274/1920, I.II.113).
10. Aquinas (1274/1920, I.II.109.7).

God becoming human in the person of Jesus Christ is presented as God, in Jesus, taking on human nature or joining human nature to himself (John 1:14–16; Hebrews 2:14–15). Because of the fallenness of the world, human nature is corrupted; the body is subject to aging, decay and death; and the imperfect reason, will, and passions are often in conflict with one another. God's taking on human nature in Jesus Christ is sometimes depicted as a joining of human nature with God's nature, thereby somehow allowing or facilitating the restoration of human nature and enabling it to ultimately have full communion with God.[11]

Jesus's life is also often presented as an overcoming of sin by providing a perfect example of a life lived with God, in obedience to God, and in love for God and for neighbors. Jesus provided an example, a model of what our own lives should be like. He is the perfect exemplar. He showed us how we are to be in this fallen world. He showed us the nature of perfect love in his life and his teachings. He showed us how to love others and how to do good to others, and in his love, he prompts love in us.[12] His perfect example and teachings revealed God's intent for our lives, how to avoid sin and address sin in the world when we encounter it and how to live in union with God in love.

Jesus's life and teaching also enable us to understand more deeply the nature of God and God's love. The New Testament teaches that Jesus is "the image of the invisible God" (Colossians 1:15), that it is Jesus—God the Son—"who has made [God] known" (John 1:18), and that it is by Jesus's coming to us that God's love is revealed (1 John 1:9). The Gospel of John records Jesus as teaching, "Whoever has seen me has seen the Father" (John 14:9; see also Matthew 11:27). Jesus is referred to as God's

---

11. In Aquinas's *Summa Theologica*, the incarnation—God joining human nature with himself in Jesus Christ—is described as helping accomplish the restoration of the human race through a variety of means: strengthening our faith since in Jesus Christ, God himself communicated to us; strengthening our hope because the incarnation was proof of God's love; strengthening our love or charity because God's love kindles our own; promoting our doing good to others because Jesus was an example for us to follow; withdrawing us from sin because we are taught the greatness of man's dignity and that we should not disgrace it with sin; doing away with presumption and making us humble since it is clear that the incarnation occurred not through any merit of ours; and allowing full participation in divinity that is bestowed upon us by Christ's humanity (1274/1920, III.1.2).

12. Aquinas (1274/1920, III.1.2, III.49.1).

word (John 1:14) and the way that God has spoken to us (Hebrews 1:1–4), and much of his ministry is occupied with teaching about God and about how God desires us to live. Jesus's life and teachings help reveal to us the nature of God and God's intent.

Jesus's suffering and death is often presented as being central in God's accomplishing salvation in Jesus. This too is depicted in a variety of ways.[13] His death is sometimes portrayed as the ultimate act of love. Jesus's death was the costly result of God becoming human but a cost that Jesus willingly accepted so that God could be present with us in Jesus and prompt similar love within us.[14] His suffering and the intensity of his suffering for us in love further helps us to turn away from sin.[15]

Perhaps most centrally, Jesus's death is presented as a destroying of or a doing away with our sin, our sinful nature, and our guilt. Theological accounts and New Testament accounts of Jesus's death interpret it as a taking of our sins upon himself and suffering the consequences in order to free and heal us: "He himself bore our sins in his body on the cross, so that, free from sins, we might live for righteousness; by his wounds you have been healed" (1 Peter 2:24). Several accounts relate Jesus's taking away of our sin and guilt to our being united with Jesus in his death. The New Testament likewise speaks of "being united with him in a death like his" (Romans 6:5) or of "being buried with him by baptism into death" (Romans 6:4; Colossians 2:12). Sin separates us from God and has led to a corruption of human nature that ultimately results in death. There is something of

---

13. Although the various prominent theories of the atonement—moral exemplar, Christus Victor/ransom, substitutionary atonement, satisfaction, etc.—all have more paradigmatic presentations in other authors, each of these is arguably present, with varying degrees of emphasis, in Aquinas's exposition of Jesus's Passion and death (Aquinas (1274/1920, III.46–52).

14. Romans 5:8; 1 John 4:9–10. See also Aquinas (1274/1920, III 46.3, III.47.2, III.48.3, III.49.1).

15. Aquinas comments that the intensity of Christ's suffering was greater than any other because the cause of it was the sins of the world and because of Christ's perfect perception (1274/1920, III.46.6). The intensity of this suffering is portrayed powerfully when Jesus cries out, "My God, my God, why have you forsaken me?" (Matthew 27:46). Aquinas indicates the possibility that Christ's suffering will turn us away from sin as one of several reasons why there was no means more suitable than Christ's Passion for delivering the human race (1274/1920, III.46.3).

human nature that is now corrupted; there is something of human nature and individual and corporate guilt that must be done away with if it is to be completely restored to wholeness. God in Jesus Christ mysteriously unites us to himself. His death is the death of our fallen nature and the doing away with our individual and collective guilt (Colossians 2:12–14; Romans 6:3–7).[16]

St. Paul wrote in his Epistle to the Romans that "we have been buried with him by baptism into death . . . we have been united with him in a death like his. . . . We know that our old self was crucified with him so that the body of sin might be destroyed, and we might no longer be enslaved to sin. For whoever has died is freed from sin. But if we have died with Christ, we believe that we will also live with him. We know that Christ, being raised from the dead, will never die again; death no longer has dominion over him" (Romans 6:4–9). There is a corporate solidarity in Jesus Christ that frees us from sin in Jesus's death and gives us new life. It is a restoration of human nature that applies to each person in union with Jesus Christ through faith in him.[17] It is in union with Jesus Christ in his death that we are ultimately freed from sin and brought to new life and new wholeness.

---

16. With regard to St. Paul's letter to the Romans (6:6–11), Aquinas comments, "Now the oldness of sin can refer to the guilt of sin or to the stain of actual sins or even to the habit of sinning. . . . Thus, therefore, our old self is said to be crucified together with Christ, inasmuch as the aforesaid oldness is removed by the power of Christ; either because it has been entirely removed, as the guilt and stain of sin are entirely removed in baptism, or because its force has been diminished, i.e., the force of the 'fomes' or even of the custom of sinning" (Aquinas, 1272b, 6:6–11, 480). Similarly, "Now by Christ's Passion we have been delivered not only from the common sin of the whole human race, both as to its guilt and as to the debt of punishment, for which He paid the penalty on our behalf; but, furthermore, from the personal sins of individuals, who share in His Passion by faith and charity and the sacraments of faith" (Aquinas, 1274/1920, III.49.5). See also Colossians 1:21–22.

17. As discussed in section III.4g, the union of the body of the Church with Christ is accomplished by faith. That incorporation into his mystical body, which is the Church (Ephesians 5:29–32; see also Aquinas, 1274/1920, III.8.3), in baptism includes union with him in his death (Romans 6:3–4; Aquinas, 1274/1920, III.49.5); Christ's satisfying God by offering himself belonging to us also (Hebrew 7:24–27; Aquinas, 1274/1920, III.48.2.ad 1); Christ's merits and righteousness being referred to us (2 Corinthians 5:21; 1 Corinthians 1:30; Aquinas 1274/1920, III.48.1); the promise of union in his resurrection (Romans 6:5–9); and ascending with him to heaven (John 14:2–3; Ephesians 4:8–10; Aquinas, 1274/1920, III.57.6).

Because it was Jesus's death and his freely offering himself that accomplished our salvation, the New Testament also speaks of Christ's death as a "sacrifice" (Hebrews 9:26; 10:10–12; 1 Corinthians 5:7; Ephesians 5:2). It was the offering up of one great good, the life of Jesus Christ and his love and obedience, for the sake of another, the salvation of humanity.[18] This sacrifice was an honoring of God that was carried out from Christ's perfect love, and thereby it was satisfying or pleasing to God.[19] It was a sacrifice that Jesus Christ himself made: "Christ loved us and gave himself up for us, a fragrant offering and sacrifice to God" (Ephesians 5:2; see also Hebrews 7:27). The New Testament presents this sacrifice as what removed sin: "He has

---

18. A sacrifice might be understood as the offering up of some good for the sake of another. Augustine (417/2019, iv.14; quoted in Aquinas, 1274/1920, III.48.3) notes that "four things are to be considered in every sacrifice—to whom it is offered, by whom it is offered, what is offered, for whom it is offered." In sacrifices offered to God, there is an honoring of God (Aquinas, 1274/1920, III.48.3). Christ offered himself and his love and obedience to God on our behalf. When something is offered up in response to some offense and the offering is of equal or greater compensatory value than the offense, that offering might also be understood as a propitiation. The New Testament describes Jesus's offering of himself and his love and obedience on our behalf in response to our wrongdoing as a propitiation or sacrifice of atonement (Romans 3:25; Hebrews 2:17; 1 John 2:2, 4:10). See also Aquinas (1274/1920, III.48.2).

19. Satisfaction might be understood as redress, a (potentially costly) acknowledgment of what went wrong in an attempt to move past and prevent subsequent instance of that wrong. The sacrifice of atonement or propitiation (see endnote 18) may thus also be understood as making satisfaction for our sin. There was in Christ's suffering and death an acknowledgment of something wrong and an offering of Christ's love and all that he suffered in being with us in love. Aquinas sometimes refers to the need to redress the wrong and reestablish justice after an offense as the "debt of punishment" (Aquinas, 1274/1920, I.II.87.1). He also says that with respect to the offense to God of our sins, Christ's Passion was "was sufficient and superabundant satisfaction for the sins of the whole human race" (Aquinas, III.49.3; see also III.49.5, III.50.1). That this is appropriate is in part because we are united with Christ (III.48.2.ad 1). This offering of Jesus Christ is thus also described as a "demonstration of justice" (Romans 3:25; see also Aquinas, 1274/1920, III 46.1.ad 3, III.48.4.ad 2), since the offense to God of our sins has been properly addressed. However, we still may accept our suffering in this life as a sort of satisfactory punishment to help turn our will to God, which is indeed what God desires of us (Aquinas, III.49.3.ad 2, I.II.87.6; Colossians 1:24; Romans 5:3–5; James 1:2–4; see also Van Nieuwenhove, 2005; and sections II.6f–g and III.5e–g). In such cases, suffering takes on less of the aspect of punishment and is of a more voluntary or medicinal character (Aquinas, 1274/1920, I.II.87.6–7).

appeared once for all at the end of the age to remove sin by the sacrifice of himself" (Hebrews 9:26).[20]

Because we are freed from sin by Jesus's death, that suffering and death is sometimes also referred to as the means of our redemption (Ephesians 1:7) or as a "ransom" (Matthew 20:28; Mark 10;45; 1 Timothy 2:6), the price paid to free us from sin.[21] Relatedly, Jesus's death is sometimes also portrayed as a victory over or the overcoming of the powers of sin, evil, and death and is sometimes portrayed as the confounding of the powers of evil or the devil (Hebrews 2:14–15; Colossians 2:15).[22] Although certain portrayals of Jesus's death that presuppose that God owed a debt to evil or needed to resort to deceit are problematic, there is a sense in which God uses sin itself to overcome sin. Jesus's death is portrayed as a means of salvation and deliverance from sin. However, it was sinful human action—envy, hatred, betrayal, lying, and murder—that brought about the death that God uses for our salvation.[23] God used human sinful acts to ultimately triumph over sin. By doing away with our guilt and by empowering us to love, Jesus's death frees us from bondage to sin, from being entrapped by our own wrongdoing; Jesus's death redeems us.[24]

Because Jesus's death saves us from sin and death, that death is also sometimes described as a substitution, as Jesus's death somehow substituting for our own.[25] In the first Epistle of St. Peter we read, "For Christ also

---

20. Likewise, in the Gospel of St. John, an account is given of John the Baptist declaring, "Here is the Lamb of God who takes away the sin of the world" upon seeing Jesus (John 1:29).

21. See 1 Peter 1:18–19; Revelations 5:9; Aquinas (1274/1920, III 48.4, III.49.2). The term "price" might be used to refer to the "the atonement by which one satisfies for self or another . . . by which he ransoms himself or someone else from sin and its penalty" (Aquinas, 1274/1920, III.48.4). See also footnotes 18 and 19 above.

22. Aquinas (1274/1920, III 46.3, III.49.2).

23. Acts 2:22–24; see also Aquinas (1274/1920, III.46.3.ad 2). Likewise, in the Gospel of St. Matthew, when those who accuse Jesus and want him to be put to death cry out "His blood be on us and on our children" (Matthew 27:25), the gospel author arguably wants to suggest that although their action is wrong, that blood, that death, will also be the means of salvation.

24. Titus 2:11–14; Aquinas (1274/1920, III.48.4).

25. See 1 Peter 3:18. The Old Testament text of Isaiah 53 is also generally understood within Christianity as being prophetic of Jesus: "However, it was our sicknesses that He Himself bore, And our pains that He carried. . . . But He was pierced for our offenses, He was crushed for our wrongdoings; The punishment for our well-being was laid upon Him, And by His wounds we are healed" (Isaiah 53:4–5). Aquinas writes, "It was fitting for Christ to die . . . to satisfy for the whole human race, which

suffered for sins once for all, the righteous for the unrighteous, in order to bring you to God" (1 Peter 3:18). Sometimes concerns are raised about the morality and logic of such theories of substitution. Is it just for one person to bear the consequences for the action of another?[26] The theories of such substitution that arguably best address these concerns relate back to a union with Christ. By our union with Jesus Christ, accomplished by God, his death does away with our sin, our sinful nature, and our guilt. In some mysterious way, we, along with our sin and guilt, die in his death. It is not that the guilt is somehow transferred away from us to him, but rather that our guilt is done away with in our union with Jesus Christ in his death.[27] It is thus in our union with Christ that it makes sense to say that Jesus "bore our sins in his body on the cross" (1 Peter 2:24). Although guilt is done away with, Jesus Christ's suffering and death can still be said to have been *substituted* for our spiritual death and Jesus can be said to have died *for* our sins or as a consequence of our sins. Full union with God would not be possible without the doing away of our guilt and of that part of our nature that is sinful and contrary to God's intent. By our union with Jesus Christ in his death, we are freed from sin, guilt and death, and, in some ultimate sense, his death is thus effectively substituted for ours.[28]

---

was sentenced to die on account of sin. . . . Now it is a fitting way of satisfying for another to submit oneself to the penalty deserved by that other. And so Christ resolved to die, that by dying He might atone for us" (Aquinas, 1274/1920, III.50.1).

26. Aquinas several times argues that it can be just for someone to be punished for another when there is corporate solidarity or when punishment takes the aspect of a medicine intended to accept some loss for the greater benefit of another's soul or by way of taking on another's debt, but no one is punished with respect to spiritual goods except by or for their own sin (Aquinas, 1274/1920, I.II.87.7–8, II.II.108.4, Supplement 13.2).

27. Guilt pertains to an act that has already taken place, and guilt concerning what has already taken place effectively remains even after punishment. See Aquinas (1274/1920, I.II.87.2, I.II.87.6, Supplement 13.2.ad 2).

28. We might refer to this as "unitive substitution": because of our union with Jesus Christ, his death does away with our corporate and individual guilt and his death effectively substitutes for ours. Although union with Christ and his suffering and death are all part of the efficacious means of salvation, the "substitution" is really the *outcome*, rather than the *mechanism*, of God's work. Jesus Christ's death might be considered "substitution" because the natural consequence of sin is eternal separation from God. Jesus's death on the cross, an act that helped accomplish our salvation, substituted for this. Aquinas, citing Augustine (417/2019, iv), writes: "The one death of our Saviour," namely, that of the body, "saved us from our two deaths," that is, of the soul and the body (Aquinas, 1274/1920, III.50.6).

In the New Testament, Jesus's resurrection also plays an important role in our restoration and freedom from sin. Jesus's resurrection is depicted in the New Testament as having an essential role in salvation, in our deliverance from sin, and in our restoration to wholeness as God intended. The resurrection is pictured as a triumph over death. In his resurrection, Jesus is no longer dead. As noted also above, solidarity with Jesus Christ, our union with him, has the potential to empower and restore our nature (Romans 6:5–9). The New Testament depicts the resurrection of Jesus Christ and our solidarity with him as pointing to and guaranteeing our eventual resurrection by God (1 Corinthians 15). Jesus's resurrection furthermore grounds both our faith and our hope.[29] In doing so, the resurrection empowers us to better conform to God's intent here and now, to better overcome sin in this life, and ultimately to be entirely freed from sin and death in the life to come.[30]

Likewise, Jesus's ascension into heaven and ruling over all things,[31] Jesus's sending the Holy Spirit, and the formation of the Church are all pictured as important means by which our lives are transformed to be in greater conformity with God's will.[32] As will be discussed further in the next section, God's action in our lives through the Holy Spirit and through the Church helps guide us to obey God, to love others, and to live life according to God's intent. This process, sometimes called sanctification in Christian theology, is also a part of salvation, a part of our being freed from sin and the consequences of sin, a part of our restoration to God's intent. To further accomplish this process of transformation we can, in seeing what Jesus did for us, in seeing the adverse

---

29. Aquinas (1274/1920, III.53.1) argues that it was fitting for Christ to rise from the dead for five reasons: first, for the demonstration of divine justice and the exalting of Christ, who had humbled himself; second, for our instruction in the faith, since our belief in Christ's Godhead is confirmed by his rising again; third, for raising our hope that we shall likewise rise again; fourth, to help us order our lives away from sin; and fifth, to complete the work of our salvation, as the resurrection is the beginning and exemplar of all good things.

30. Aquinas (1274/1920, III 56.2); Romans 6:8–14. See Craig (2000), Wright (2012), Pannenberg (2013), and VanderWeele (2017e) for arguments supporting the historicity of the resurrection.

31. Aquinas (1274/1920, III.57.6); John 14:2–3; Ephesians 4:8–10; Hebrews 12:5–11.

32. Romans 8:2–11; Ephesians 4; Aquinas (1274/1920, I.II.68.5, I.II.106.1, I.II.114.3).

consequences of our sin, and in our own experience of suffering resulting from sin, continuously turn our will to God in love.[33]

Thus, in Jesus's conception and birth and God taking on human nature, in Jesus's life and example, in Jesus's death in love for us, in Jesus's resurrection and ascension to heaven, and in his sending the Spirit and forming the Church, God overcomes sin. He does so by taking on and redeeming our nature, by providing us an example of love, by doing away with our guilt and re-creating our corrupted nature, by empowering us now to live more as God intended, and by promising a new resurrected life wherein full restoration can take place. God addresses the problem of sin and brings salvation in these various ways through Jesus Christ.

Our final end of communion with God is beyond natural human capacity. It requires God's help and God's grace. Our nature is empowered in Jesus's incarnation and resurrection. What is corrupted in our nature is done away with in Jesus's death, and we are guided to who we are meant to be in love by God's Spirit and in the life of the Church. As the human person is restored to God's intent and as that intent is fulfilled by Jesus's life, death, resurrection, and Spirit, there a restoration of health of the person. Communion with God is enabled by the restoration of the person to God's intent and by their deliverance from sin. Moreover, that communion and the deliverance from sin empowers a wholeness that enables a person to flourish throughout life. It empowers a person to find happiness in God. It alleviates fear, anger, and sadness, thus bringing about mental and emotional health. As a person conforms more to God's intent, his or her purpose, as rooted in the pursuit of God and God's love and the service of others, becomes firm. The overcoming of sin and the greater conformity to God's intent empowers relationships and facilitates the healing of broken relationships. The overcoming of sin and

---

33. See Aquinas (1274/1920, I.II.87.6, III.48.2). The sufferings we experience in this life as a consequence of or punishment for sin, if accepted as such, can help us turn our will to God and away from sin (1 Peter 4:1–2). It is the offering up of our wills that is satisfying to God. Suffering, accepted as punishment for sin, that enables us to turn our will to God may be viewed as "satisfactory punishment" (Aquinas (1274/1920, I.II.87.6). See also Van Nieuwenhove (2005). Jesus's offering of himself in obedience to and love of God was likewise satisfying to God (Aquinas, 1274/1920, III.48.2). His death was a consequence of our sin, but one that can be an occasion, in recognizing Jesus's obedience and the consequence of sin, for turning our will to God. See also footnotes 10 and 12 in section II.6 and footnote 19 above.

greater conformity to God's intent itself constitutes a growth in character. Salvation, or deliverance from sin, thus helps bring about the health of the person. It facilitates human flourishing here and now and prepares us for, and transforms us into, who we are to be in the life to come.

However, the relation between salvation and deliverance from sin to bodily health in this life is arguably more complex. Certainly by promoting happiness, good relationships, the formation of character, and a sense of purpose, the social and psychological context is established for good bodily health. However, good health is not assured by these things, and everyone eventually confronts aging and infirmity in this life. A greater conformity to God's intent can help facilitate bodily health but can also lead to persecution, suffering, and even martyrdom. Good bodily health is not guaranteed in this life. Various aspects of the wholeness of the person can contribute to the wholeness or health of the body, but it does not guarantee this, and indeed we do eventually die. However, even in our death, in union with Jesus Christ in his death, God accomplishes a freedom from sin. We can still experience his love, and we are brought toward the life to come. Full bodily health, the resurrection and perfection of the body, is promised only in that life to come.

3.3d. The individual receives God's gift of salvation and is delivered from sin through faith in Jesus Christ.

There are mysteries in the Christian teaching on Jesus Christ and salvation. There is mystery in God becoming human, in Jesus Christ being understood as fully God and fully human, as having two natures but being one person. There is a mystery in the mode by which Jesus's death and resurrection delivers the human person from sin and its consequences. There is mystery in the relation between God and Jesus during Jesus's life and death and in the very doctrine of the Trinity as God being Father, Son, and Holy Spirit. There is a mystery in how God, in Jesus Christ, overcomes sin and restores us to wholeness.

However, it perhaps should not be entirely surprising that there is mystery in the working of God's salvation, in God's deliverance from sin and its consequences. If the cause of ill health is sin and sin came about by voluntary human action contrary to God's will but was allowed by God in order to sustain the possibility of human freedom and free response to him in love, then it is perhaps not surprising that the answer to the seemingly impossible goal of ensuring a free response to God in love involves mystery. It is that mystery of God's action in Jesus Christ that is embraced in faith.

It is through faith, through trust in God's action and in the message of salvation through Jesus Christ that each person appropriates God's salvation.[34] Faith is the acceptance of the gift of salvation, the forgiveness and deliverance of sins, that was accomplished in Jesus Christ. Receiving God's grace in faith allows that salvation to begin to be actualized in a person's life.[35] It is not a blind faith; it is a faith rooted in the historical events of Jesus's life, death, and resurrection. It is a faith rooted in the biblical testimony of God's action in the world. It is a faith described by the biblical authors and the Christian tradition and in the life and teaching of the Church. Grounded in these sources of evidence for faith, we come to believe in God and in all that God has revealed.[36] We come to believe more deeply in the biblical testimony and in what the Church teaches. We come to more fully trust in God.

---

34. The New Testament speaks of being "justified by faith" (Romans 3:28, 5:1; Galatians 2:15, 3:24). The object of faith that brings justification is Jesus Christ (Galatians 2:15). Faith involves a trust in God's salvation in Jesus Christ. In the New Testament, that faith and that justification are related both to the death (Romans 5:9) and resurrection (Romans 4:25, 10:9–10) of Jesus. Faith involves a belief and trust in what God has done in Jesus Christ to bring salvation (Aquinas, 1274/1920, I.II.113.4). There is a necessity for faith in salvation, both because our final goal, a full restoration to wholeness, is communion with God (Hebrews 11:6; Aquinas, 1274/1920, II.II.2.3) and because in Jesus Christ, God provides the means for achieving this goal (Romans 1:16–17; Aquinas, 1274/1920, II.II.2.7).

35. Salvation is spoken of in the New Testament as a gift of God's grace (Ephesians 2:8–10) and justification as having been accomplished by God's grace (Romans 3:23–25; see also Aquinas, 1274/1920, I.II.113.2). However, this salvation involves a transformation of the person, who goes on by God's grace to have his or her will reoriented to God and to do good works (Ephesians 2:8–10; Romans 6; James 2:14–26). Once this process has been set in motion by God's grace, it becomes appropriate to speak immediately of "justification" (see Aquinas, 1274/1920, I.II.113.7).

36. Faith itself, taken as a theological virtue, involves the habit of believing in God and all that God has revealed and all that follows from that (Hebrews 11:1–2; Aquinas, 1274/1920, II.II.1–4). However, the faith that is needed for justification does not necessarily initially entail all articles of faith, only faith that God justified humanity through the mystery of Jesus Christ (Aquinas, 1274/1920, I.II.113.4).

However, some mystery remains. The work of God extends beyond our full understanding.[37] Faith—that trust in God that believes that God is able to accomplish what is promised in salvation in restoring us to wholeness and our receiving of that salvation—reorients our life to God with his help.

Nevertheless, even in faith, we reach the limits of our understanding of God, his intent, and his action when we contemplate how God can provide deliverance from sin while still also maintaining human freedom. That central mystery is grounded in the life, death, and resurrection of Jesus Christ. By these things, God brought salvation, a deliverance from sin, a restoration of the human person to God's intent. It is this salvation that is embraced in faith and lived out in the life of the Church.

Propositional Summary 3.3: God has brought healing and salvation through Jesus Christ.
3.3a. God is the principal agent of healing.
3.3b. Sin cannot be fully dealt with through human efforts.
3.3c. God has dealt with the problem of sin in the person of Jesus Christ.
    3.3c.i. Jesus Christ restored human nature by uniting it to the divine.
    3.3c.ii. Jesus's life and teaching enables us to better know God.
    3.3c.iii. Jesus Christ demonstrated God's love, which can in turn prompt love in us.
    3.3c.iv. Jesus provided a model of a life lived in love for God and neighbor that we are to imitate.
    3.3c.v. Jesus did away with sin and guilt in uniting us to himself in his suffering and death.
    3.3c.vi. Jesus's resurrection empowers our life and guarantees we too will be raised from the dead and restored to complete wholeness.
    3.3c.vii. Jesus's sending his Spirit and the formation of the Church enables our lives to conform to God's intent both here and now and in the life to come.
3.3d. The individual receives God's gift of salvation and is delivered from sin through faith in Jesus Christ.

---

37. 1 Timothy 3:16; Aquinas (1274/1920, II.II.1.4–5, II.II.2.3).

III.4. The Church, Community, and Healing

Proposition 3.4. The Church and its members are both agents and recipients of healing, and that healing comes about by means of communal life, forgiveness, prayer, fasting, the sacraments, growth in character, and the care of others, including the work of medicine.

3.4a. The Church is called to bring healing and the message of salvation to the world.

The Church is the community that is founded upon and has arisen out of God's work of salvation in Jesus Christ. The Church may be understood as "the whole universal community of believers . . . the assembly of those whom God's word . . . gathers together to form the People of God."[1] The Church, as this community, is centered on salvation in Jesus Christ,

---

1. Catholic Church (2000, 752, 777). The *Catechism of the Catholic Church* uses "Church" to designate this universal community of believers. The unity of the Church is derived from the unity of its source in God—Father, Son, and Holy Spirit (Catholic Church, 2000, 810, 813; Paul VI (1964a, 4); Paul VI (1964b, 2.5). The catechism distinguishes this more general use of "Church" from the more specific use of the term "Catholic Church," which is understood as "the Church established by Christ on the Foundation of the Apostles, possessing the fullness of the means of salvation which he has willed: correct and complete confession of faith, full sacramental life, and ordained ministry in apostolic succession" (Catholic Church, 2000, 870). The profession of one faith, common celebration of worship, and apostolic succession are referred to as the visible bond of communion. The ultimate bond of unity is charity, which binds "everything together in perfect harmony" (Catholic Church, 2000, 815; see also Colossians 3:14). The understanding presented in the catechism, however, is also that there are Churches and ecclesial communities separated from or outside the visible confines of the Catholic Church that "Christ's Spirit uses . . . as a means of salvation, [and] whose power derives from the fullness of grace and truth that Christ has entrusted to the Catholic Church" (Catholic Church, 2000, 819; see also Paul VI, 1964a, 15; Paul VI, 1964b, 3.2). Protestant theologies may share much of the Catholic understanding of the "Church" universal without giving the Catholic Church the central place it has in Catholic theology.

entrusted with the message of salvation and healing it has received, and empowered by God's grace and Spirit to carry out its work. The Church is both the means and the goal of God's plan of salvation.[2] The Church is in some sense the goal of salvation because it is constituted by all of the people that God gathers in the world, who find salvation in Jesus Christ. However, the Church is also the means. The Church is called to bring healing and a message of salvation to the world.

The Church offers numerous pathways to healing and numerous opportunities for the operation of God's action and grace. It is within the Church that Christian communal life is experienced. It is within the Church that members are instructed to love and support one another and to use their complementary gifts to serve others (1 Corinthians 12). It is within the Church that communal prayer to God and worship of God takes place. It is the Church's responsibility to administer the sacraments—celebrations and rites that signify and make present God's grace.[3] The Church is thus referred to as the "body of Christ" (1 Corinthians 12). The Church furthermore cares for the material, financial, and health-related needs of its members and of the world at large. It is especially concerned with the needs of those who are poorest or in greatest difficulty.[4] It is principally the work of the Church to proclaim the message of God's salvation in Jesus Christ and to invite others to receive it in faith and to join the Church in seeking God and in its work of bringing healing to the world. The Church also encourages and promotes character formation as well as the spiritual formation of its members, helping them carry out their individual callings and make use of their gifts to serve others. The Church contributes to and offers healing for both bodily health and the health or wholeness of the persons, both for its members and for the world. The Church, given that its life and calling are founded upon the love of God, and given that it is a community whose members are to love one another, and given its calling to

---

2. Catholic Church (2000, 778).

3. Catholic Church (2000, 1131).

4. Catholic social teaching concerning the principle of the "preferential option for the poor" is that "the poor, the marginalized and in all cases those whose living conditions interfere with their proper growth should be the focus of particular concern" (Catholic Church, 2004, 182). Jesus taught that he was especially present when his followers cared for those in severe need (Mathew 25:31–46).

love and serve and bring a message of God's loving salvation to the world, might thus be understood as a "community of love."[5]

3.4b. The Christian is called to bring healing and the message of salvation to the world.

The Christian, as part of the Church community, is called to bring healing to the world and to share the message of God's salvation in Jesus Christ with others. Part of Jesus's teaching on the greatest commandment to love is to love one's neighbor. That love is the seeking of their good, the seeking of their flourishing, the seeking of a complete restoration to wholeness as God intended. Because that wholeness cannot be attained apart from God and cannot be attained without addressing the problem and consequences of sin, true love of one's neighbor includes telling others of God's salvation in Jesus Christ. This may be done in various ways: by sharing one's own experience, by attempting to explicate the message of God's love and God's salvation in Jesus, and by inviting others into the experience of the Christian community. It is in part by telling others of God's salvation and encouraging them to receive that salvation through faith in Jesus Christ that the Christian can help others and can love others.

The love of others does not simply end at the proclamation of the good news of God's love. It extends to providing the material, emotional, and social needs of others, to seeking the full flourishing of others. Loving one's neighbor results in acts of love or works of love to help bring healing to the world. In the epistle of James, the author writes: "What good is it . . . if you say you have faith but do not have works? . . . If a brother or sister is naked and lacks daily food, and one of you says to them, 'Go in peace; keep warm and eat your fill,' and yet you do not supply their bodily needs, what is the good of that? . . . Show me your faith apart from your works, and I by my works will show you my faith. . . . For just as the body without the spirit is dead, so faith without works is also dead" (James 2:14–26). The Christian's calling is to invite others toward healing and wholeness as God intended through faith in Jesus Christ, but the Christian is also called to provide for their needs in

---

5. See Sarah (2011).

this life. The Church and its individual members are called to bring healing and the message of salvation to the world and thereby always to promote, wherever possible and appropriate, flourishing in the lives of others, including their happiness, their health, their relationships, their character, the formation of a system of meaning, and the material and financial means to sustain these. The Church and its members are called to bring both spiritual and physical healing.

3.4c. Healing comes through community life.

From the standpoint of Christian theology, God is the principal agent of healing and salvation, and restoration to wholeness is ultimately accomplished in the life, death, and resurrection of Jesus Christ and in God's continuing work by the Spirit and in the life of the Church. However, community life is one of the principal means by which that salvation and restoration are worked out.

Community is thus given strong emphasis in Christian theology. Throughout the biblical account, the community was understood to be the central context within which salvation, forgiveness, and healing would come. The community was instructed to provide for the needs of its members (Romans 12:13; 1 John 3:16–18; James 2:14–17). Its members were instructed to hold one another accountable and issue rebuke for wrong action when necessary (Matthew 18:15–18). They were told to participate together in religious life and ritual (Hebrew 10:23–25), to work together using their various gifts and strengths (1 Corinthians 12), and to love, support, and encourage one another (Hebrews 10:23–25; 1 John 4:7–12). The community was thus an important part of the process of salvation and healing. Spiritual healing through faith in Jesus Christ would bring one into this community, and the Church community was a source of healing. In Jesus's healings of those with leprosy or hemorrhaging, the healing was not only physical; it also constituted a full restoration to community and religious life that illness had prevented.[6] Jesus's life, death, and resurrection, and the healing and salvation they brought, were to be remembered within the community by a common meal following the model of the last supper of Jesus with his disciples

---

6. Pilch (2000).

(Luke 22:14–20; 1 Corinthians 11:23–26). Love was to be the central defining feature of this community, following Jesus's life and example (John 13:34–35). Jesus also summarized the whole of the law as love of God and love of one's neighbor (Matthew 22:35–40). Paul's writing described love as a central goal of communal and religious life (1 Corinthians 13; Romans 13:8–10).

Numerous studies testify to the power of community life and close relationships to promote and sustain health and well-being, including their role in sustaining health, creating meaning, and fostering character.[7] In practical terms, participation in community provides a forum for the formation of friendships and close relationships. This is constitutive of flourishing, but such close relationships can also promote bodily health through the social support that is available during times of need and through a sense of social connection and its effects on the body.[8] Community life also provides opportunities for the formation of character. The members of the community can hold one another accountable, provide guidance, and admonish against wrong behavior. A shared communal sense of service and a call to help others both builds up, helps, and supports the community and those in it and provides further opportunities for character formation. A number of these benefits and pathways to healing can also be found in other forms of community life, such as the family, the workplace, or educational institutions.[9] These other communities also provide important opportunities for relationships to form, for holding one another accountable and forming character, for providing

---

7. Large, well-designed research studies have indicated that attending religious services is associated with greater longevity, less depression, less suicide, less smoking, less substance abuse, better cancer and cardiovascular disease survival, less divorce, greater social support, greater meaning and purpose in life, greater life satisfaction, more charitable giving, more volunteering, and greater civic engagement (see Idler, 2014b; VanderWeele, 2017a, 2017c; Koenig et al., 2023; Balboni et al., 2022; and references therein).

8. See Holt-Lunstad et al. (2015). Although social support is undoubtedly an important pathway by which participation in religious community affects physical health, studies indicate that it may only account for about a quarter of the protective effect of participation in religious community on mortality risk. Other possible pathways may include lower depression, greater optimism or hope, less smoking and improved health behaviors, and greater purpose (Li et al., 2016; Kim and VanderWeele, 2019).

9. See VanderWeele (2017a) for a review of the empirical literature.

support, and possibly for providing a shared purpose. These are all important goods and ends that Church communities and other forms of community life share.[10] The Church additionally proclaims a message of faith, hope, and love; it provides a system of meaning grounded in God's love and God's grace; and it provides communal opportunities to find communion with God in love.

Within the context of the Christian Church, the message of faith and of hope can also help alleviate sadness, fear, and depression. The understanding of God, of the world, and of the place of the human person in it provides a rich framework of meaning for making sense of life. Moreover, each member's pursuit of final communion with God in love gives a strong sense of shared purpose. The Church provides a shared communal worship of God, and an appreciation of the beauty of God, facilitating communion with God as the purpose of human life. The proclamation of the message of God's love and salvation is furthermore the principal means by which a person enters into the Church community. Community life brings wholeness and healing.

Communal life thus helps bring about a fuller flourishing; it helps bring about a healing of the body and a healing of the person. Relationships and communal life were part of God's original intent. They also are intended as a powerful way of restoring health, flourishing, and wholeness.

3.4d. Healing comes through forgiveness.

Relationships are central to human well-being, to the wholeness of the person. God's intent was for the human person to be in relationship. It is within relationships that love is given and received. Due to sin and wrong actions, relationships are disrupted and often broken. Such broken relationships often contribute to declines in health and to a decline in well-being in other ways. The restoration of relationships can thus constitute a powerful form of healing and restoration of the wholeness of the person

---

10. Although studies indicate important effects of other forms of community participation on health and well-being (Holt-Lunstad et al., 2015; Shor and Roelfs, 2013), the effect sizes tend to be smaller. For cardiovascular disease, all-cause mortality risk, and suicide, attendance at religious services had stronger protective associations than any other social support variable examined, including marital status, time spent with friends, time spent with family, time spent in other community groups, or even a summary of all of these components (Chang et al., 2017; Li et al., 2016; VanderWeele et al., 2016).

as God intended. Forgiveness is the principal means by which relationships are healed.

The New Testament emphasizes the importance of forgiving others, which is to be done irrespective of the number of past offenses, and is essential within community and religious life (Matthew 18:21–35). Forgiveness of others follows from God's forgiveness, a connection that is explicitly made in Jesus's parables and in the Lord's Prayer (Matthew 6:9–15; 18:23–35). The book of James presents forgiveness an important pathway to healing (James 5:15–16). Forgiveness helps overcome evil and helps propagate love and goodwill and good actions toward others. St. Paul wrote in his Epistle to the Romans, "Do not be overcome by evil, but overcome evil with good" (Romans 12:21). Healing and forgiveness are spoken of in parallel in the prophetic books, with forgiveness enabling healing (2 Chronicles 7:14; Psalm 103:3; Hosea 14:4). The New Testament presents Jesus's life and death as the forgiveness of sins and restoration of the person to wholeness and communion with God. In some of the Gospel healing accounts, Jesus ties healing to the forgiveness of sins (Mark 2). In the Epistle of James (2:15–16), healing is tied to confession and the forgiveness of sins in the context of congregational life. The various writings thus suggest that forgiveness from God brings healing, wholeness, and salvation; one's forgiveness of others brings healing to oneself, to the offender, and to the community.

Forgiveness may be understood as the replacing of ill will toward the offender with goodwill. Because forgiveness orients the person toward the good of the other, it is a restoration of love.[11] Forgiveness is not the same as forgetting or ignoring the offense or not pursuing justice. One can forgive and ultimately desire the good for the offender while still pursuing a just outcome.[12] Forgiveness can open possibilities of reconciliation and the restoration of a relationship, but it does not necessarily entail this.[13] However, for two people to reconcile and to have a

---

11. Stump (2006).

12. See footnote 24 in section III.2 for a discussion of the compatibility of love with justice and with punishment of the offender when the intention is to accomplish good for the offender and for the community. If just anger is understood as a desire for just punishment ultimately aimed at the good of the offender, then even anger and forgiveness may be seen as compatible. See also Potts (2022) for an account of how forgiveness is compatible with anger.

13. In cases, for example, of repeated domestic abuse, while forgiveness, viewed as desiring the good of the offender, may be appropriate, a restored relationship

healthy restored relationship following a major offense, forgiveness will generally be needed. Forgiveness is a pathway to healing because forgiveness promotes love and restored relationships.

Many studies indicate that forgiveness can promote health—certainly mental health and possibly also physical health.[14] Forgiveness serves as an important alternative to unhealthy responses to an offense such as rumination or suppression.[15] Forgiveness provides a release from anger and rumination. Although forgiveness is in some sense fundamentally an act of the will, a replacing of ill will toward the offender with goodwill, the place of forgiveness with respect to emotion is more complex. It can take time for the emotions to heal, for anger to subside. A distinction is sometimes drawn between what might be called decisional forgiveness and emotional forgiveness, the former being an act of the will, but the latter concerning emotions that are not fully within one's control.[16] Decisional forgiveness will often precede and help bring about emotional forgiveness.

---

without reform on the part of the offender may not be appropriate. Forgiveness as a replacing of ill will toward the offender with goodwill might be understood as only necessarily entailing a desire for reconciliation in this life provided appropriate conditions are met, but as always entailing, from the perspective of Christian theology, a desire for the offender's repentance and ultimate reconciliation in the life to come (see Stump, 2006).

14. For a review of the literature on forgiveness and health, see Toussaint et al. (2015). The effects of forgiveness in reducing depression and anxiety and in increasing hope are now clear from both experimental (Wade et al., 2014; Ho et al., 2024) and rigorous observational (Long, Worthington, et al., 2020) evidence. However, the effects of forgiveness on physical health are not yet as definitely established and may vary by context (Long, Worthington, et al., 2020; see also Toussaint et al., 2015).

15. Unforgiveness and rumination may sometimes adversely affect one's physical health, possibly damaging cardiovascular and immune systems. See Toussaint et al. (2015).

16. See Worthington (2013) for further discussion of the distinction between decisional and emotional forgiveness and implications of this distinction for efforts to bring about forgiveness. The distinction between decisional and emotional forgiveness can help make sense of the experience of believing one has forgiven the offender but then finding that feelings of anger have returned only a few days later: while decisional forgiveness may have taken place, emotional forgiveness may remain incomplete. The distinction between decisional and emotional forgiveness also clarifies the appropriateness of a command to forgive (Matthew 18:21–22; Colossians 3:13; Ephesians 4:31–32). Decisional forgiveness can be commanded because it is an act of the will; emotional forgiveness, in contrast, is not entirely within one's control.

Forgiveness can also help restore and preserve relationships more broadly in a community. In a community, relationships are often tightly interwoven, and a damaged relationship between two people may affect not only the two individuals but many others connected to them. Forgiveness can thus also help preserve and sustain community life. Specific actions can help bring about forgiveness and emotional healing.[17] Confronting the offender and publicly stating that the offender is forgiven can sometimes be helpful. Apologies and restitution on the part of the offender can help bring about emotional forgiveness. Sometimes simply the passage of time and letting wounds heal can enable emotional forgiveness. However, none of this is necessary for making the decision to forgive, for making a commitment to replace ill will toward the offender with goodwill. That decision to forgive is the beginning of the restoration of one's own peace and healing from anger. It is potentially the beginning of a restored relationship, and it is a movement toward love for the other. Forgiveness of others is thus an important path to healing. If forgiveness were more actively promoted, it would bring about greater healing within society and greater health for its members.[18]

Being forgiven is also an important path for healing. Being forgiven for an offense can, when appropriate, help restore and strengthen a relationship with the one who was offended. Being forgiven can relieve sadness and guilt over the wrong that was committed. Being forgiven can bring about a greater awareness of the needs of others and of one's own

---

17. See Enright and Fitzgibbons (2000) and Worthington (2013) for different models of facilitating forgiveness. See also section III.7f for further discussion.

18. The principles from the various forgiveness interventions that have been developed and evaluated in randomized trials (Wade et al., 2014) have been distilled into a workbook format (Worthington, 2021; Ho et al., 2024) that can be done on one's own. Evidence from randomized trials (Harper et al., 2014; Ho et al., 2024) suggests that these modalities are effective in promoting forgiveness and improving mental health and well-being. Since interventions are indeed effective not only for promoting forgiveness but also for reducing anxiety and depression, a compelling case can be made that forgiveness should be taken seriously as a public health issue (VanderWeele, 2018a; Ho et al., 2024). The experience of being wronged is common and the effects of forgiveness on mental health are substantial, so community-level or even national or international campaigns to promote forgiveness and distribute workbook resources to enable forgiveness could substantially affect mental health at the population level, in addition to giving rise to restored relationships and more forgiving communities. See also section III.7f.

shortcomings and can lead to a growth in humility and in character. Being forgiven and experiencing the love of the other can help empower one to love. Moreover, salvation in Jesus Christ necessarily entails the forgiveness of sins, as God no longer allows our sins, our voluntary actions contrary to his will, to separate us from him.[19] The knowledge and experience of God's forgiveness can bring us into deeper communion with him and can empower us to better forgive others and live more as God intended; it can empower us to love. Both forgiving and being forgiven by God and by others can bring healing to the person and may help bring healing to the body.

3.4e. Healing comes through prayer.

Prayer is depicted in the biblical accounts as an important pathway to healing. In several biblical stories, someone is healed directly as a response to prayer (Genesis 20; Number 12; 1 Kings 17; Mark 9). In some of the healing accounts, such prayer is accompanied by the laying on of hands; it is often tied to faith in God. Prayer does not always result in

---

19. God's forgiveness of us might still be understood as "replacing ill will toward the offender with goodwill," although when God's forgiving is in view, the "replacing" must be interpreted with certain qualifications. Aquinas distinguishes between God's antecedent will and God's consequent will (Aquinas, 1274/1920, I.19.6.ad 1). God's will does not change in an absolute sense (Aquinas, 1274/1920, I.19.7). However, Aquinas argues that the will is directed to things as they are in themselves under their particular qualifications, and thus something that is good when considered absolutely may be good or evil when some additional circumstance is taken into account. What is willed apart from, or prior to, the circumstances is willed antecedently, but what is willed taking the additional circumstances into account is willed consequently or simply. God wills antecedently that all will be saved (1 Timothy 2:14; Aquinas, 1274/1920, I.19.6). However, the consequent will of God follows from our response to God's offer of salvation. If we turn our will to God, we experience God's consequent will as salvation; if we do not turn to God, we experience God's consequent will as punishment. Aquinas writes, "Hence that which seems to depart from the divine will in one order, returns into it in another order; as does the sinner, who by sin falls away from the divine will as much as lies in him, yet falls back into the order of that will, when by its justice he is punished" (1274/1920, I.19.6). The "replacing" of ill will with goodwill in God's forgiveness of sin is our experience of his consequent will, even though the good that God wills absolutely does not change. However, our experience of God's consequent will depends on our response to his offer of forgiveness.

healing in the biblical accounts, but it is presented as a pathway to healing by asking God to act.

In the Christian tradition, prayer is effectively any being with or communion with God or speech to or hearing from God. Prayer thus includes but extends beyond intercessory prayer, asking God for various goods for oneself or others. Biblical stories and personal testimony suggest that God sometimes provides physical healing as a result of prayer, but direct physical healing does not always occur.[20] Different Christian

---

20. Although somewhat controversial, there have in fact been randomized trials of intercessory prayer. The standard design of these trials is that patients are randomized to receive intercessory prayer from someone else. Patients are often blinded in the sense that they don't know whether or not they are being prayed for. Some of these randomized trials have suggested an effect of prayer; other studies have suggested no effect. Two reviews have attempted to synthesize all available evidence, but their findings are divided. Astin et al. (2000) conducted a systematic review with fairly broad inclusion criteria. They included twenty-three randomized trials and concluded that there was some evidence for an effect. Meta-analysis carried out by the Cochran Collaboration has been repeated a number of times (Roberts et al., 2000, 2007, 2009). Using stricter inclusion criteria than the Astin et al. (2000) study, the Cochran meta-analysis of 2000 was inconclusive. In 2007, their meta-analysis suggested an effect on mortality but no effect on clinical state or complications. In 2009, the meta-analysis still had a protective effect estimate, but one that was not "statistically significant." The conclusion seemed to depend somewhat on which studies were included. Reasonable objections to this research on intercessory prayer have come from both those who practice a religious faith and those who do not. It is often thought that those engaged in such research almost always have an agenda—for or against—and that the research may be less credible for that reason. Theological objections include that the forms of prayer examined in these blinded trials do not correspond to the forms of prayer that are actually practiced within religious communities, which often occur within the context of a relationship and involve the laying on of hands. Other theological objections include that the research design effectively presumes that God is somehow not aware that the trial is taking place and is constrained to act as would ordinarily be the case. For further discussion of the results, controversies, and objections around these randomized trials, see VanderWeele (2017c). Beyond randomized trials, observational studies of prayer frequency generally do not manifest the same beneficial associations with health as one finds with attending religious services (VanderWeele et al., 2017; see also footnote 7 above). However, it is also possible that higher frequency of prayer is, for some, in fact a marker of health problems or threats already present, thus partially confounding the association. One exception to this general pattern seems to be practices of prayer and meditation among adolescents that are associated with better subsequent health and well-being (Chen and VanderWeele, 2018). This result might be because adolescence is a particularly formative time or it may be that observational studies of prayer

traditions emphasize and hope for direct physical healing to varying degrees and believe it to regularly take place to varying degrees, but many across different Christian traditions believe that God can and sometimes does provide physical healing as the result of prayer.

Even when physical healing does not come about as a result of prayer, prayer can result in spiritual, emotional, relational, or communal healing. Although the absence of physical healing can be disappointing and can result in a questioning of God's love, it can, like suffering, be an opportunity to reflect on what is most important, to reassess priorities, to grow in character, to seek new meanings and possibilities, and to renew faith and trust in God. Both prayer for others, and knowing one is being prayed for by others, can strengthen and heal relationships. Communal prayer for someone who is ill can strengthen community bonds. All of these forms of spiritual, emotional, relational, and communal healing can happen even if physical healing does not take place.

However, the role of prayer in the Christian life extends beyond direct physical healing or deepening of relationships or growth in character. Prayer is an essential part of friendship with and communion with God. Prayer is fundamentally relational, connecting the one praying to God. In its more meditative and contemplative forms, prayer is a being with, an awareness of, and an experience of God.[21] Prayer thus is central in bringing about spiritual healing, a restored and fuller relation with and being with God. It is constitutive of, and leads toward, one's final end of full communion with God.

3.4f. Healing comes through fasting.

Fasting is abstaining from food or drink or some other material good or pleasure in order to free one's attachment to it and free one for greater prayer. Fasting is known to have various benefits with regard to physical

---

among adolescents are less subject to confounding by health status because severe illness is less common at younger ages. See also Brown (2012) for further discussion of various other aspects of the study of prayer. Perhaps more compelling evidence for supernatural healing comes from well-documented accounts of healings that defy naturalistic explanations in the context of existing medical knowledge (Duffin, 2009).

21. Pieper (1998); Garrigou-Lagrange (1937).

health.[22] However, from the perspective of Christian theology, its primary purpose is to promote spiritual health and well-being, to promote a restoration to a greater wholeness with less psychological dependence on material comforts. The practice of fasting can remind one that one's ultimate sustenance comes from God. Fasting can free one's time and mind for greater prayer and contemplation. Fasting can weaken attachment to material goods and pleasures, thereby building temperance and fortitude and a certain self-mastery that is motivated and empowered by God. Fasting can also be a means of penance and an expression of sorrow for what one has done wrong, thereby providing a self-imposed discipline that will help one to avoid wrongdoing. In these ways, fasting helps bring about healing and restoration to God's intent.[23] Fasting is not to be done to such an extent that a person has insufficient sustenance to fulfill his or her duties in loving or serving others. However, when it is carried out in the right time and in the right proportion, fasting can facilitate wholeness. Fasting can help bring about restoration of the body and, more centrally, of the person. Fasting can help a person attain spiritual well-being.

Closely related to fasting is voluntarily giving up other goods such as riches, pleasures, and honors in order to obtain higher spiritual goods. Although these things are not bad in and of themselves, excessive attachment to them can distract one from the spiritual life and the pursuit of God. It is possible to make use of riches, pleasures, and honors in the process of serving others and even in seeking spiritual well-being and one's final communion with God so long as these things do not become the final goal one is pursuing. However, voluntarily giving up and seeking detachment from these things can also allow for a greater increase in charity and a more unified pursuit of spiritual well-being and communion with God.[24] Jesus's counsel to the rich young ruler who approached him concerning how to go about attaining eternal life was this: "If you wish to be perfect, go, sell your possessions, and give the money

---

22. See De Cabo and Mattson (2019) for a review of the effects of intermittent fasting on health, aging, and disease.

23. Aquinas (1274/1920, II.II.147.1).

24. Giving up riches, pleasures, and honors has sometimes been referred to as the "evangelical counsels" (Catholic Church, 2000, 944). The gospel does not require such renunciation for all individuals, but it counsels it for some as a way to move toward greater perfection. See Aquinas (1274/1920, I.II.108.4).

to the poor, and you will have treasure in heaven; then come, follow me" (Matthew 19:21). The monastic vows of poverty, chastity, and obedience constitute a more formal renunciation of these goods for greater pursuit of the spiritual life, often within the context of a communal religious life.

Thus, while fasting may indeed have important effects on the health of the body, its primary role from the perspective of Christian theology is the health of the person—a growth in temperance and fortitude, a spiritual growth, and a freeing of the person to be oriented toward and to be better able to pursue higher spiritual goods.

3.4g. Healing comes through the sacraments.

The Church practices various liturgical celebrations that signify and make present God's grace. These celebrations or rites are sometimes referred to as sacraments.[25] Christian theology draws a connection between these sacraments and the healing of persons, including the various modes of healing, such as community, forgiveness, and prayer, in the previous sections.[26] The Catechism of the Catholic Church (2000) connects the sacrament of the Eucharist to community, forgiveness, and healing and restoration. It relates the sacrament of the anointing of the sick to prayer, forgiveness, caregiving, and healing. It relates the sacrament of penance and reconciliation to forgiveness, prayer, community, and conversion and healing. Each of the traditional sacraments of the Church can bring about healing in profound ways.[27]

---

25. The sacraments may be understood as "efficacious signs of grace, instituted by Christ and entrusted to the Church, by which divine life is dispensed to us" (Catholic Church, 2000, 1131) or "an outward and visible sign of an inward and invisible grace" (often attributed to Augustine, although the phrase does not seem to appear in any extant text; see Cary, 2008; and Letourneau, 2019). Some Protestant theologies diverge from the traditional Catholic understanding in restricting the role of the sacraments to a sign of grace rather than necessarily also as an efficacious means of grace.

26. The very cursory exposition that follows is in no way intended to provide an overview of sacramental theology or a theology of the individual sacraments, but only to highlight some of the ways that each of the sacraments is connected to healing. Although the sacrament of penance and reconciliation and the sacrament of the anointing of the sick are sometimes referred to as the two "sacraments of healing" (Catholic Church, 2000), each of the other sacraments arguably also has the potential to bring healing, understood as a restoration to the wholeness of the person.

27. Although a number of Protestant theologies may not consider marriage, holy orders, confirmation, penance, or the anointing of the sick to be sacraments, many of

Baptism is an incorporation into the Church. It is symbolic of union with Christ and in a profound and mysterious way accomplishes that union, the being united with Jesus Christ in his death and thereby the washing away of sin and being given new life.[28] Catholic teaching is that the rite of baptism conveys grace, empowers the one baptized, and anticipates final redemption and resurrection.[29] However, as incorporation into the Church, it also is the initiation into Christian communal life and the community, love, forgiveness, prayer, and grace that is present there. The sacrament of baptism thus brings healing.

Healing also comes through the celebration of the Eucharist. This sacrament, the celebration and remembrance of Jesus Christ's giving his life for us and the sharing together of bread and wine as his body and blood, is central to the life of the Church. The remembering of Jesus Christ's love and work refocuses the life of the community on God's salvation accomplished through Christ (see section III.3c). Celebrating this by sharing the bread and the wine unites the community, restores relationships, makes Christ present to us, points to the future, restores our hope, and conveys to the Christian God's grace. The sacrament of the Eucharist thus brings healing.

Healing also comes through the confirmation of faith. It is by faith that God's salvation in Jesus Christ is received (see section III.3d). Faith brings about the forgiveness of sins and reconciliation with God, a receiving of the Spirit that prompts a growth in character and an orientation of one's life to one's final communion with God. It is by faith in God's work in Jesus Christ by the Spirit that we are saved and are ultimately restored to complete wholeness in God. The sacrament of confirmation thus brings healing.

Healing comes also through the confession of sins. Sin separates us from God. The first Epistle of St. John indicates that God has promised that if we confess our sins, we will be forgiven (1 John 1). The confession of sins, and reconciliation with God and with the Church, helps remove sin and its consequence in our lives. The removal of sin helps restore our

---

these theologies may still acknowledge God's grace in these rites and practices, along with their potential power to bring wholeness and healing.

28. Romans 6:3–4; Aquinas (1274/1920, III.49.5); Catholic Church (2000, 1262–1266).

29. Catholic Church (2000, 1266, 1274).

relationship with God and thereby helps bring fuller healing of the person. In the epistle of St. James, the author writes: "Confess your sins to one another, and pray for one another, so that you may be healed" (James 5:13–20). By confessing our sins, we are healed in our relationship to God. Confession can bring about the healing of the person in other ways. By confessing our sins, we are more fully restored to the life of the Church. We are more fully able to receive God's grace within it. The sacrament of penance and reconciliation can bring healing.

As discussed above, healing can also come through prayer. In the sacrament of the anointing of the sick, those prayers take place within the life of the Church in more particular contexts. They may take place at the end of life, in the case of serious illness, or in various other circumstances. They may take place in conjunction with the confession of sins and reconciliation. In these prayers, God can heal. The author of the Epistle of St. James writes: "Are any among you sick? They should call for the elders of the church and have them pray over them, anointing them with oil in the name of the Lord. The prayer of faith will save the sick, and the Lord will raise them up; and anyone who has committed sins will be forgiven" (James 5:13–20). In these prayers and in the anointing of the sick, God can heal the physical body, the soul, and the whole person. The sacrament of the anointing of the sick thus brings healing.

Healing can also come through marriage. Marriage forms a close relationship and brings union. It can lead to a growth in love and in character. It can lead to new life and the raising of children in love. It can provide a purpose and a sense of meaning in the common pursuit of the mutual support of one another, the upbringing of children, and the strengthening of the family in love. It can bring happiness, but it can also bring suffering, further building character and love. Marriage can thus bring healing and wholeness to the body and to the person.[30] Marriage moreover points to the union of Christ and the Church (Ephesians 5), pointing to the fuller restoration of wholeness to come. The sacrament of marriage thus brings healing.

---

30. See Wood et al. (2007), Manzoli et al. (2007), VanderWeele (2017a), and Chen et al. (2023) for some of the empirical research literature on marriage and subsequent health and well-being.

Healing can also come about through ordination to Christian ministry, through the sacrament of holy orders. Although the whole Church is a priestly people, some are called to a ministerial priesthood in which they give their time and service to teaching the faith, facilitating worship, and governing the Church. This work is essential for the life of the Church for sustaining the community, for the formation of faith, for promoting love and forgiveness, for proclaiming the good news of God's salvation, for administering the sacraments, for promoting prayer, and for facilitating all of the members of the Church in their own callings. All of these things bring healing. Although a calling to healing is part of the work of the whole Church, that work is facilitated by those called to holy orders. The sacrament of holy orders and the calling to the ministerial priesthood thus facilitates healing.

All of the sacraments of the Church thus bring healing and restoration.

3.4h. Healing comes through growth in character.

Healing can come about through growth in character. Good character is itself constitutive of the wholeness of the person. However, growth in character facilitates the healing of the person in numerous other ways. Growth in character can bring about healing by contributing to other dimensions of the health of the person, including promoting happiness, bodily health, meaning, relationships, and a greater communion with God.[31] A growth in practical wisdom, justice, temperance, and fortitude can help improve our relationships and help orient our own actions to what is healthy and what is good for ourselves and for others. A growth in character helps orient the whole of our lives to what is most meaningful and gives us purpose as we better pursue the good of ourselves and of others and as we pursue God. A growth in character helps us clarify and prioritize our pursuits and appreciate more fully that our final end is communion with God. A growth in

---

31. Plato (4th C BCE/2004) argued that virtue is constitutive of flourishing. Aristotle (4th C BCE/1925, I.7–9) and many others, including subsequent virtue theorists, have made similar arguments. See Garrigou-Lagrange (1999) for an analysis of the importance of the virtues for spiritual life. See VanderWeele (2022a) for a review of some of the empirical longitudinal and experimental evidence for the effects of character on other aspects of flourishing and on some of the challenges in empirically studying the effects of character.

character allows us to find happiness in goodness, in right action, and in God, even in the midst of disappointment and suffering. In these various ways, growth in character can sometimes help bring about the healing of the body and the healing of the person.

Growth in character can be facilitated by our own efforts, by the formation of good habits and continually seeking what is good. However, growth in character is perhaps more profoundly facilitated by the work of the Spirit, by the life of the Church and participation in community, the receiving of the sacraments, and the experience of forgiveness and love. These things enable us to experience what is good and to better pursue it.

Growth in character is also facilitated by a right orientation to and response to suffering.[32] By seeing suffering as an opportunity to turn to God, to let go of our less important desires and pursuits, to clarify our purposes, to strengthen our resolve, we can allow suffering to bring about a transformation of character. St. Paul wrote in his Epistle to the Romans, "We also boast in our sufferings, knowing that suffering produces endurance, and endurance produces character, and character produces hope, and hope does not disappoint us, because God's love has been poured into our hearts through the Holy Spirit that has been given to us" (Romans 5:3–5). Suffering can thus be a pathway to healing through growth in character. God's grace, our cooperation with it, our approaching life and suffering with an openness to grow all thus help facilitate a growth in character. That growth can then bring about a fuller healing of our person in numerous ways.

3.4i. Healing comes through the care of others.

Healing can also come through the care of others. Healing is in part brought when the needs of others are met. In the biblical accounts, care and healing take place through prayer and through community, but they also take place in ways that are more physical and direct, through caregiving (Luke 14:13; Acts 2:44–47; 6:1–5; 28:7–8; Colossians 4:14; James

---

32. See Brady (2018) for a philosophical analysis of the role of suffering in the formation of virtue. In the New Testament, see, for example, Romans 5:1–5 and 1 Peter 4. See also section II.6.

5:14–15; Sirach 38:1–15). The prophets command care for the sick and rebuke the people and the leaders when they fail to do so (Ezekiel 34:1–4). Jesus expected that his followers would be involved in healing and in the care for the sick (Matthew 10:5–8; 25:31–46; Luke 9:1–6). In the epistles of St. Paul, healing is spoken of as one of the gifts of the Spirit (1 Corinthians 12:9–10, 29–30). In the biblical accounts, giving care to those in need is an important pathway for healing. Healing can take place when material needs are met, when physical wounds are healed, when food and sustenance are provided, when someone is given rest. Healing also can take place when we help address emotional wounds or help restore relationships. Healing can take place when someone's existential or spiritual struggles are being addressed or when a person is helped in their decisions to do what is right or in their growth in character. Each of these things helps restore the health of the person. We restore the health of the person when we care for others. Such care can also be a form of love. Such care can strengthen the relationship between the caregiver and the recipient of that care. That love, that strengthening of the relationship, that deepening of community is a form of healing.

Such caring for and loving of others also helps fulfill one's calling as a person. It constitutes a restoration to life as God intended. The act of loving others, of providing for their needs, of bringing healing to the world also brings healing and restoration to the caregiver (see sections III.2b and III.2c).

Moreover, those acts of love that the Christian and the Church carry out not only fulfill the call to love and thereby bring the Christian and the Church closer to God's intent, they can also constitute an experience of God. God in Christ is mysteriously encountered in the person in need. In serving the person in need, one is in some respect serving Christ himself. In his teaching on appearing before God in judgement, Jesus instructed his listeners: "All the nations will be gathered before him, and he will separate people one from another as a shepherd separates the sheep from the goats, and he will put the sheep at his right hand and the goats at the left. Then the king will say to those at his right hand, 'Come, you that are blessed by my Father, inherit the kingdom prepared for you from the foundation of the world; for I was hungry and you gave me food, I was thirsty and you gave me something to drink, I was a stranger and you welcomed me, I was naked and you gave me clothing, I was sick and you took care of me, I was in prison and you visited me.' Then the righteous will answer him, 'Lord, when was it that we saw you hungry and gave you food, or thirsty and gave you something to drink? And when was it that we saw you a stranger and welcomed you, or naked and gave you clothing? And when was it that we saw you sick or in prison and visited you?' And the king will answer them, 'Truly I tell you, just as you did it to one of the least of these who are members of my family, you did it to me'" (Matthew 25:32–40). Christ, in solidarity with the world, identifies with the "least of these." Care for those in need, for their material and spiritual needs, is an experience of caring for Christ himself. By bringing healing and a message of salvation to the world, the Christian and the Church are healed. They are healed by being restored to life as God intended and they are healed by an encounter with God himself.

3.4j. Healing comes through the work of medicine.

Restoring bodily health is the primary domain of medicine. The practice of medicine provides healing to the body. Medicine aims at restoring the parts and systems of the body to their normal functioning or mitigating the malfunction when full restoration is not possible. Through various interventions, therapies, surgeries, prescriptions, and medications, the practice of medicine can help restore the body to its normal functioning.[33] Public health efforts have the primary role in preventing ill health, and medicine has the primary role in restoration from ill health,[34] and both are important and contribute to preservation and restoration.

---

33. Of course medicine will also work in conjunction with other forms of and pathways to healing. This is applicable generally but perhaps especially so in the practice of psychiatry. See Kheriaty (2012) for discussion of various biological, psychological, and spiritual pathways to healing for depression.

34. See Rozier (2017, 2020) for some discussion of how and why the Church has been more involved in the work of medicine than in public health efforts and for an argument that the Church could play a stronger role. However, as noted throughout this present section and as documented in considerable empirical evidence (see footnote 7 above and footnote 12 in section III.7), the Church makes a considerable contribution to population health in that, by carrying out its primary spiritual and religious functions, it brings about the maintenance and restoration of both bodily health and health of the person. Nevertheless, there are further opportunities to expand the role of the Church beyond medicine to more substantially engage with public health. See also section III.7b.

Medicine uses science, knowledge, and reason to promote human health, and these require human intellect and creativity. These also may be viewed as given by God. Much of the work of medicine makes use of the body's remarkable ability to often heal on its own.[35] Medicine often helps facilitate or guides and directs such healing.[36] However, the capacity of the body to heal is a gift from God in the goodness that God created. Many theological accounts of medicine thus picture the clinician working with God to bring about healing.[37]

Giving care to those in need is an important pathway for healing. It is one that the Church is to engage in, empower, and facilitate. The emergence of hospitals in the West largely arose from the hospitality and the care of those in need by the Church and by monasteries.[38] Many hospitals have since been founded by religious institutions and orders and much of medical care throughout the world is provided by religious hospitals and medical mission efforts.[39] The work of medicine is an important pathway to bodily healing that is facilitated by and empowered by the work of the Church. The Church is to bring healing and the message of salvation to the world. That work includes both the healing of souls and the healing of bodies.

> *Propositional Summary 3.4: The Church and its members are both agents and recipients of healing, and that healing comes about by means of communal life, forgiveness, prayer, fasting, the sacraments, growth in character, and the care of others, including the work of medicine.*
> 3.4a. The Church is called to bring healing and the message of salvation to the world.
> 3.4b. The Christian is called to bring healing and the message of salvation to the world.
> 3.4c. Healing comes through community life.
> 3.4d. Healing comes through forgiveness.

---

35. Aquinas (1274/1920, 1.3.157); Gadamer (1996, chapter 8).

36. Aquinas argues that "many are healed by the operation of nature without the art of medicine. In these things that can be done both by art and nature, art imitates nature" (1274/1920, 1.2.75).

37. Larchet (2002); Balboni and Balboni (2018).

38. See, for example, Crislip (2005), Ferngren (2016), Balboni and Balboni (2018), Miller (1997), Porterfield (2005), Avalos (1999).

39. Mwenda (2011); Idler (2014a); Olivier et al. (2015).

3.4e. Healing comes through prayer.
3.4f. Healing comes through fasting.
3.4g. Healing comes through the sacraments.
- 3.4g.i. Healing comes through the Eucharist.
- 3.4g.ii. Healing comes through baptism.
- 3.4g.iii. Healing comes through confirmation of faith.
- 3.4g.iv. Healing comes through the sacrament of reconciliation.
- 3.4g.v. Healing comes through the anointing of the sick.
- 3.4g.vi. Healing comes through marriage.
- 3.4g.vii. Healing comes through ordination to the priesthood.

3.4h. Healing comes through growth in character.
3.4i. Healing comes through the care of others.
- 3.4i.i. The care of others can bring health and healing through the provision of material needs, the addressing of wounds and disease, the meeting of spiritual and emotional needs, and through the experience of love.
- 3.4i.ii. Care and healing constitute acts of love and bring healing and wholeness to the person providing care.
- 3.4i.iii. The Christian experiences Christ in the other when caring for those in need.

3.4j. Healing comes through the work of medicine.
- 3.4j.i. Wounds and disease can be healed by the practice of medicine.
- 3.4j.ii. The practice of medicine is facilitated by God in his creating the body's natural capacity to heal and in granting human intellect and creativity endowed by God.
- 3.4j.iii. The Church is to empower and facilitate the practice of medicine.

III.5. The Limits of Healing

Proposition 3.5. There are limits to healing in this life, but healing in relation to God can come about in the midst of and sometimes even through ill health.

3.5a. Salvation does not, in this life, free the body from illness and death.

There are limits to healing in this life. The practice of medicine, the restoration of relationships, participation in community, a right orientation to life and character, and better practices can all help bring about healing of the person and of the body. However, there are limits to this healing. Diseases are still manifest, aging still takes place, infirmity sets in, and eventually all still face death. Salvation, the deliverance from sin and its consequences, is a process. Because that process is not complete in this life, because sin and its consequences still persist, so also does ill health. All do still eventually face ill health and death. There are thus limits to the healing that takes place in this life. These limits must be accepted with humility, but also in hope that a fuller restoration and fulfillment of health will eventually come.

3.5b. Salvation in this life gradually, but not completely, frees the person from sin.

Salvation, the deliverance from sin and its consequences, is a process. Freedom from sin and its effects does not take place fully in this life.[1] By the help of God's grace, there can be an increasingly greater conformity to God's will and intent. By means of prayer, a right orientation to God,

---
1. The Catholic doctrine of purgatory concerns the further transformation of the will and of the human person that is needed after the present life is over before there can be full communion with God. See also section III.6e.

repentance, the work of the Spirit, participation in communal life and a receiving of the sacraments, the Christian is assisted in this freedom from sin. Yet sin and its consequences still persist in this life. Perfection is not entirely achieved. The sins of others are present, often prompting sin within ourselves. Although there can be growth and an increasing freedom from sin, the process never seems to be brought to full completion in this life. In his Epistle to the Romans, St. Paul wrote of this experience of struggling with sin: "So I find it to be a law that when I want to do what is good, evil lies close at hand. For I delight in the law of God in my inmost self, but I see in my members another law at war with the law of my mind, making me captive to the law of sin that dwells in my members. Wretched man that I am! Who will rescue me from this body of death? Thanks be to God through Jesus Christ our Lord! So then, with my mind I am a slave to the law of God, but with my flesh I am a slave to the law of sin" (Romans 7:7–25), and later, "We ourselves, who have the first fruits of the Spirit, groan inwardly while we wait for adoption, the redemption of our bodies. For in hope we were saved. Now hope that is seen is not hope. For who hopes for what is seen? But if we hope for what we do not see, we wait for it with patience" (Romans 8). There is a struggle for freedom from sin. That freedom is brought about here and now through Jesus Christ and is aided by God's grace and the work of Jesus through the Spirit and the life of the Church. Through God's work in Jesus Christ, the Spirit, and the Church, the ultimate conclusion of this work has been secured, and yet here and now that process is ongoing. There is an aspect of salvation that is already present and an aspect that has not yet fully been attained. However, we are in some sense becoming who we will ultimately be. There is hope that freedom will be brought to completion through the work of Jesus Christ in the life to come, but there appear to be limits to that freedom from sin in the world at present. In this life, we are gradually, but not completely, freed from sin and its consequences.

3.5c. Salvation does not, in this life, completely free the Church from sin.

If the individual is not fully freed from sin in this life, it follows that the Church, which is constituted by its members, will also not be free from sin. The wrong actions of individuals—actions contrary to God's intent, contrary to love—will be manifest in the life of the Church and will influence the life of the Church, both as it pertains to the community of its members and in its relations with the world.

History testifies to the ways the Church has failed to live up to the standard of love to which it is called and to which it is to call others. Although contributing enormous good in the promotion of both temporal and eternal flourishing, the Church and its members have also sometimes wrongly brought about harms. There have been instances of violence, of abuse, of injustice. These cause harm to victims and to the Church's witness and its message of love. The recent abuse scandals within the Church have caused considerable harm to victims and have led many to withdraw from participation in the life of the Church. Such wrongs need to be addressed. Although there will inevitably be sin in individuals' lives, that sin cannot and ought not be sanctioned by the Church. When sin and harm are left unaddressed, it is more likely to be perpetuated and is more likely to be perceived as having the Church as its source. This damages the message of the Church and its role as an agent of healing. Thus, while sin will persist in this life, it cannot be left unaddressed.

3.5d. The Church, as an agent of healing, must seek to limit the presence and influence of sin.

Although sin will persist, the Church, as an agent of healing, must seek to limit its presence, spread, and influence. The disciplinary practices taught by Jesus (Matthew 18), and embedded in the life of the Church in various ways, are essential for limiting sin and its consequences and ensuring that the Church's ministry of healing and its message of love and of God's salvation in Jesus Christ are preserved. Such discipline may range from private rebuke to public rebuke to expulsion or excommunication from the Church. Importantly, even such discipline is to be done out of love—love of God and love of one's neighbor.[2] Love of one's neighbor includes love for the victim and efforts to address the harm done. Love of one's neighbor also includes love of the community, love of those who might be directly harmed or morally scandalized if actions to prevent and address wrongdoing do not take place. Love of one's neighbor also requires preventive action.

---

2. Aquinas (1274/1920, II.II.33).

Love of one's neighbor also involves love for the perpetrator. That does not preclude and may indeed entail discipline and punishment. Discipline and punishment may help prevent the perpetrator from taking further wrong action, protecting both future victims and the perpetrator from committing further evil. Such discipline can also be the means of repentance, correction, and change for the perpetrator. In Jesus's teaching on discipline (Matthew 18), if someone is privately and publicly rebuked and still will not change, Jesus comments, "let such a one be to you as a Gentile and a tax collector" and yet in Jesus's own ministry these were often precisely the individuals with whom he spent his time, trying to help them alter their patterns of thinking and behavior. If someone persists in wrong in spite of public and private rebuke, the attitude toward him or her is not to be hatred but rather a sober realization that such a person is effectively no longer acting as part of the Church community and is in need of the message of God's salvation in Jesus Christ and of repentance. And when such repentance occurs, the response is to be one of forgiveness, even if there is not a full restoration to the person's original role or office or place within the community.

The attitude toward someone who persistently does wrong is thus to continue to be one of love even in the midst of discipline. It is by such discipline, carried out in love, that it is possible to limit the presence and influence of sin, even as sin continues to persist in various forms in the lives of individuals and communities. Love, even in the midst of discipline, will help prevent sin and hatred from spreading. It will also help preserve trust in the healing ministry of the Church. It will help the Church continue its important work as an agent of healing through its communal life, forgiveness, prayer, fasting, the sacraments, and the care of others. The Church limits the presence and influence of sin by ensuring discipline, by loving in the midst of that discipline, and by carrying out its ministry of healing to those harmed, even to the perpetrators of those harms, in love.

3.5e. Even in the midst of ill health and suffering, there can be personal growth and healing.

Even in the midst of ill health and of sin, there can be growth in character, growth in communion with God, and growth in healing as persons.

Often ill health and suffering can bring about a growth in character. As we try to act rightly and seek God even in the midst of ill health, our character and resolve are strengthened, our fortitude is increased, we develop a temperance and a capacity to forgo pleasure, our sense of justice and humility can be strengthened, and we can develop practical wisdom. Moreover, as we confront our limitations, we also turn to God. As we struggle with ill health and suffering, our desires are set more firmly, in hope, upon the life to come. As the things of this world cease to please, we become more and more devoted to friendship with God, to charity, to loving God and our neighbor. Ill health and suffering can bring a growth in character and thus a healing of the person.

3.5f. Even in the midst of ill health and sin, there can be a greater communion with God.

Moreover, even our struggles with sin can sometimes bring about a greater communion with God. Our struggles with sin and the seeming limits of what we can attain can bring about a greater humility.[3] Our struggles with sin, and the realization that we cannot free ourselves from sin on our own, help us turn to God in greater dependence and with a sense of greater need.[4] Our struggles with sin lead us to turn to God in prayer. Our struggles with sin and our repentance and our turning away from sin further open us to the work of the Spirit, of the Church, and of the sacraments in order to empower us to seek God more fully with all our hearts. That pattern of struggle, of growth, and, in humility, the realization of our limits increases our dependence, our trust, our faith, and our hope in God's action and work in our lives. That pattern can bring about a greater charity, a greater friendship and communion with God.

In some sense, then, God triumphs even in the midst of sin and ill health. God uses even sin and ill health, that which has come about because of free action contrary to his will, to bring about healing, to bring

---

3. Aquinas notes that sin can offer the opportunity to repent and rid oneself of pride (II.II.162.6).

4. St. Paul concluded his exposition on struggles with sin (Romans 7:14–25) with "Who will rescue me from this body of death? Thanks be to God through Jesus Christ our Lord!" (Romans 7:24–25).

about greater conformity to his will. St. Paul wrote in his Epistle to the Romans, even after his discussion of the struggles with sin: "We know that all things work together for good for those who love God, who are called according to his purpose.... Neither death, nor life, nor angels, nor rulers, nor things present, nor things to come, nor powers, nor height, nor depth, nor anything else in all creation, will be able to separate us from the love of God in Christ Jesus our Lord" (Romans 8:18–39). God works in all things—even in our struggles with sin—to bring about a fuller restoration to himself, a fuller conformity to his intent, a fuller communion with himself.[5]

3.5g. Those with faith in Jesus Christ are to hope for a fuller restoration and fulfillment of wholeness in the life to come.

Although we are faced with limits to healing in this life, limits to our freedom from sin and its consequences, nevertheless there is still hope.[6] There is hope for growth and healing as a person even in the midst of ill health and suffering. There is hope for a greater communion with God even in the midst of ill health and sin. There is hope for the restraining of evil and the promotion of good. There is hope also for a more final restoration in the life to come—of oneself, of others, and of creation.[7] The

---

5. Concerning Romans 8:28 and God working all things for the good, Augustine comments that, for the elect, God ultimately works "even sins" to their advantage (Augustine, 426/427, chapter 24); cf. Aquinas (1274/1920, III.89.2.ad 1).

6. In Aquinas's writings, hope as a passion is understood as a "movement of the appetitive power ensuing from the apprehension of a future good, difficult but possible to obtain; namely, a stretching forth of the appetite to such a good" (1274/1920, I.II.40.2). Aquinas also considers hope to be one of the three theological virtues (I.II.62). Concerning hope as a theological virtue, Aquinas comments, "Wherever we find a good human act, it must correspond to some human virtue.... Now the act of hope, whereof we speak now, attains God. For, as we have already stated (I-II:40:1), when we were treating of the passion of hope, the object of hope is a future good, difficult but possible to obtain... in so far as we hope for anything as being possible to us by means of the Divine assistance, our hope attains God Himself, on Whose help it leans" (II.II.17.1). The theological virtue of hope might thus be understood as the habit of having the will moved toward God by the apprehension of the future difficult but possible good that is God.

7. See Aquinas (1274/1920, II.II.17.3) on our hope for the eternal happiness of others with whom we are united in love. St. Paul spoke of the hope of a restoration of creation, of setting it "free from its bondage to decay" (Romans 8:19–23).

Christian message is one of healing and salvation. It is a message received in faith and lived out in love. It is also a message of hope.[8] Our faith leads to our hope that evil will not have the last word and that in the midst of our struggles and in the midst of the limitations we face at present, a fuller restoration to and even fulfillment of wholeness lies ahead.[9] The complete fulfillment of health is a completion of the wholeness of the person, bringing about a full communion with God. But the attaining of that for which we hope cannot be accomplished on our own. Our hope requires the action of God—action that has taken place and will take place by Jesus Christ and in the work of the Spirit. We cannot obtain that for which we hope without God. The object of our hope is thus both a full communion with God and God as the agent who will bring this about.[10] As we face the limitations of this life, of sin, of suffering, of death, we can be tempted to despair.[11] Hope in God and hope for a better future sustains us.[12] It helps us along the way. It helps us to find growth amid suffering, to restrain evil whenever possible, to address the ills of this world, and to wait patiently for God's final action.

---

8. Aquinas in several instances distinguishes hope from charity. Both hope and charity relate to the will and to union with God (1274/1920, I.II.62.3, I.II.66.6). However, charity pertains to adhering to God for God's sake, while hope pertains to union with God for one's own sake. Charity additionally wills the divine good in the union with God (II.II.17.8). Hope regards this union as something principally future, whereas charity regards this union as both present and future (I.II.66.6). Charity regards the future union absolutely, whereas hope regards it under the aspect of difficulty and uncertainty (II.II.17.1, II.II.18.1). Whereas hope is principally for the desired end of union of the will with God, charity transforms the will to that end (I.II.62.3).

9. Aquinas (1274/1920, II.II.17.7–8).

10. Aquinas (1274/1920, II.II.17.1–2,7).

11. Pieper (1986) comments that it is only the theological virtue of hope, the object of which is God, that can properly be said to be a virtue. We otherwise might hope for things that are bad, or our hope might be without adequate grounds if our hope is not in God.

12. The empirical literature on hope suggests important effects of hope on various aspects of health and well-being (e.g., Long, Kim, et al., 2020). Much of this empirical literature in the field of psychology has been dominated by a conceptualization and measure of hope proposed by Snyder (2000). It is questionable whether Snyder's proposed approach captures hope even as a disposition, and its contrast with theological hope is notable (Kinghorn, 2013).

Propositional Summary 3.5: There are limits to healing in this life, but healing in relation to God can come about in the midst of and sometimes even through ill health.

3.5a. Salvation does not, in this life, free the body from illness and death.

3.5b. Salvation in this life gradually, but not completely, frees the person from sin.

3.5c. Salvation does not, in this life, completely free the Church from sin.

3.5d. The Church, as an agent of healing, must seek to limit the presence and influence of sin.

3.5e. Even in the midst of ill health and suffering, there can be personal growth and healing.

3.5f. Even in the midst of ill health and sin, there can be a greater communion with God

3.5g. Those with faith in Jesus Christ are to hope for a fuller restoration and fulfillment of wholeness in the life to come.

III.6. God, Resurrection, and Salvation

Proposition 3.6. The fulfillment of wholeness, a communion with God and a completion of God's intent, comes only in the resurrection in the life to come and will be accomplished by God.

3.6a. God has promised a full healing of and restoration of creation.

Although there are limits to healing in this life, God has promised a fulfillment of and a final restoration of all things to his intent. This is spoken of in various ways in the biblical accounts: as "resurrection of the dead" (1 Corinthians 15), as a "new heavens and a new earth" (Isaiah 65; 2 Peter 3; Revelation 21), as the ending of all "death . . . mourning . . . crying . . . pain" (Revelation 21). The biblical account suggests that this state of affairs concerns the future, although its anticipation and its partial realization at present are accomplished in the work of God and of the Church in ushering in the kingdom of God.[1] The final restoration and fulfillment to come is linked to an anticipated return of Jesus Christ. Christian theologies have pictured that return in various ways. Among theologies that picture a more literal return, the timing and relation of Jesus's return to full restoration are pictured differently. What is common throughout the Christian tradition, however, is a promise of restoration and fulfillment by God. In the description of that restoration and fulfillment provided in the final chapters of the book of Revelation, the author recounts a vision wherein Jesus declares, "See, I am making all things new" (Revelation 21:5). It is this making all things new, this restoration and fulfillment of all things to God's intent, this complete healing, that is the Christian hope.

---

1. The *Catechism of the Catholic Church* describes the Church as being given gifts of the Holy Spirit to fulfill her mission of proclaiming and establishing among all people the Kingdom of Christ and thus being the seed and the beginning of that kingdom (Catholic Church, 2000, 768, 1049).

3.6b. God's restoration of all creation will come about through Jesus Christ and is received by faith.

The promise of restoration and fulfillment of wholeness, of complete healing, is closely tied to the work of God in Jesus Christ. As described in section III.3, healing and the salvation of the human person are ultimately brought about by the life, death, and resurrection of Jesus Christ. Freedom from sin comes about through God taking on human nature in the person of Jesus Christ and thereby redeeming that nature. Salvation comes about by Jesus's providing a model of life lived in conformity to God's will, a life lived in love and his giving his life in love for us. Salvation comes about from Jesus's removing of sin and the doing away with our sinful nature in his death and by his restoring to us a new nature in his resurrection. Salvation comes about by his ruling over all things in his ascension and his empowering us by his Spirit and helping and healing us through the life and work of the Church. All of this God accomplishes in Jesus Christ to help conform our will to God and to prepare us for final healing and transformation that is to take place upon his return. God offers all of this as a free gift. This gift is received by faith, by trust in Jesus Christ. The restoration is partial in this life and is only brought about in full at the end of time in the return of Jesus Christ, in judgment and the establishing of justice, in the resurrection of the dead, the restoration of creation, and the subsequent perfect and eternal communion with God.

3.6c. God's restoration of all creation requires the establishing of justice and thus a judgment of good and evil.

The restoration of all things requires a recognition of what has been done for good and for evil and the establishment of a justice wherein all things are put right. The Christian teaching is that at the end of time, when Jesus Christ returns to restore all things, there will be a judgment.[2] Each person's actions will be exposed for what they are.[3] The good and the

---

2. Catholic Church (2000, 1038–1040); see also John 12:44–50.
3. Catholic Church (2000, 1021–1022); see also 1 Corinthians 3:12–15.

evil that each person has done will be made manifest before God to each person and to all (Matthew 25).

In principle, sin, voluntary deviation from God's intent, has separated the human person from God, and were it not for the work of Jesus Christ in his life, death, and resurrection, there would be nothing to bring about restoration. However, in Jesus Christ's life, death, and resurrection, sin and the corruption of human nature and the resulting separation from God are done away with. By our union with Christ, God brings about a restoration. Although a person's deeds, both good and evil, are manifest in judgment, because of the work of Jesus Christ, a person's sin no longer separates him or her from God.

However, while God's gift of grace is available to all who will receive it in faith, it must indeed be received. If it is definitively rejected, there is permanent separation from God. That permanent separation from God, that rejection of God's gift of grace and salvation, is what the Christian tradition understands as hell.[4] Sin is the voluntary deviation from God's intent. This sin has corrupted human nature and has led to separation from God. To be restored to God's intent, there must be a renewed nature and a freely coming to God in love, a receiving of his gift of restoration and of grace.[5] Without that turning to God, it is not possible to be present with God forever in love. Without receiving the gift of God's grace, there is permanent separation from God. When one receives God's grace in Jesus Christ through faith, there is deliverance from sin and its consequences, a restoration and fulfillment of God's intent and subsequently a communion with God forever.

However, our deeds in this life are not irrelevant. They affect others. They can cause harm, but they can also bring others love and joy. The final judgment is one that both makes deeds of the past manifest but also sets things right.[6] It is ultimately an establishing of justice, a justice that is both judged by, and made right by, by Jesus Christ.[7]

---

4. Catholic Church (2000, 1033, 1035, 1037); see also 1 John 3:14–5; Matthew 5:22, 29, 10:28, 13:42, 50.

5. See Aquinas (1274/1920, I.II.109.5–7).

6. See Case (2021) for an exposition of the importance of accountability in the final judgment and in our interactions in human life more generally.

7. See Benedict XVI (2007, 43–44).

3.6d. God will bring about a final and perfect bodily health in the resurrection of the dead.

The restoration to health and the fulfillment of wholeness of the human body is brought about in and depicted as the resurrection of the dead. The Christian belief is that following Jesus Christ's crucifixion, God raised him from the dead on the third day after his death. This resurrected body is pictured as a transformed body but with similarity to and in continuity with Jesus's body prior to death (Luke 24:39; John 20:25–27). The biblical reflection on Jesus's resurrection and the Christian's union with Jesus by God's taking on human nature in Jesus Christ suggest that Jesus's resurrection ensures the resurrection of those who are united with him (Romans 6; 1 Corinthian 15).[8] St. Paul depicted the resurrected body as one that is imperishable, glorious, powerful, and spiritual, a body that resembles Jesus's resurrected body; he depicts it as a body that is transformed and immortal and is no longer subject to death (1 Corinthians 15). It is a body that is fully restored to health, to wholeness. Thus, in the final chapter of the book of Revelation, the author writes that because of this restoration and transformation, "death will be no more" and "mourning and crying and pain will be no more" (Revelation 21:4). In the resurrection of the dead, God will bring about a final and more perfect health of the body, a life everlasting.

3.6e. God will bring about a fulfillment of healing of the person and complete freedom from sin.

Along with the resurrection of the body, full restoration of health will include complete freedom from sin. That deliverance from sin is understood as the consequence of the work of God in Jesus Christ through the Spirit. As discussed in section III.3, the deliverance from sin and its consequences are depicted in Saint Paul's writings as being accomplished by the union of the Christian with Jesus Christ in his death on the cross (Romans 5–6). In Jesus's death, Jesus took our nature and sin upon himself,

---

8. Aquinas (1274/1920, III.56.1). See Craig (2000), Wright (2012), Pannenberg (2013), and VanderWeele (2017e) for arguments supporting the historicity of the resurrection.

and did away with it. In the resurrection, our nature is transformed to what God ultimately intended. In this life, freedom from sin arises further from the work of the Spirit and the Church, through our cooperation with God's grace and our efforts to live a life more as God intended, through prayer and communal life and love, and through the sacraments (see section III.4). Gradually we are freed from sin and we more closely conform to what it is that God intended.

However, final deliverance from sin awaits the resurrection of the dead and the new resurrected body and nature that accompanies it.[9] A transformation occurs that frees us at last to avoid sin, to freely conform in every way to God's will. That transformation is a gift of God's grace that we freely receive in faith.[10]

How it is that at the end of this life we are not yet entirely freed from sin and yet in the resurrected life we are thus restored is understood differently in different parts of the Christian tradition. It is clear that further purification or transformation is required. Some understand the resurrected body as accomplishing that final transformation. The Catholic doctrine of purgatory concerns the further transformation of the will and of the human person that is needed after the present life is over before there can be complete communion with God. Purgatory is the accomplishing of that transformation and the purification of the will so that it can freely choose to be present with God forever.[11]

The final state that is accomplished by God is in the end a complete freedom from sin. It is a state united with God in Jesus Christ in love. In contemplating this final state, the author of the first Epistle of St. John wrote: "Beloved, we are God's children now; what we will be has not yet been revealed. What we do know is this: when he is revealed, we will be like him, for we will see him as he is. And all who have this hope in him purify themselves, just as he is pure" (1 John 3:2–3). Our final state is the full healing of the person, the restoration and fulfillment of the human person to God's intent, in full conformity to God's will, and thus with full freedom from sin.

---

9. Aquinas (1274/1920, III.56.2).

10. Aquinas (1274/1920, I.II.113); see also Philippians 3:20–21; 1 Corinthians 15:20–28.

11. Catholic Church (2000, 1030–1032); see also 1 Corinthians 3:15; 1 Peter 1:7.

3.6f. God will bring about a full restoration and transformation of all of creation.

The Biblical and Christian tradition also affirms that God will restore and transform all of creation, that he will create a "new heavens and a new earth" (Revelation 21).[12] The images provided for this are diverse and, perhaps of necessity, all metaphorical or visionary. Communal celebration is consistent among the images provided. The new creation is sometimes pictured as a banquet (Matthew 25) or as a city (Revelation 21). The celebration is sometimes pictured as a wedding or wedding feast (Matthew 25; Revelation 21), and as a union between Christ and the Church (Ephesians 5). This union will include a unity among people and union with God. The restoration of all creation thus includes the fulfillment of community, the establishing of perfect communal well-being with peace among all people and peace and union with God.

Many of the prophetic passages in the Old Testament are interpreted within Christian theology as pertaining to this restoration and fulfillment. The ruler of this renewed community is interpreted as being Jesus Christ, who will usher in a new era of peace (Isaiah 11). All of creation will be transformed so that the "wolf shall live with the lamb . . . the leopard shall lie down with the kid, the calf and the lion . . . together" (Isaiah 11:6–8). In St. Paul's Epistle to the Romans, the whole creation is described as awaiting this restoration from the corruption brought about by sin: "For the creation waits with eager longing . . . for the creation was subjected to futility, not of its own will but by the will of the one who subjected it, in hope that the creation will be set free from its bondage to decay and will obtain the freedom of the glory of the children of God. We know that the whole creation has been groaning in labor pains until now" (Romans 8:19–23). The ultimate fate of creation is intimately tied to that of the human community. Human sin caused disruption and corruption of creation, but the full restoration, healing, and fulfillment of the human person will be accompanied by the restoration and transformation of all of God's creation.

---

12. Catholic Church (2000, 1043–1047); see also Romans 8:19–23. For discussion of the "cosmic" dimension of salvation and its relation to health, in Christianity and in other religions, see Tillich (1981).

3.6g. God will be fully present, and there will be full communion with God.

The transformation of the human body and the human person, the complete deliverance from sin and its consequences, will also allow for full and eternal communion with God.[13] This is the life of heaven. God's salvation, God's grace, and the free receiving of that gift of grace by faith allow the human person to forever choose to be with God and to be in accord with God's will and love.[14] Sin, that which separates the human person from God by voluntary deviation from God's will, will be no more. The mystery of salvation is the accomplishing of this transformation in Jesus Christ by the work of the Spirit. However, with this accomplished, a complete, full, final, and everlasting communion with God is then possible. That final state, that full restoration to the wholeness of the body and of the person, is beyond full comprehension. St. Paul wrote, "no eye has seen, nor ear heard, nor the human heart conceived, what God has prepared for those who love him" (1 Corinthians 2:9). However, that final state of blessedness, of wholeness, of eternal flourishing, that final state that is not fully comprehensible, will include a full communion with God. In the final chapter, the author of the book of Revelation writes, "And I heard a loud voice from the throne saying, 'See, the home of God is among mortals. He will dwell with them; they will be his peoples, and God himself will be with them" (Revelation 21:3). This final communion with God is described in various ways in Christian theology; for example, as a union with God, or as a complete and perfect vision of God, a loving gazing upon God's beauty.[15] There is a full healing and a full restoration to and completion of God's intent. But this salvation extends beyond restoration.[16] It is a fulfillment of wholeness as God intended, a complete attainment of all that is good. It is a participation in God's goodness, a participation, in some sense, in God's own flourishing. This is the final end of the human person as intended by God, to be fully with God in love.

---

13. Catholic Church (2000, 1023–1027).
14. Catholic Church (2000, 1029); Aquinas (1274/1920, I.II.62.3).
15. Aquinas (1274/1920, I.II.3.8, I.II.5.7, II.II.180.1); Catholic Church (2000, 360, 1028, 1045); Pieper (1998). See also 1 John 3:2.
16. Aquinas (1274/1920, I.II.109.3, I.II.109.5, I.II.114.2).

Propositional Summary 3.6: The fulfillment of wholeness, a communion with God and a complete restoration to God's intent, comes only in the resurrection in the life to come and will be accomplished by God.

3.6a. God has promised a full healing of and restoration of creation.

3.6b. God's restoration of all creation will come about through Jesus Christ and is received by faith.

3.6c. God's restoration of all creation requires the establishing of justice and thus a judgment of good and evil.

3.6d. God will bring about a final and more perfect bodily health in the resurrection of the dead.

3.6e. God will bring about a fulfillment of healing of the person and complete freedom from sin.

3.6f. God will bring about a full restoration and transformation of all of creation.

3.6g. God will be fully present, and there will be full communion with God.

III.7. The Implications of Healing and Salvation

The previous section concluded with a vision of restoration to wholeness for all things, a vision that Christians believe will ultimately be accomplished by God. Yet the difficulties and struggles of the present life continue. We continue to face and struggle with ill health. In the midst of these difficulties and struggles, we seek healing and restoration and wholeness. We seek to bring healing of the body through the practice of medicine. We seek to prevent ill health by good public policy and public health measures. We seek to bring about the wholeness of the person that is human flourishing. We seek to love others well. In considering this search for wholeness in the present life with an eye also toward more ultimate horizons, this section will consider the implications of an understanding of healing as a full restoration to wholeness of the body and of the person. Although some of the insights here arise most clearly from considerations of Christian theology and a Christian vision of full restoration, these insights are perhaps of importance and interest in more pluralistic contexts. Many of the aims for the restoration of health and for the healing of persons and for flourishing are shared across traditions, perspectives, and cultures and we can seek them together. This concluding implications section will explore various psychological, social, and spiritual pathways to health and healing; the critical role of community in healing; the possibilities for partnerships between religious communities and public health communities in promoting health; the possibility of promoting forgiveness, love, and character development at local, national, and international scales; the need for love to ensure the highest attainable standard of health; and the importance of freedom, the pursuit of truth, and respectful exchange as different communities contemplate and share what they consider their most important and ultimate goals and ends.

3.7a. Medicine and public health need to pay greater attention to psychological, social, and spiritual pathways to health and healing.

Medicine and public health institutions have developed an array of approaches to promoting health and healing. On the side of prevention, some of this is focused on health behaviors: having a good diet, getting exercise, having enough sleep and rest, not smoking, and so forth. Public health efforts extend in critical ways to community-level approaches and interventions related to sanitation, mitigating air pollution, ensuring access to clean water, and providing vaccinations. Medicine has furthermore developed a vast range of surgical, pharmacological, biologic, radiation, or physical therapies that are useful in bringing healing to address a host of diseases. This work of public health and of medicine has advanced population health in astounding ways.

However, this success has led to a neglect of other psychological, social, and spiritual pathways to health and healing. Evidence clearly suggests that positive psychological states such as having a sense of purpose contribute to physical health and longevity, that social connectedness and community contribute to both physical and mental health, and that attending religious services contributes to a host of positive physical, mental, psychological, and social outcomes.[1] Although these psychological, social, and spiritual outcomes do not principally fall within the purview of medicine and public health, these various other pathways should be considered important health resources and assets because of their profound effects on health outcomes. There should be an awareness of their importance and of their role in a patient's life in the context of medicine; and efforts should be made to support and promote these other pathways when appropriate. Not to do so is to neglect important pathways to health and healing. Although medical and public health efforts can continue to focus on more material and physical pathways, there

---

1. See, for example, Martín-María et al. (2017), Hernandez et al. (2018), Trudel-Fitzgerald et al. (2019), and Steptoe (2019) for reviews of empirical evidence for the effects of psychological states; Berkman et al. (2014) and Holt-Lunstad et al. (2015) for social connectedness; and Chida et al. (2009), Koenig et al. (2023), Idler (2014b), VanderWeele (2017a, 2017c), and Balboni et al. (2022) for attending religious services.

needs to be greater awareness of and attention paid to the various other psychological, social, and spiritual pathways to health and healing if the institutions of medicine and public health are to most effectively serve the health of the public. As described in the sections that follow, the institutions of public health and medicine might better promote these various psychological, social, and spiritual pathways to healing in numerous ways.

3.7b. Institutions of public health and medicine should partner with religious communities to promote health and healing.

Religious communities can contribute substantially to the promotion of physical health, and that goal could be further advanced if the institutions of public health and medicine more often partnered with religious communities in their work. Some of the contribution religious communities make to physical and mental health comes through the life of the religious community itself, through social support, a common purpose, a sense of hope, and shared set of values and healthy behaviors. However, religious communities often contribute to physical and mental health in numerous other ways, including to those both within and outside of the community, by means such as soup kitchens and food pantries, Alcoholics Anonymous meetings, financial and material assistance, and the provision of health care. Religious groups have often also provided material resources and infrastructure for hospitals, clinics, and medical missions.[2] Such work and activities effectively carry out the calling to love one's neighbor. Religious communities that provide such services are effectively allies in the promotion of health and healing and should be appreciated as part of the public health and medical landscape.

---

2. Most nineteenth-century homes for the aged in the United States were started by Christian and Jewish religious groups. As late as the mid-twentieth century, most remained religious (Maves, 1960). L'Arche communities for the disabled had religious origins (see Idler, 2014a). A relatively recent report (Brown, 2014) indicated that the Catholic Church, as one of the largest global health care providers, operated 5,246 hospitals, 17,530 dispensaries, 577 leprosy clinics, and 15,208 houses for the chronically ill and handicapped worldwide. In a number of African countries, it is estimated that faith-based organizations provide from 30 to 50 percent of health-related facilities (Mwenda, 2011).

Research has also been conducted on religious communities as settings for pursing health promotion activities.[3] These activities include promoting healthy diets, breastfeeding, cancer screening programs, exercise groups, and vaccination programs and providing mental health services and church-based health promotion/prevention programs for diabetes, maternal and child health, and hypertension.[4] Having such efforts take place in the context of religious communities has the advantages of including a physical space to meet in, a network of existing relationships, and a sense of trust. These things can be of considerable value when promoting public health programs or trying to expand the reach of clinical care. Religious communities that are grounded in the love of others—the love of neighbor—often have a service-oriented focus that can be useful in reaching out to those outside the religious community and that has the potential to further facilitate clinical and public health promotion efforts. Partnerships between religious communities and medical and public health institutions thus have considerable potential to advance the goals of health and healing.

Religious groups have also provided a powerful moral message and advocacy in the context of public health. Important examples include the role of religious institutions in civil rights advocacy in the

---

3. In the literature on health-promoting interventions in religious contexts, a distinction is sometimes drawn between "faith-based" and "faith-placed" interventions, the former involving some sort of spiritual or religious approach and the latter indicating that the intervention is merely taking place at a religious institution (DeHaven et al., 2004; see also Lasater et al., 1997). Much of the literature on these interventions is descriptive. There is a much smaller literature on empirically assessing the effectiveness of such interventions (Campbell et al., 2007). Many of the studies that have an evaluative component have been conducted in African American churches. There is evidence from various randomized trials that interventions can increase fruit and vegetable consumption, lead to smoking cessation, and perhaps promote weight loss and increase cancer screening (see Chatters, 2000; Allen et al., 2014). Campbell et al. (2007) discuss five important elements of the design of such interventions: cultivating true partnerships and trust, forming accurate membership lists, understanding the social and environmental context of the religious community when designing the intervention, incorporating the appropriate spiritual/religious content and involving community members in delivery of services, and leaving something behind, e.g. providing training, leaving materials behind, or helping churches find funding to continue the program. See also Evans (1999) for healing ministries within churches.

4. Idler (2014a) discusses in detail a number of such partnerships. See also Levin (2014, 2016), Idler et al. (2019), Olivier et al. (2006), and Chatters (2000).

United States,[5] in the Truth and Reconciliation Commission in South Africa,[6] and in community advocacy concerning the link between environmental pollution and leukemia in Massachusetts.[7] The Church has a powerful moral message concerning the importance of care for the poor, of promoting the common good, and of advocating for love and solidarity.[8] Public health institutions can partner with the Church to more powerfully convey these important moral teachings.

The responsibility for attaining greater partnership extends in both directions. Medical and public health institutions should seek ways that clinical and population health can be advanced by partnering with religious institutions, and the Church and other religious institutions should seek greater partnerships and find ways to contribute to medical and public health efforts. As noted above and in section III.4j, over centuries, religious institutions have provided medical care and have established hospitals and clinics for care. However, the role of the Church and other religious institutions in public health has arguably been somewhat weaker than in medicine.[9] New partnerships ought to be sought and the Church should continue to act as an agent of healing both through its own community life and practices and through the resources it can bring to aid public health efforts.

Although there have been some very effective partnerships between religious groups and public health institutions, there have also been tensions. Examples include questions about handling the spread of HIV/AIDS, distributing condoms, access to abortion, and religious meetings during the COVID-19 pandemic.[10] There have also been important

---

5. Morris (1986).
6. Tutu (2000).
7. Van Ness (1999); Harr (1996).
8. Catholic Church (2004, chapter 4). See also Rozier (2020) for some discussion concerning the potential role Catholic social teaching might play in global public health.
9. See Rozier (2017, 2020) for some discussion of why the Church has perhaps historically been more engaged in medicine than in public health efforts and for further reflections on what might be possible going forward.
10. See Levin et al. (2021) for discussion of various issues related to religious communities during the COVID-19 pandemic. An example with a much longer history is the role of religious organizations in providing care for HIV/AIDS patients. Within the United States, some Christian commentary suggested that AIDS was a divine punishment for the sins of homosexuality, adultery, or premarital or

examples of partnerships between religious communities and public health institutions that have persisted even in the midst of irreconcilable tensions because the participating groups perceived that continuing with such partnerships and navigating the disagreements was important for the promotion of health.[11] Although tensions might in principle be circumvented in clinical settings by the development of tradition-specific practices as discussed in section I.7d, such options are often not available with regard to public health and public policy in pluralistic contexts. Finding ways to navigate tensions and different understandings of the good and of human well-being will be important for the fullest promotion of health. Future work on developing guidelines, principles, and approaches to advancing the goals of health through partnerships even in the midst of tensions would be a valuable contribution.

The principal goal of religious communities is generally not physical health. As discussed in section III.7j, religious communities should be

---

extramarital sex. It has been argued that this may have affected government funding and policy (Dalmida and Thurman, 2014). However, faith-based hospitals also provided much of the care early in the epidemic and provided considerable institutional support. In the United States, the Episcopal Church sponsored a national AIDS-related faith gathering in 1986. In 1989, various Catholic programs came together in the United States as the National Catholic AIDS Network. In the 1990s, an AIDS National Interfaith Network was formed in the United States. Globally, early faith-based efforts focused on care and support for those with HIV/AIDS, but later programs have focused more on education and prevention (Derose et al., 2011). There is some evidence that faith-based organizations may have at first contributed to increasing discrimination and stigmatization in Uganda, but such groups later made important contributions to decreasing discrimination and stigmatization (Otolok-Tanga et al., 2007). Religious groups have focused more on providing care, raising awareness, and testing.

11. An example of one such partnership is that between the Catholic Church and Brazil's National AIDS Program (Murray et al., 2011). The use of condoms was one of the most important controversies in this regard. Public health groups advocated for their use in preventing the spread of HIV, but religious groups sometimes advocated against condom use, arguing either that they encourage more promiscuous sexual activity or that they are wrong in and of themselves. See Murray et al. (2011) for discussion of how these tensions were handled, but not eliminated, in this partnership, with some willingness on each side to tolerate different ideological perspectives. In a number of instances, partnerships between religious organizations and public health institutions have been powerful and effective, but they have certainly not been without various tensions. See Trinitapoli and Weinreb (2012) and Idler et al. (2019) for further discussion.

free to continue to pursue their own more central spiritual ends. Nevertheless, often the pursuit of these spiritual ends, including the love of neighbor, is consonant with the ends of population health. Greater efforts at partnership between religious communities and the institutions of public health and medicine could go a long way in advancing health.

3.7c. Participation in religious communities should be encouraged for those who already positively self-identify with a religious tradition to promote health and healing.

As noted in section III.4c, evidence has become increasingly clear that participation in religious community contributes to the health of the body and the health of the person. Rigorous studies have indicated that attending religious services is associated with greater longevity, less depression, less suicide, greater survival from cancer and cardiovascular disease, and numerous other important outcomes.[12] The evidence strongly suggests that attending religious services plays an important role in preserving health and in healing.[13] The mechanisms for

---

12. See Chida et al. (2009), Koenig et al. (2023), Idler (2014b), VanderWeele (2017a, 2017c), Chen et al. (2020), Rosmarin and Koenig (2020), and Balboni et al. (2022). Evidence for the effects of attending religious services on reducing all-cause mortality and depression risk is now available from meta-analyses of rigorous longitudinal studies (Chida et al., 2009; Garssen et al., 2021). The sensitivity of this evidence to potential unmeasured confounding is robust (VanderWeele et al., 2022; Balboni et al., 2022) and is furthermore either supported by a fairly clear understanding of the mechanisms (Strawbridge et al., 2001; Li et al., 2016; Kim and VanderWeele, 2019) or, in the case of depression, by quasi-experimental designs (Fruehwirth et al., 2019). See also Levin and Meador (2012) and VanderWeele (2017c) for some theological reflection on these associations.

13. Although the evidence indicates that attending religious services has an important role in maintaining health, its role in healing from ill health may be even more powerful. For example, the evidence for an effect of attending religious services on surviving cancer or cardiovascular disease is more substantial than for such effects on the incidence of cancer or cardiovascular disease (Li et al., 2016). Likewise, it may be the case that the effects of attending religious services on recovery from depression or drug use are greater than on preventing depression or drug use, although there is at least some evidence for both; see VanderWeele (2018b) for further discussion. If this is so, this would be in concordance with various theological teachings that faith may not keep one from suffering but perhaps better allows one to find meaning and wholeness even within it (John Paul II, 1984).

these effects that empirical research has uncovered include social support, hope and optimism, health behaviors, and a sense of purpose.[14] From a theological perspective, these effects in some sense are not surprising, given the importance of community life as a pathway to physical, mental, social, and spiritual healing. As discussed in section III.4, from the perspective of Christian theology, healing through the Church can come about by means of communal life, forgiveness, prayer, fasting, the sacraments, growth in character, and the care of others, including the work of medicine. Moreover, the Church promotes and provides the context for communal and interpersonal love, which constitutes a central pathway to health and healing, as section III.2 discussed. Regardless of how the mechanisms are understood, the evidence for powerful effects of participation in religious community on health is clear, and this has important implications for public health and medicine. The implications need to be nuanced, but they are important.

The links between participation in a religious community and public health do not imply that there ought to be a universal "prescription" for attending religious services in public health or clinical settings.[15] Religious commitments and beliefs are not principally shaped by concerns about physical health but rather reflect values, relationships, experiences, systems of meaning, truth claims, and evidence. A potentially more reasonable and nuanced approach to the implications of the existing research on the connections between religion and health would be to promote attending religious services for those who already positively self-identify with a religious tradition and to promote other forms of community life for those who do not.[16]

---

14. See, for example, Li et al. (2016) and Kim and VanderWeele (2019).

15. In a provocative commentary entitled "Should Physicians Prescribe Religious Activities?" Sloan et al. (2000) set up a "straw man" position concerning the notion of a universal prescription of religious activities that they then effectively critique. See Koenig (2000a) for a rebuttal to the piece that argues that even though a universal prescription is unreasonable, no one is arguing for that and that this does not mean that the empirical literature on religion and health does not have clinical implications.

16. See VanderWeele et al. (2022) for further discussion and development of this proposal, from which the brief discussion in the next few paragraphs is taken and summarized.

This more sensitive nuanced approach also helps address prior objections about such discussions of religion in clinical contexts[17] concerning clinicians and patients having different beliefs, the topic being too sensitive, the instrumentalizing of religion, lack of clinician training, and concerns about proselytization and abuse of power.[18] Instead of instrumentalizing religion, the approach acknowledges that religious commitments are typically shaped by concerns other than health but also recognizes that with respect to communal participation for those who already positively self-identify with a religious tradition, there will generally be consonance between health-related, social, and spiritual goals.

---

17. Sloan et al. (1999, 2000); Bishop (2009).

18. To determine whether such discussions might be appropriate, clinicians could pose neutral questions such as "Is religion or spirituality important to you in thinking about health and illness, or at other times?" and "Do you have, or would you like to have, someone to talk to about religious or spiritual matters?" (VanderWeele et al., 2022; Balboni et al., 2022). These two simple questions could be integrated into a social history and could be asked even if the clinician and the patient view religious matters very differently. Longer assessments of spiritual history are also available, but they require more time (Koenig, 2000b; Puchalski and Romer, 2000). For patients who positively identify with a religious or spiritual tradition, clinicians could also inquire about and even encourage involvement in religious community when appropriate. For patients without such beliefs and affiliations, other forms of community involvement could be encouraged. Such conversations during clinical care must also be sensitive to those who may have suffered past negative experiences or even abuse from religious communities. The relatively neutral questions above may help uncover such painful past experiences, which can then prompt empathy, support, and referrals to appropriate specialists. Both anecdotal evidence and studies of patient experiences suggest that when these issues are handled in a patient-centered fashion, raising questions of religion or spirituality within the clinical context can be nearly universally positive (Nicklin, 2000; Phelps et al., 2012). Moreover, it is desired by a large proportion of patients (Balboni et al., 2013; Steinhauser et al., 2000; Silvestri et al., 2003). Lack of clinician training certainly requires attention, since prior training in spiritual care is one of the strongest predictors of clinicians providing such care (Balboni et al., 2013). Although many medical schools now offer electives in spiritual care (Koenig et al., 2010), this is not likely sufficient because few participate. As part of the core curriculum, a one-session training module that reviews neutral spiritual-assessment questions in the context of epidemiological evidence may more powerfully facilitate an approach to raising issues of attending services and other forms of community participation in clinical contexts (Balboni et al., 2022).

A sensible approach to navigating these challenging issues in a clinical context is thus arguably possible. For the roughly half of all Americans (and many others around the world) who report a religious affiliation but do not participate in a religious community, such discussions of religious community may be appropriate and help promote health. For those who remain unconvinced, one might also turn the question around: Given the strength of the evidence on service attendance and health, are we doing harm if this information is withheld? It is arguably time for clinical practice to start taking these issues seriously and begin wrestling with the implications.

3.7d. Other forms of community participation should be encouraged and supported to promote health and healing.

Similar efforts to promote community participation could also be made in public health contexts for other forms of community. Although the research suggests that the effect sizes on health for other forms of social participation are not as strong as for attending religious services,[19] they are still meaningful and important.[20] However, in the public health context, more complex and nuanced considerations may need to be considered. When outreach efforts are made at the community level, it may no longer be possible to have the more nuanced assessment concerning an individual's specific religious affiliation, or lack thereof, that is possible in a clinical context.

Other efforts to promote community participation more broadly might be pursued by community or public health organizations putting forward the health benefits of community participation and providing a list of local community opportunities that include but are not restricted to attending religious services.[21] Alternative approaches could include such organizations providing an array of more targeted tradition-specific or activity-specific community promotion activities.[22]

---

19. Li et al. (2016); VanderWeele et al. (2016); Chang et al. (2017).
20. Shor and Roelfs (2013).
21. See Holt-Lunstad et al. (2015); Berkman et al. (2014); Hong et al. (2023).
22. There is some evidence that arts communities and religious communities are especially powerful with regard to effects on health and well-being (Fancourt and Steptoe, 2018; Fancourt and Finn, 2019; Balboni et al., 2022; Koenig et al., 2023). With regard to attending religious services, materials could be tailored to each

In the United States, at present such efforts are limited, but the practice of "social prescribing" has increased significantly in clinical and public health contexts in the United Kingdom in recent years.[23] Neglect of these opportunities and of community life as a social determinant of health is irresponsible. Promoting community participation has the potential to contribute substantially to population health; neglecting efforts to promote community participation and attending religious services, when these are appropriate, does not serve the public's health.

3.7e. Character development should be promoted at local, national, and international scales to foster health and healing.

Both physical health and the health of persons can also be advanced by efforts to promote character development at local, national, and even international levels. As discussed in part I of this book, good character,

---

specific religious or cultural tradition, describing the research on community and on attending religious services, noting various theoretical or theological understandings of the importance of community within that tradition, listing local communities that invite participation, and ideally also offering resources or contact information for those who have experienced abuse within religious or other community contexts. Such promotional material could be sent to lists of those who have previously indicated a particular religious affiliation and could also be a part of more general efforts to promote community. A number of future research directions may facilitate efforts to promote community participation and attending religious services. Randomization of religious participation would generally be unethical and infeasible. However, person-centered interventions to *encourage* participation in some kind of community, such as those described above, could be amenable to evaluation in randomized trials (VanderWeele, 2017c). Within clinical contexts, practice-level randomized trials could involve interventions that study providing training to implement assessment of patients' spiritual history and, when appropriate, encouragement to engage with a community. Likewise, individual-level randomized trials of tradition-specific outreach materials or community-level randomized trials of encouraging people to engage in social participation could be implemented. Because these efforts to promote engagement with some kind of community would likely change participation for only a small minority, relatively large sample sizes would be required in order to have adequate power to detect effects. Any concerns that promoting religious participation would have negative spillover effects on nonreligious individuals (Krieger, 2017; Aksoy et al., 2022) could be evaluated by collecting outcome data on other members of the community, though that would require even larger sample sizes.

23. NHS England (2019).

or virtue, is constitutive of the health of persons; it is a part of what it means for all aspects of a person's life to be good, for a person to flourish. Moreover, evidence continues to accumulate that character can contribute to physical health as well.[24]

Numerous interventions are now available for promoting various aspects of character. A number of these have been successfully evaluated in randomized trials, including activities to promote gratitude, forgiveness, compassion, patience, and perseverance.[25] These randomized trials have indicated that such character interventions have also promoted other aspects of well-being, including increasing happiness, promoting better sleep, and improving physical health; lowering depression and anxiety; increasing hope; and even improving education test scores.[26] Such interventions could be employed in local contexts in schools, workplaces, families, religious communities and elsewhere. Campaigns to make use of these evidence-based interventions could also be carried out at local, national, and international scales. Existing evidence indicates that such interventions could be effective both in promoting these various aspects of character and in promoting physical health.[27]

Character is developed and shaped over the course of a lifetime. Relationships, communities, and institutions play a critical role in the development and formation of character. From the standpoint of Christian theology, spiritual transformation, the life of the Church, and the work of

---

24. See section I.3e and Emmons and McCullough (2003), Long, Kim, et al. (2020), Węziak-Białowolska et al. (2021), and VanderWeele (2022a, 2022b).

25. As examples, interventions that have been evaluated in randomized trials have promoted gratitude (Davis et al., 2016; Cregg and Cheavens, 2020), forgiveness (Wade et al., 2014), compassion (Kirby et al., 2017), patience (Alan and Ertac, 2018), and perseverance or grit (Alan et al., 2019).

26. Evidence is now available from individual randomized trials or, in several cases, meta-analyses of randomized trials for effects of these character interventions on happiness, sleep, and physical health (Emmons and McCullough, 2003; Kirby et al., 2017; Davis et al., 2016); depression and anxiety (Wade et al., 2014; Kirby et al., 2017; Cregg and Cheavens, 2020); hope (Wade et al., 2014); and education test scores (Alan et al., 2019).

27. As noted in section I.3d, good character and virtue can facilitate physical health, but they might not always do so. Right or virtuous action can also sometimes involve sacrifice and might thus, in some circumstances, promote the good of others but entail some loss of one's own physical health. Because of the fallenness of the world, the goods of virtue and of physical health are not always consonant in this life.

the Spirit can powerfully shape character, assisting in the development of virtue and the infusing of virtues with an orientation toward more ultimate and supernatural ends.[28] Efforts to promote character development at local, national, and international scales can make use of evidence-based character interventions. However, because of the important role that communities, relationships, and institutions play in the formation of character, efforts to promote character should also foster and encourage community participation and acknowledge their critical role in development and formation.[29] These various efforts to promote character development have considerable potential to foster the health and healing of the person and the body.

3.7f. Forgiveness should be promoted at local, national, and international scales to foster health and healing.

One way the brokenness of our lives is manifest concerns our social relationships. We frequently wrong or hurt other people. To restore and heal these relationships and to restore and heal communities, we need forgiveness. As argued in section III.4d, forgiveness can be a powerful means to healing. There is notable evidence that it can bring healing related to struggles with mental health, including healing from depression, anxiety, and hopelessness.[30] Forgiveness may also have a role to play in the shaping of physical health.[31] And forgiveness can go a long way in bringing healing to relationships.

---

28. See Aquinas (1274/1920, I.II.63.3–4. I.II.65.2–3) and Garrigou-Lagrange (1999) for further discussion of the relation between so-called acquired and infused virtues, the latter being the work of the Spirit arising from the theological virtue of charity.

29. See Rozier (2016) for discussion of the potential for "structures of virtue" (Daly, 2011) to promote population health and to have a role in public health and public health ethics. As argued in section III.4, the Church constitutes one such structure of virtue that has the capacity to promote the development of character. The family, educational institutions, and the workplace likewise also arguably have such potential (VanderWeele, 2017a).

30. Wade et al. (2014); Ho et al. (2024).

31. See Toussaint et al. (2015), but see also Long, Worthington, et al. (2020) and footnote 14 in section III.4.

Forgiveness interventions have been developed to help enable forgiveness for those who want to forgive but are struggling to do so.[32] Such interventions involve recognizing the hurt, working to better understand the offender, deciding to forgive, working through the difficult emotions, and holding on to the commitment to forgive. Numerous randomized trials have indicated that such interventions can be effective for promoting forgiveness and for reducing depression and anxiety and increasing hope.[33] These interventions have also been converted into do-it-yourself workbook formats,[34] which evidence suggests are likewise effective.[35]

Such forgiveness interventions have the potential for wide dissemination at local, national, and international scales. The experience of being wronged is very common and many people struggle with anger that often leads to depression, anxiety, and possibly worse physical health. Since these forgiveness interventions can be powerful and effective, broadly disseminating them has the potential to make major contributions to mental and possibly physical health and to bring healing to relationships.[36]

---

32. Various models of enabling forgiveness have been developed (Enright and Fitzgibbons, 2000; Worthington, 2013). In the Enright Process Model of Forgiveness (Enright and Fitzgibbons, 2000), therapeutic intervention to promote forgiveness takes place over twenty steps organized into four phases: uncovering negative feelings about the offense, deciding to pursue forgiveness for a specific instance, working toward understanding the offending person, and discovering unanticipated positive outcomes and empathy for the forgiven person. Interventions using this model have been shown to be effective with groups as diverse as adult incest survivors, parents who have adopted special needs children, and inpatients struggling with alcohol and drug addiction. In Worthington's REACH model (Worthington, 2013), each letter of "REACH" represents a component of the process: *recall* the hurt one has experienced and the emotions associated with it; *empathize* with the offender and take the other's perspective in considering reasons for action (without condoning the action or invalidating one's feelings); make the *altruistic* gesture of recalling one's own shortcomings and realizing that others have offered forgiveness; *commit* to forgiving; and *hold* on to or maintain the forgiveness through times of uncertainty or through the returning of anger and bitterness.

33. Wade et al. (2014); Ho et al. (2024).
34. Worthington (2021); Ho et al. (2024).
35. Harper et al. (2014).
36. VanderWeele (2018a).

In considering efforts to promote forgiveness at national and international scales, it is important to consider the morality and appropriateness of forgiveness. As argued in section III.4d, forgiveness, conceived of as replacing ill will toward the offender with goodwill, should be distinguished from excusing or forgetting the action. It should be distinguished from not demanding justice, and it should be distinguished from reconciliation. One can forgive and hope for the ultimate good of the offender while still pursuing a just outcome. Moreover, in certain circumstances, as for example with repeated intimate partner violence, one might forgive without restoring the relationship. Forgiveness thus does not entail foregoing justice and does not necessarily entail reconciliation in this life. With these distinctions in mind, both philosophical and theological arguments have been put forward that forgiveness—as the replacing of ill will with goodwill toward the offender—is always morally appropriate provided the victim does not deny the wrongdoing and provided the above distinctions are kept in mind.[37] If this is indeed so, then promoting forgiveness, even at national and international scales, could arguably be carried out in an ethically responsible manner and doing so has the potential to make substantial contributions to population mental health and, when appropriate, to the restoration of relationships and communities. Forgiveness is thus arguably a public health issue.[38] Forgiveness can and should be promoted at local, national, and international scales to foster health and healing.

3.7g. Love should be promoted at local, national, and international scales to foster health and healing.

If, as discussed in section III.2, love is a central pathway to health and healing, then it arguably follows that love can and should be promoted at local, national, and international scales. Love involves seeking the good of another, seeing the good in the other, and seeking to be with the other. Love involves an affirmation of the other's being. As discussed in section III.2, various forms of love have the potential to bring health and healing, both to the beloved and to the one who loves. From the perspective of

---

37. See, for example, Holmgren (1993), North (1987), Stump (2006), or VanderWeele (2017c) for summaries.
38. VanderWeele (2018a).

Christian theology, love for God and love for one's neighbor also ultimately bring one to final communion with God. Promoting love thus has the potential to bring health and healing of the body and of the person.

Interventions have been developed to promote various aspects of love. As noted in the previous section, interventions are available to promote forgiveness, which has the potential to facilitate love and to improve mental health. Other interventions have focused on developing compassion for others. These have been evaluated in randomized trials that have found beneficial effects on compassion for others, on increasing happiness and emotion regulation and on decreased depression and anxiety.[39] Other interventions focus on specific relationships and on

---

39. See Jazaieri et al. (2013, 2014), Galante et al. (2014), and Kirby et al. (2017) for evidence from randomized trials. Many of these trials have focused on some form of training to develop compassion or meditation to develop loving-kindness. Although a number have not examined the effects of such training on compassion or love, a few have, and have found effects (Kirby et al., 2017). A number of the programs that provide training for compassion focus specifically on love or compassion in the context of suffering (see also Hordern, 2020, for a discussion of what compassion ought, and ought not, to look like within the context of medicine), but the meditation interventions to develop loving-kindness are usually more general. Meditation to develop loving-kindness as typically examined in these trials often comes out of Buddhist practices. Although these are, in principle, applicable to more secular or pluralistic contexts, they could be adapted to more explicitly Christian contexts. Meditation to develop loving-kindness often involves four steps (see Wiebel, 2007): sitting or lying down with closed eyes and mindfully focusing on the breath and the body; imagining receiving love, kindness, and compassion from a person who loves, or has loved, one deeply; attempting to send the same feelings of kindness, love, acceptance, and unconditional regard to oneself; imagining sending those same loving feelings outward sequentially to different recipients who are increasingly removed from oneself (e.g., family and friends, one's community, all people, all beings). One could envision adaptations of this to more explicitly Christian contexts in which the person from whom one imagines receiving love extends beyond friends and family to include God, Jesus Christ, or the Holy Spirit. One could also envision adaptations in which the final step involves extending or offering up love to God. The first step in the loving-kindness meditation described above typically involves some form of mindfulness. Although certain aspects of mindfulness meditation practices, such as judgment-free acceptance of all thoughts and feelings (see Bishop et al., 2004), are arguably contrary to Christian moral understanding, other aspects of mindfulness such as awareness or centering are practiced in Christian prayer and could reasonably constitute the first step of a loving-kindness meditation. See Brinkmann (2017) for further reflections on compatibilities and tensions between mindfulness practices and Christian prayer. Further reflection on and development of Christian loving-kindness meditation

improving love within relationships, such as love within marriage.[40] Each of these types of interventions has the potential to bring health and healing, and each of these could in principle be disseminated widely in local, national, and international contexts.

One might envision future interventions and campaigns to promote love at local, national, and international scales. Love ultimately requires a recognition of the goodness of the other—this involves seeing a dignity that makes them worthy of good and deserving of companionship. Promoting love can thus be facilitated by drawing attention to the dignity and worth of each person. This can be done by focusing on the extraordinary complexity and splendor and capacities of the human person or, from the perspective of Christian theology, on the fact that they were created by God, are loved by God, and have their final end in communion with God. Drawing attention to these matters can make the dignity and worth of each person more apparent. Even the deficiencies of the other person can then be viewed more in light of something to be corrected and healed in love and of their being worthy of such healing and change rather than seeing them as the object of dislike or hatred. Love can transform one's vision from aversion and hatred to the seeking of the good for the other and the good that is the other. Further research could be carried out to determine how best to bring about such understanding and in what contexts different interventions, activities, and campaigns are effective. However, promoting love at local, national, and international scales arguably has tremendous untapped potential to foster health and healing. Love arguably ought to be taken as an important matter from the perspective of public health and public policy. Love brings health and healing of the body and of the person.

3.7h. Love needs to be promoted in order to ensure that the right to the highest attainable standard of health is upheld as best as possible.

The 1946 constitution of the World Health Organization puts forward the principle that "the enjoyment of the highest attainable standard of health

---

practices, or alternative methods of promoting love through prayer, could be a promising direction for future work.

40. See, for example, Doss et al. (2016).

is one of the fundamental rights of every human being without distinction of race, religion, political belief, economic or social condition." This "highest attainable standard of health" is a high bar, and attention has been given to the question of what is meant by "attainable."[41] The notion that this is a right also requires some consideration about who is to ensure that this right is upheld and by what means.

A commitment to the highest attainable standard of health for all is a laudable goal, one that the WHO's constitution declares is "basic to the happiness, harmonious relations and security of all peoples." Rights entail responsibilities, and the constitution appears to recognize various roles for different constituencies in ensuring this right. The constitution states that "the health of all peoples is fundamental to the attainment of peace and security and is dependent on the fullest cooperation of individuals and States. The achievement of any State in the promotion and protection of health is of value to all. Unequal development in different countries in the promotion of health and control of disease, especially communicable disease, is a common danger." The constitution further notes the importance of the "healthy development of the child," perhaps implicitly acknowledging the role of the family in ensuring this right to the highest attainable standard of health, and emphasizes the importance of disseminating health-related knowledge to all people, active cooperation on the part of the public, and the responsibility of governments.[42] The constitution establishes the World Health Organization and states that its objective is "the attainment by all people of the highest possible level of health." The World Health Organization's constitution also seems to recognize that the responsibility for attaining the "highest attainable standard of health" lies in part with the individual but also with

---

41. The notion of the "highest attainable standard of health" can be interpreted in a way that recognizes that perfect health and perfect equality of health may not be attainable. What is attainable may be understood as respecting the constraints of nature. What is attainable can also be understood in a way that respects the freedom of individuals to act in ways that may be contrary to their health, thereby altering what is attainable. What is attainable may also be relative to the resources that are available (Hunt et al., 2015). The United Nations Committee on Economic, Social and Cultural Rights has gone some way toward specifying what the right to the "highest attainable standard of health" might be understood, in practice, to entail (UNCESCR, 2000).

42. See also section I.4e.

the broader community, perhaps including the family, the public health community, the state, and the World Health Organization.[43]

One interpretation about what is being envisioned is that this right to "the highest attainable standard of health" arises from some combination of both human rights and legal rights. Each person arguably has the natural right to not be intentionally harmed by other individuals acting as individuals. Parents have both rights and responsibilities to care for their children. A well-functioning state will arguably establish legal rights to various health-related resources. The World Health Organization's constitution seems to use language that effectively establishes rights conferred by agreement of the World Health Organization and member states. The combination of these might be taken as establishing a right to the "highest attainable standard of health," which is ultimately constituted by various natural rights, legal rights, and conferred rights.

However, if public health is ultimately aimed at achieving the "highest attainable standard of health" for all, then it is not clear that a focus on rights and justice alone will suffice. A person acts justly by acting to render each what is his or her due. This will entail not intentionally doing harm to others and doing what is within one's reasonable ability to help others in one's community. Attaining health for all will require justice, both in avoiding harm and as a constitutive part of what is entailed by the wholeness or well-being of a person and of a community.[44] However, if health is to be understood as a state of complete physical, mental, social, and spiritual well-being, then it is not clear if the actions of individuals and the well-intentioned policies and interventions of institutions will suffice.

If health includes social well-being, more than this will be needed. As discussed in section III.2, social relationships are generally most powerfully and adequately formed out of love, out of a disposition to desire the good for the other and union with the other.[45] Love for another will entail justice,[46] but love entails more than justice; it also entails a disposition toward willing the other person's good and toward being with

---

43. Hunt et al. (2015).
44. See also section I.4d.
45. Aquinas (1274/1920, I.II.Q26.4); Stump (2006).
46. See Wolterstorff (2015).

them, resulting in an affirmation of the goodness of their being.[47] This love is what almost all persons seek. It is the fabric of social well-being. It is needed for health. As discussed in section III.2, love is also the foundation of spiritual well-being. From a Christian understanding, attaining spiritual well-being requires charity—a love for God—along with the presence of God's grace and love, which is characteristically mediated in and through the Church community. Health, understood as the wholeness of the person, requires love. The New Testament and Christian teaching put love—love for God and love for one's neighbor—at the foundation of all of law, of all of ethics (Matthew. 22:37–40; Romans. 13:9–10). The wholeness of persons requires justice, but it also requires love.

Love—love for God and love for neighbor—is also needed for health because it is a powerful resource for physical and mental well-being. There is evidence that the experience of loving and being loved contributes to physical and mental health.[48] Moreover, as discussed above, there is now ample empirical evidence that social relationships and participation in religious community (i.e., social and spiritual well-being) profoundly contribute to both physical health and mental health.[49] Social and spiritual well-being are perhaps among the most powerful forces for attaining physical and mental health. A commitment to trying to achieve the "highest attainable standard of health" for all will require love because love is the foundation of social and spiritual well-being and because love powerfully shapes physical and mental well-being. The only way to adequately attempt to preserve and support the right to the "enjoyment of the highest attainable standard of health" is to look beyond rights and beyond justice—to love. We must seek a just society—yes—but we must also seek to create a "civilization of love."[50] Our love is needed to bring about physical, mental, social, and spiritual well-being. God's love and forgiveness is needed as well for spiritual well-being and to bring about a complete restoration to wholeness. The highest attainable standard of health cannot be brought about without love.[51]

---

47. Pieper (1974).
48. See footnote 5 of section III.2 for discussion of the empirical evidence.
49. Holt-Lunstad et al. (2015); Hong et al. (2023); VanderWeele (2017a, 2017c).
50. John Paul II (1991); Catholic Church (2004, 580–583).
51. Although the argument here is that love is needed to ensure that the right to the highest attainable standard of health is upheld as best as possible, the same thesis

Love is important in and of itself. It is important because it makes us fully human. It is important because it fosters good relationships. It is important because it can bring health and healing both to oneself and to others; it contributes to the good of others and allows us to enjoy the presence of others. Love is also important because it both enables and is constitutive of our final end of communion with God. From the perspective of public health, love is important because it facilitates what in the public health community has come to be understood as a "right to health"—the highest attainable standard of health. This right cannot be upheld as best as possible unless we also facilitate a civilization of love.

3.7i. In the context of a pluralistic society, there should be open dialogue concerning how different communities understand well-being and what is ultimately most important.

This book has offered a theology of health of the body and health of the person. The health of the person is effectively synonymous with human flourishing. A Christian understanding of human flourishing, or the health of the person, is distinctive in a number of respects, including an emphasis on conformity to God's intent; in its understanding of human nature, sin, and the fall; in the centrality of Jesus Christ, of God's grace, of the work of the Spirit, and of the life of the Church in the restoration to health and wholeness; in the possibility of suffering as a pathway to healing; in the centrality of love as a pathway to healing; in an understanding of complete happiness as ultimately rooted in a final vision of and communion with God. Although other traditions, including with those with more secular perspectives, share numerous aspects of what it means to flourish in this life, in Christianity, there is a subordination of temporal flourishing to eternal flourishing—that final communion with God—or to spiritual well-being constituted by one's life at present being good with respect to that final end in God.

Within a pluralistic context, it is important to come to as broad a common understanding as possible of human health and human

---

might be argued concerning the upholding of all other rights or concerning a position that justice cannot be adequately upheld without love (John Paul II, 1980, 14; Catholic Church, 2004, 583).

well-being. This is important because many public health and public policy efforts affect the whole of society. The more we can reach agreement about what is good and what we can and should pursue together, the easier it will be to promote that good.[52] It was argued in section I.1c that most understandings of human flourishing include various domains of life that most religious and cultural traditions value and emphasize. Such domains arguably include happiness and life satisfaction, physical and mental health, meaning and purpose, character and virtue, and close social relationships.[53] Most also include some notion of communal well-being. Religious and spiritual traditions also include, and often make central, tradition-specific notions of spiritual well-being. These will generally differ in important ways across different traditions and communities. Complete agreement on what constitutes the good in general will not be feasible here and now.

However, in order to attain consensus that is as broad as possible and to understand differences, open dialogue is essential concerning how different communities understand well-being and what it is that they consider most important.[54] Such discussions and such understanding will facilitate finding common ground; they will also make clear what is not shared and perhaps facilitate reflection on approaches and policies for navigating life in a pluralistic society whose members have different visions of what constitutes the good. No solution will be perfect; conflicts will arise. But loving one's neighbor requires appreciating that the people one disagrees with also have particular understandings of the good that they aspire to and seek. Within a pluralistic context, there needs to be a reciprocity in understanding the views of others if society is to be structured as best as possible so that individuals and communities are able to pursue their visions of the good.

In many or most cases, one believes that one's vision of the good is the right or best one. These beliefs are often shared and shaped, to varying

---

52. See also section I.7e.
53. VanderWeele (2017a).
54. In such dialogue, one can both put forward arguments and positions rationally grounded in more universally accessible terms and present what is distinctive about one's own view and the grounds for it. See, for example, International Theological Commission (2009) or Biggar (2011) for further discussion of these points from a Christian perspective. See also Volf (2015).

degrees, by a specific tradition or community. Although one can acknowledge that those one disagrees with also believe that their own vision or that of their community is right, one retains one's own perspective. Competing truth claims can be in conflict. The right approach here is not to abandon the notions of truth or objective good, but rather, through dialogue, to consider the reasons and evidence for one vision and set of truth claims over another.[55] Such dialogue may include an attempt at persuasion. After all, if one truly believes that the vision of the good embedded in one's tradition or understanding is right and best, then true love for one's neighbor would arguably entail helping them to come to that understanding as well so they can pursue what is good—the health of persons, human flourishing—as best as possible. There needs to be an acceptance of the freedom of the other—freedom of action and freedom of intellect. However, as with other truth claims, truth claims about what is good, about human flourishing, and our disagreements over these matters, are arguably best navigated through dialogue, in community, and in the weighing of evidence and arguments concerning the truth claims themselves.

Sharing these truth claims as carried out by the life of the Church is often what is referred to as evangelism or apostolate. In the contemporary West, these terms and the corresponding phenomena and attempts to engage in dialogue around these issues are often met with suspicion. Evangelism or apostolate is sometimes viewed as an imperialistic attempt to impose one's will and view on another. However, ultimately when these attempts to share the Christian vision of the good life and of human flourishing—both temporal and eternal—are carried out rightly, they should be viewed as attempts to love, to help others better attain what is good and to flourish as persons, and, from the perspective of Christian theology, to pursue and find their final end in God. The Christian gospel—the good news of Jesus Christ—is precisely that: it is meant to be good news. It is the teaching that in the life, death, and resurrection of Jesus Christ, God has brought salvation and that in the life of the Church, in a life of love, in a life in which God, by his Spirit, acts to bring healing, full human flourishing is eventually possible with the help of God's grace. In some sense, if one truly believes in a particular vision of

---

55. Even those who would reject the notion of an objective good are making a particular truth claim.

what constitutes the good, of what constitutes human flourishing, one will want others to attain that more complete flourishing as well, at least from the Christian understanding of love. As noted above, many others from different religious traditions may well share that perspective of wanting others to come to their own particular understanding of the good so as to be able to better attain it and will thus want to have the capacity to share their vision of the good—to evangelize.

The most promising way to navigate these competing visions of the good is through dialogue. Having opportunities to discuss these matters, to present these competing visions, to present truth claims, arguments, and evidence, will facilitate different traditions having the opportunity to make their case. Such dialogue, even when others are not persuaded, can help facilitate an understanding of and appreciation for the visions of the other. Such dialogue can sometimes also lead one to a deeper understanding of and appreciation for one's own tradition. Such understanding and such dialogue may also facilitate a better sense of what is shared across traditions and how to navigate the competing visions each community, tradition, and individual has in order to facilitate a better and freer pursuit of how each envisions the good. Such dialogue—a free exchange concerning how different communities understand well-being and understand what is ultimately most important—is needed to facilitate deeper understanding of one another, a fuller pursuit of truth, and a greater freedom for individuals and communities to pursue the ends they deem most important.

3.7j. Religious individuals and communities should be free to pursue their ultimate goals and ends in promoting the health and the healing of persons.

From the understanding of Christian theology and from the understanding of many other religious traditions, spiritual well-being ultimately is what is central. From a Christian standpoint, spiritual well-being includes a transformed character; a life that allows for growth through suffering; a life grounded in faith, hope, and love; a life in the Church; a life of prayer; a life with God. The health of the body is important but cannot, in this life, be sustained indefinitely; the body faces aging, deterioration, and decline. The health of the person includes happiness, bodily health, meaning, character, and good relationships. All of these are goods that are to be pursued. However, there are limits also to these other aspects of flourishing and, as the body and mind decline, we are impeded in the pursuit of many of these goods. All ultimately also face death. A Christian understanding of the health of persons values all of these goods but ultimately sees them as subordinate to, as pointing toward, and as finding their fulfillment in a final union with God. A Christian understanding thus values all of these goods but gives priority to the seeking of spiritual well-being.

To that end, the Church encourages participation in the life of the Church community, living out life as best as possible according to God's intent, turning one's will toward God, living in accord with one's conscience concerning right and wrong, experiencing God in prayer, and living out a life of love. To achieve this, it is important that the Church community—and thus, in a pluralistic context, other religious communities too—be free to pursue their ultimate spiritual goals. It is important that there be freedom to meet and freedom of association. It is important that there be free practice of religion. It is important that there be freedom of speech and a free exchange of ideas and understandings of what constitutes the good, of what constitutes human flourishing. To not grant this is to deny the pursuit of what religious communities and of what countless individuals worldwide consider most important. To facilitate the health of persons—human flourishing as it is understood across traditions—it is important that individuals and communities be free to pursue their spiritual goals.

This does not mean other goals should be neglected. Considerable progress can and has been and should be made toward common understandings of the good—of bodily health and of the health of person, of human flourishing. What can be pursued together we should pursue together. However, many—perhaps most—religious and cultural traditions have also pointed toward more transcendent aims, and these too should be taken into account. There ought to be freedom for individuals and communities to pursue these more ultimate aims.

From the Christian standpoint, our final transcendent end is a vision of and communion with God, attained by God's action in Jesus Christ, through the life of the Church, and lived out in love. It is in this that the true health of the person consists. This final transcendent end is attainable only in the resurrection in the life to come—in the perfecting of full bodily health and the full health of the person. That end is a bringing of health, of human flourishing, to completion. Our ultimate end is a final attainment, freely pursued and enabled by God's grace, of that complete wholeness that God intended, for the body and for the person, in communion with others and in communion with God.

Propositional Summary:
- 3.7a. Medicine and public health need to pay greater attention to psychological, social, and spiritual pathways to health and healing.
- 3.7b. Institutions of public health and medicine should partner with religious communities to promote health and healing.
- 3.7c. Participation in religious communities should be encouraged for those who already positively self-identify with a religious tradition to promote health and healing.
- 3.7d. Other forms of community participation should be supported and encouraged to promote health and healing.
- 3.7e. Character development should be promoted at local, national, and international scales to foster health and healing.
- 3.7f. Forgiveness should be promoted at local, national, and international scales to foster health and healing.
- 3.7g. Love should be promoted at local, national, and international scales to foster health and healing.
- 3.7h. Love needs to be promoted in order to ensure that the right to the highest attainable standard of health is upheld as best as possible.
- 3.7i. In the context of a pluralistic society, there should be open dialogue concerning how different communities understand health and what is ultimately most important.
- 3.7j. Religious individuals and communities should be free to pursue their ultimate goals and ends in promoting the health and the healing of persons.

A NONTHEOLOGICAL POSTSCRIPT

This book has put forward a distinctively Christian theological view of health, wholeness, and healing. Although much of the book draws upon various positions within Christian theology, much of its content might also be of interest and relevance to those who do not embrace the Christian faith. Some of the positions and arguments that are put forward do not necessarily require the suppositions of Christian theology. Likewise, some of the implications of the positions put forward do not require a distinctively theological perspective. In this postscript, I would like to attempt to briefly explore and describe what I see as the relevance and implications of the material in this book for those who do not hold Christian perspectives on these topics.

In part I, I put forward the idea that when we use the word "health," two related but distinct concepts may be in view: the health of the body or the health of the person (section I.0).[1] I argued that the health of the person is synonymous with human well-being or flourishing. Such an understanding of health is embedded in the World Health Organization's definition of health as "a state of complete physical, mental, and social well-being, and not merely the absence of disease or infirmity."[2] The health of the body, in contrast, is a narrower concept pertaining to the body's parts and systems being and functioning so as normal to allow for the full range of activities characteristic of the human body. Both concepts of health are embedded in our ordinary language; we can even use them in the same sentence. One might, for example, say of someone, "Every day he just sits in his room; he is physically healthy, but he is not a healthy

---

1. VanderWeele et al. (2019a, 2023b).
2. WHO (1946).

person." Here the idea of "not healthy" is used to indicate that something is not right or whole about the person, even though the body may be intact and functioning well. I argued in part I that many of the conceptual disputes over the meaning of health might be resolved by more clearly distinguishing between the health of the body and the health of the person and acknowledging that our language includes both concepts.

I also argued in part I (section I.7b) that these distinctions might be helpful in clarifying the proper purview of medicine. I put forward the position that complete well-being or flourishing was much too broad a focus for medicine but that health of the body was, in most cases, too narrow a focus for medicine, since many decisions about medical interventions affect not only the body but also other aspects of a person's life and that this was especially the case when various interventions or treatments may have substantial side effects. I thus argued that the proper purview of medicine might be understood as including both the health of the body and those aspects of the health of the person that pertain to decisions concerning the health of the body.[3] This keeps the focus of medicine principally on the health of the body but recognizes the implications of decisions made about the health of the body for the person more generally.

The purview of psychiatry ought to be somewhat broader (section 1.7c). Although mental health is affected by the health of the brain, it relates to other aspects of a person's life. There will be varying levels of comfort across psychiatrists concerning their willingness to engage in helping a patient work through challenges and difficulties in their life more generally. Moreover, value systems may differ between a patient and the psychiatrist. A reasonable purview for psychiatry might thus be taken to be the wholeness of the mind as it pertains to the proper functioning of the brain along with those aspects of flourishing that the patient and clinician agree through dialogue to address.

Matters become more complex when we turn to public health and public policy. The reality of our pluralistic context and our different and potentially competing value systems become even more clear. Bodily health and adequate material and financial resources are important goals almost everyone shares. As a result, much of public policy and public

---

3. VanderWeele et al. (2019a, 2019b, 2024).

health are shaped around trying to promote these goods. This is important, but human well-being consists of more than just bodily health and financial stability. Policy and public health efforts and decisions have the potential to shape a host of other aspects of a person's life. In principle, it would be desirable for public health and public policy efforts to contribute to well-being more generally.[4] However, differing values and conceptions of what is good potentially make such efforts problematic. A reasonable course might be to focus on promoting the aspects of well-being that it is possible to obtain a reasonable consensus about. In section I.1, I argued that although well-developed conceptions of well-being or flourishing may differ across various philosophical, cultural, and religious traditions, many of these traditions have a great deal in common. Much of what people seek after is shared across cultures and traditions. Although nearly everyone wants to be healthy and to have adequate financial resources to sustain life, people care about more than this. Almost everyone also wants to be happy, to have a sense of meaning and purpose, to be a good person, and to have good relationships. These are things we all seek. Although conceptions of flourishing will vary across traditions, almost any reasonable conception of flourishing will include a number of different goods within human life, including happiness, health, meaning, character, and relationships.[5] These are goods around which it may be possible to attain considerable consensus. I thus proposed (section I.7e) that the proper purview of public health and public policy ought not to be restricted to health and economic considerations but ought to include the health of persons and the aspects of human flourishing around which consensus can be attained.

All of this has implications for measurement (section I.7f). What we measure shapes what we discuss, what we know, what we aim for, and what policies are put in place to achieve those aims.[6] If the proper purview of public policy and public health is the health of persons, or human well-being, then we should begin to measure or assess these various other aspects of well-being. Measuring gross domestic product alone is

---
4. See Diener et al. (2009), Adler and Fleurbaey (2016), Trudel-Fitzgerald et al. (2019), Stiglitz Fitoussi, and Durand (2019), and Plough (2020) for discussions of creating a public policy of well-being or a public health of well-being.
5. VanderWeele (2017a).
6. Stiglitz Sen, and Fitoussi (2009); Hall and Rickard (2013).

not sufficient.[7] Discussion was given to a variety of measurement and assessment approaches for aspects of well-being such as happiness, meaning, character, and social connections in addition to bodily health and financial stability.[8] If these measures are embedded in communal and national assessments and in our studies, we will be better able to evaluate the effects of our actions, promote well-being, understand trends over time, and see who needs help and in what ways. Such assessment could, when appropriate, be carried out in clinical care and clinical research as well and would be especially important when treatment involves substantial side effects that affect other aspects of life or when the goals of bodily health and other aspects of human well-being come into conflict (section I.7g).[9]

Good relationships and good community are goods that are nearly universally sought. Good community is both constitutive of and instrumentally related to well-being (section I.4).[10] If flourishing or the health of the person is understood as living in "a state in which all aspects of a person's life are good," then flourishing includes having good community.[11] To pursue complete human well-being, we must pursue good, healthy, welcoming, and just communities, whether at the level of the family, the state, or the numerous intermediate communities that make up society. This is part of what it means to flourish. Communities are critical for sustaining the well-being of individuals and bear responsibility for sustaining health and well-being (section I.6). We should thus seek to promote and assess both social and communal well-being. Clinical, public health, and public policy decision-making should take relational and communal considerations into account (section I.7i).[12]

Although happiness, health, meaning, character, and close relationships are all part of the health of persons, or flourishing, these aspects of life would generally not be considered exhaustive of human well-being

---

7. Stiglitz, Sen, and Fitoussi (2010); Stiglitz, Fitoussi, and Durand (2019); VanderWeele (2017a).
8. VanderWeele (2017a); Węziak-Białowolska et al. (2019).
9. VanderWeele et al. (2019b).
10. See, for example, Berkman et al. (2014) and Holt-Lunstad et al. (2015) for reviews of the empirical evidence for the effects of social connection and social support on health.
11. VanderWeele (2017a, 2019a).
12. Holt-Lunstad (2022); VanderWeele (2019a).

for many well-developed conceptualizations of flourishing. However, fuller, more comprehensive understandings of flourishing, or the health of persons, are likely to vary across cultural, religious, and philosophical traditions. These differences and nuances are important, along with what we hold in common. One aspect of well-being that is important in many traditions but that will differ across traditions is spiritual well-being. For much of the world's population, some notion of religious or spiritual well-being may be what the person considers very important or most important.[13] Because understandings of spiritual well-being will vary across religious and cultural traditions, any reasonable assessment or study of spiritual well-being will require tradition-specific understandings and measures of spiritual well-being.[14] In principle, such assessments could be carried out even in pluralistic contexts (section I.7j), acknowledging that the assessments across traditions will not be commensurable but also acknowledging that such assessments and efforts to help promote spiritual well-being will be considered important to numerous persons and communities around the world. Because understandings of spiritual well-being (and values more generally) may vary across cultural and religious traditions, it may be reasonable to allow some space for tradition-specific practices of medicine (section I.7d), taking into account individuals' and communities' priorities and values.[15]

Traditions that include spiritual well-being as a part of flourishing might understand the health of the person, or human flourishing, as a "state of complete physical, mental, social, and spiritual well-being" (sections I.1 and I.5). This extends beyond the World Health Organization's definitions of health as "a state of complete physical, mental, and social well-being, and not merely the absence of disease or infirmity." It includes a spiritual dimension. The World Health Organization's definition of health has been criticized as being too broad (section I.0) but if one distinguishes between health of the person and health of the body, it is reasonable to take the former as synonymous with complete human well-being or flourishing (section I.0) and in principle to include spiritual well-being.

---

13. Pew Research Center (2012); Diener et al. (2011).
14. VanderWeele et al. (2021).
15. Balboni and Balboni (2018).

Considerations of both concepts of the health of the body and the health of the person are important. Consideration of both also acknowledges the unity of the human person (section I.3) and the interconnectedness of the body, the mind, and the human person considered as a united whole (section I.2). The distinction allows us to seek to promote health of the person in various ways even when bodily health is poor or is in decline and cannot be fully restored (section I.7k).

Part II of the book considered causes of ill health. In a Christian understanding, the cause of ill health is sin, not necessarily an individual's own wrongdoing but possibly that of others, or past or present injustices. Although the notion of sin typically assumes a religious interpretation concerning some sort of deviation from God's intent, the notion of wrongdoing is shared by religious and more secular perspectives alike. Wrongdoing affects human health—the health of bodies and the health of persons (section II.1). We do not often consider wrongdoing in discussions of public health, or at least do not often describe it as such.[16] However, if we are to understand the full scope of the various forces that shape health and illness, it is important to consider wrongdoing. Wrong actions toward others, whether consisting of verbal or physical abuse, assault, or violence, can bring ill health. Wrong actions toward others also damage social relationships and community life, which is harmful in and of itself but can also bring about the ill health of persons and the ill health of bodies, since social relationships affect health. Wrong actions can also bring about ill health for oneself, whether this be directly through harm done to one's body or psychologically through guilt and shame over one's actions.

Wrongdoing is also a cause of ill health because it can create or perpetuate or sustain injustices and structures of injustice (section II.2). Such injustice may take the form of discrimination or decisions that disadvantage entire communities. It may involve more direct violence, oppression, or war. Injustice may also involve restrictions of freedoms of association, of speech and thought, or of the practice of religion. Each of these impede the health of the person and the health of the body.[17] In

---

16. Jeffrey and Levin (2020).
17. See Berkman et al. (2014) for summaries of empirical evidence of how working conditions, social capital, and discrimination can affect physical and mental health. See also Grim and Finke (2011), Chetty, Friedman, and Rockoff (2014),

many cases, unjust structures established by wrongdoing in the past may persist, if left unaddressed, without any further individual intentional wrongdoing. This makes it particularly important to be attentive to these injustices and to take action to address them. Unjust structures and communal relations can actively diminish human flourishing, can give rise to lack of opportunities for flourishing, and can prevent each person from receiving what is their due. Thus, unjust structures are constitutive of the ill health of communities. Wrongdoing and injustices disorder our relations to one another, to our communities, and to our environment and world (section II.3), ultimately also giving rise to mortality and death (section II.4).

Because wrongdoing so profoundly affects the health of persons, the health of bodies, the health of communities, and the health of our world, ultimately ill health cannot be addressed without addressing issues of wrongdoing (section II.5). We need to pay attention to wrongdoing as a cause of ill health (section II.7a). We need to address unjust structures of the past and present (section II.7c). We need to address the moral injury that can occur to persons when their deepest moral understandings, values, and intuitions are violated by their own actions or by that of others, and we need to try to bring healing when moral injury has occurred (section II.7h). We need greater attention to questions of character and the promotion of good character in order to prevent human wrongdoing (section II.7b). We need respect for all life (section II.7d) and care for the environment (section II.7e) in order to maintain health, prevent ill health, and mitigate, lessen, and alleviate the consequences of human wrongdoing.

Unfortunately, the nature of human life in this world is such that while these efforts are important and can help considerably, ill health does persist (section II.7f). Suffering continues. We need to be attentive to such suffering (section II.6).[18] We should seek to alleviate suffering when possible, but when it is not possible we should still seek to care for others and meet them in their suffering. Suffering indicates that things are still not right with our world, with human relationships, with human

---

Krieger et al. (2014), and Rand (2015) for discussion of and empirical evidence relating to effects of these social conditions on health.

18. Cassell (1982, 1991).

action. In addition to trying to alleviate suffering, we can mourn and be present with those who suffer. We can also sometimes seek transformation in suffering. A transformation in understanding, in meaning, in character, in relationships, in spiritual growth, or in life orientation might sometimes be possible.[19] This does not make the loss or suffering right, but it allows us to continue as best we can amidst suffering and to realize that more is needed to address the suffering and brokenness in our world. Medicine, public health, and public policy should thus likewise be attentive to questions of suffering (section II.7g).[20] Suffering shows us what is wrong with the world and guides us to actions we might take to address suffering.

Part III of the book was concerned with questions of healing and restoration and fulfillment of health and wholeness. This part of the book was the most explicitly theological. Nevertheless, there are insights from a Christian theological understanding that are relevant to those who do not share those particular theological commitments. Healing may be understood as a restoration to wholeness, either of the body or of the person (section III.0). The practice of medicine often allows for the healing of the body in remarkable ways; the healing of the body often also has implications for the healing of the person, by restoring functionality and capacity to engage more fully in relationships, work, and communities. However, even when it is not possible to bring about healing of the body, we should still be attentive to other ways we can assist with the healing of persons. That healing may be understood as any contribution to their physical, mental, social, or spiritual well-being. The healing of persons—and of communities—may also take place by trying to address human wrongdoing, since it is often a cause of and constitutive of the ill health of the body and of persons (section III.1).

In our search for various pathways to healing, we can use a number of psychological, social, spiritual, and communal resources that are not always adequately appreciated by medical and public health communities (section III.7a). Considerable empirical research has demonstrated important connections between social and communal participation

---

19. Tedeschi and Calhoun (2004).
20. VanderWeele (2019b).

and physical health,[21] between positive psychological states and physical health,[22] and between participation in religious community and physical health.[23] Promoting these psychological, social, and spiritual pathways thus has the potential to bring physical healing, a restoration of health to the body, as well as healing concerning mental, social, and spiritual well-being. Such psychological, social, and spiritual/religious resources and pathways to health and healing could be employed and promoted with greater frequency in medicine and public health.

Participation in community—both religious and secular—seems to be a particularly powerful and important pathway to health (sections III.7c and III.7d). Such community participation could likewise be more prominently promoted within society in general but also in clinical and public health contexts.[24] In clinical and public health contexts, questions of spirituality and religion are clearly sensitive and need to be handled carefully and appropriately. Nevertheless, studies have found that large proportions of patients would like these issues addressed in the context of medicine.[25] This can potentially be done, even if patients and clinicians do not share similar views, by simple relatively neutral questions such as, "Are religion or spirituality important to you in thinking about health and illness or at other times?" and "Do you have or would you like to have someone to talk to about religious or spiritual matters?"[26] Referrals to chaplains or other spiritual care providers could then be made as appropriate. Such questions also have the potential to uncover past abuse in religious contexts, and referrals can be made as appropriate to try to bring healing. For others, community participation could be encouraged, again when appropriate. For patients who positively self-identify with a religious tradition, encouraging participation in a religious community may promote physical, mental, and social well-being. For patients who are not religious, other forms of community participation

---

21. Berkman et al. (2014); Holt-Lunstad et al. (2015); Hong et al. (2023).
22. Martín-María et al. (2017); Hernandez et al. (2018); Trudel-Fitzgerald et al. (2019); Steptoe (2019).
23. Chida et al. (2009); Koenig et al. (2023); Idler (2014b); VanderWeele (2017a, 2017c); Chen et al. (2020); Balboni et al. (2022).
24. NHS England. (2019); Holt-Lunstad (2022); VanderWeele et al. (2022).
25. Balboni et al. (2013); Steinhauser et al. (2000); Silvestri et al. (2003).
26. VanderWeele et al. (2022); Balboni et al. (2022).

could be encouraged. Public health efforts could also be carried out to encourage greater community participation and engagement.

The effects of participation in religious community are especially notable across numerous aspects of physical, mental, and social well-being. Although much of the more rigorous research has been carried out in Western and predominantly Christian contexts, the research on all-cause mortality and longevity at least suggests that these effects extend to a number of other cultures and religious traditions.[27] The effects of participation in a religious community seem considerably more larger than those of private spiritual or religious practices.[28] Once again, the community is important for the health of the person and the health of the body. One such religious community is the Church (section III.4). One can see in the life of the Church and the spiritual and religious practices therein a number of different potential pathways or mechanisms by which participation might promote health and well-being. As noted above, social relationships contribute both to physical health and to the health of the person more generally. But religious and church communities also often promote healthy behaviors and lifestyles, they can encourage growth of character, and they promote forgiveness, which has been linked to mental health.[29] Religious communities also promote and help sustain marriage, which is also linked to health. The church community provides for the needs of their members and those outside the community. Various churches and religious organizations have supplied a substantial portion of the medical and health care services available in numerous countries throughout the world.[30] The Church understands part of the mission for itself as its members to be healing others and meeting the needs of others.

Given this understanding, it will often make sense for medical and public health institutions to partner with religious institutions to promote health and well-being (section III.7b). Although there are inevitably potential tensions in such partnerships, in many cases far more can be accomplished when the two sets of institutions work together rather than

---

27. Yeager et al. (2006); Litwin (2007).
28. VanderWeele (2017c).
29. Wade et al. (2014); Toussaint et al. (2015); Long, Worthington, et al. (2020); Ho et al. (2024).
30. Mwenda (2011); Idler (2014a); Olivier et al. (2015).

separately. Religious communities provide social networks, systems of trust, physical spaces, and participants who are willing to volunteer, all of which can potentially be used to promote health and well-being.[31] It is important that medical and public health institutions recognize the distinctive goals of religious communities, but there is potentially a lot to gain by partnerships between medical and public health institutions and religious organizations.[32]

The mission to help those in need and help provide healing to those who are ill and suffering points to another powerful pathway to health and healing that has perhaps been too neglected in public health. That pathway is love (section III.2). Love might be understood as both seeing and participating in the good that is the other person and contributing to their good.[33] Love can bring about the health of a person in numerous ways and thereby potentially contribute to the health of the body. When one loves other people by meeting their needs, this helps promote their physical, mental, social, or spiritual well-being. Love also affirms who they are as persons, and seeing the good in others and desiring to be with others likewise affirms the goodness of their being. It was noted above that social relationships that powerfully contribute to physical health and these are facilitated, enhanced, and sustained by such love.[34] Love helps bring about the health of the person and the health of the body. Loving others—loving one's neighbor—can thus bring health and healing to others. However, such love also can bring healing to the person loving.[35] The effects are reciprocal. Loving others does not always prompt love in return, but it tends to do so.[36] This has important implications for relationships. Research indicates that, for example, parental love and marital relationships help promote the health and well-being of the persons in the relationships.[37] The reciprocal nature of love also has important implications for communities. Communities are characteristically formed by

---

31. Campbell et al. (2007); Idler (2014a).
32. Gunderson and Cochrane (2012); Levin (2014, 2016); Idler et al. (2019).
33. Stump (2006); VanderWeele (2023c).
34. Berkman et al. (2014); Holt-Lunstad (2015); Hong et al. (2023).
35. Curry et al. (2018).
36. Fowler and Christakis (2010).
37. Huppert et al. (2010); Chen, Kuzansky, et al. (2019); Manzoli et al. (2007); Wood et al. (2007); Chen et al. (2023).

and sustained by relationships, so love of others—love of neighbor—is critical for communities. Given the importance of love for relationships, for communities, and for the health of persons, love could be promoted at local, national, and international scales to foster health and healing (section III.7g). Although some effective interventions have already been established, more work could be done to better understand how to promote love and thereby also health and healing.[38]

Love arguably also has a role in ensuring justice (section III.7h). Love of others—love of one's neighbor—will help prevent wrong actions against others; it will help prevent injustice; it will provide motivation to address structures of injustice that have arisen from past action. Love may help ensure that rights are respected and preserved. The World Health Organization's proposed right to "the highest attainable standard of health" requires not only that political and public health institutions be sustained; it also requires loving relationships, a fostering of communal well-being, and a world in which each person looks out for the well-being of others.[39] It will not be possible to achieve "the highest attainable standard of health" without this. Creating such communal well-being can be challenging, and the current political divisions make that manifest. Fostering love and respect for others may be helpful in trying to address these challenges. Love of one's neighbor, including even love of one's enemy, may help heal divisions and ensure better health.[40] Fostering character development more generally may likewise be of importance and might be carried out in part through evidence-based interventions in numerous community contexts to promote the health of persons and the health of communities (section III.7e).[41]

Forgiveness may be another important way to both foster love and heal division. Human wrongdoing continues and persons, sometimes intentionally and sometimes unintentionally, harm or offend one another. To foster better relationships and better communities we need forgiveness

---

38. Jazaieri et al. (2014); Galante et al. (2014); Kirby et al. (2017).
39. WHO (1946).
40. Brooks (2019).
41. See Davis et al. (2016) and Cregg and Cheavens (2020) for gratitude, Wade et al. (2014) for forgiveness, Kirby et al. (2017) for compassion, Alan and Ertac (2018) for patience, and Alan et al. (2019) for perseverance/grit.

and we need to promote forgiveness (section III.7f). Interventions to promote forgiveness have been developed and evaluated in randomized trials and have been found to have effects not only on promoting forgiveness but also on decreasing depression and anxiety and increasing hope.[42] Forgiveness can promote health and can heal relationships and communities.[43] These interventions could be more widely employed and disseminated. Forgiveness should be promoted at local, national, and international scales to foster health and healing.[44] Doing so could advance public health and create healthier and more loving—and less divisive—relationships and communities.

All of these psychological, social, and spiritual resources and pathways to health could be employed more broadly than is the case at present and could help supplement the more traditional medical and public health approaches to health promotion that often focus on physical health. The human person is a whole and what affects one part of the person—body or mind—affects other aspects of their life. We should seek to make use of the full range of resources that promote health and healing. Unfortunately, however, there are limits to what we can do (section III.5). Everyone eventually faces aging, ill health, and death. These realities need to be acknowledged and we need to try to make sense of them. How these realities and limits are understood varies across religious and cultural traditions. The Christian understanding is that God will eventually restore the human person and the world (section III.6) and that the key to that work of healing and restoration has already begun and in some sense has been ultimately secured, in the person of Jesus Christ (section III.3). Although understandings of the ultimate goal of human life and of human flourishing vary across traditions, it is important in the context of a pluralistic society that we try, as best as possible, to understand both our commonalities and our differences (section III.7i). In doing so, we will hopefully develop a greater appreciation of one another, a greater capacity to work together, a greater appreciation and understanding of our own views on these more ultimate matters, and a greater capacity to come closer to truth.

---

42. Wade et al. (2014); Harper et al. (2014); Ho et al. (2024).

43. Wade et al. (2014); Toussaint et al. (2015); Chen, Harris, et al. (2019); Long, Worthington, et al. (2020); Ho et al. (2024).

44. VanderWeele (2018a).

There should be a welcome freedom of exchange and a sharing of ideas and understandings in order to learn from others and to explain our own understandings of health and well-being and the ultimate goals of human life (section III.7j). This is arguably a critical part of promoting health—the health of the body and the health of persons.

APPENDIX

Propositional Outline

Part I. Health and Wholeness
"Thou hast made us for thyself, O Lord"
(Augustine, *Confessions*, book 1, section1)

> **Propositional Outline of Part I: Health is wholeness as intended by God.**
>
> **I.0. Health as Wholeness**
>
> **Proposition 1.0: Health can be understood as wholeness, either of the body or of the person**
>
>> 1.0a. Etymologically, the word "health" is related to wholeness.
>> 1.0b. Wholeness is to be understood as a thing being as it is meant to be.
>> 1.0c. We have two distinct concepts of health: health or wholeness of the body and health or wholeness of the person.
>> 1.0d. An understanding of wholeness requires some conception of the nature of a thing.
>> 1.0e. In a theological understanding, the nature and end of the body and of the person are found in God's intent; health of the body and of the person are thus constituted by wholeness of the body and the person as intended by God.
>> 1.0f. Health is always relative to an ideal.
>> 1.0g. God's intent for wholeness may be understood with respect to the current created order or with respect to God's final intent.
>
> **I.1. The Health of Persons and Human Flourishing**
>
> **Proposition 1.1: The health of the person consists of complete physical, mental, social, and spiritual well-being.**
>
>> 1.1a. The health of the person is physical, mental, social, and spiritual well-being.

1.1b. Health in its broadest sense, the wholeness of the person, is human flourishing, which can be understood as living in a state in which all aspects of a person's life are good.

1.1c. Human flourishing consists in part in attaining happiness, bodily health, meaning, virtue, close relationships, good community, and spiritual life.

1.1d. Various domains of human flourishing in fact constitute shared values across different traditions.

I.2. The Health of the Body

Proposition 1.2: The health of the body is constitutive of and contributes to the health of the person.

1.2a. Bodily health is constituted by the body's parts and systems being and functioning as normal so as to allow for the full range of activities characteristic of the human body.

1.2b. The health of the body constitutes and contributes to the health of the person, or human flourishing.

1.2c. Bodily health includes the health of the brain, which itself shapes, though does not fully encompass, mental health—the wholeness of the mind.

1.2d. Mental health may be understood as the wholeness of the mind, either in a narrower sense, as pertaining to the proper functioning of the brain, or in a broader sense, as pertaining to the wholeness of persons.

1.2e. God's intent for the body is to empower our capacity to love and to be united to others and to God.

I.3. Health, Unity, and Goodness

Proposition 1.3: The complete person, body and soul, was created good by God as an integrated whole.

1.3a. The human person was created good and the human body was created good.

1.3b. The natural state of the human body as created by God is health.

1.3c. The good of health presupposes the good of life, and life itself is to be respected from conception until death.

1.3d. The human person is an integrated whole, and what occurs to one aspect of the person will affect the entire person.

I.4. Health and Community

Proposition 1.4: The complete health of the person includes a flourishing community.

1.4a. The complete wholeness of a person entails the wholeness of his or her community.

1.4b. A community involves a common good, and this implies that the flourishing of one person ultimately depends on the well-being of others in the community.

1.4c. Good community includes flourishing individuals, good relationships, proficient leadership, healthy structures and practices, a welcoming environment and sense of belonging, and a common mission.

1.4d. Good community requires justice.

1.4e. Healthy families are needed for the health of bodies, the health of persons, and the health of communities.

I.5. Health and Spiritual Well-Being

Proposition 1.5: The complete health of the person includes communion with God.

1.5a. The final end of the person is communion with God.

1.5b. Communion with God requires approaching God in faith, hope, and love.

1.5c. Communion with God requires growth in character and knowledge.

1.5d. Growth in character, faith, hope, and love requires community, service, and the carrying out of one's calling.

1.5e. Communion with God requires and is found in prayer and contemplation.

1.5f. Charity, including the love of God and love of neighbor, is central in attaining communion with God.

1.5g. God's initiation and grace are necessary to bring about full communion with him.

I.6. Health and Responsibility

Proposition 1.6: Health is the responsibility of the individual and of the community but depends also on circumstances beyond the control of either.

1.6a. The causes of health are diverse.

1.6b. Fundamental approaches in sustaining health include regular use of the systems that maintain health, avoiding abuse of those systems, and seeking repair of those systems when necessary.

1.6c. Practices to sustain physical health include exercise, good diet, good sanitation, temperance, sleep and rest, and medical care.

1.6d. Mental health is sustained by the stimulation and proper use of the mind, by rest, and by mental health care as necessary.

1.6e. Human flourishing, or the health of the person, is sustained by pursuits and purposes, by commitments to relationships and institutions, by spiritual practices, by rest and balance and leisure, and by addressing the domains of life in which one is flourishing least.

1.6f. Habits that sustain the health of the mind and of the person contribute to the sustaining of bodily health.

1.6g. What we value shapes our capacity to flourish.

1.6h. Communities and their representatives also bear responsibility for maintaining health because good social relations, material resources, a safe environment, and communal practices are all needed for health and promote health.

1.6i. Facilitating flourishing at work will facilitate flourishing in life.

1.6j. The flourishing of a society facilitates the flourishing of the individual.

1.6k. The flourishing of individuals can facilitate the flourishing of society.

1.6l. Although personal and communal responsibility are necessary for maintaining health, there are limits to what can be attained and some experience of ill health is inevitable.

I.7. The Implications of Health as Wholeness

1.7a. In discussions of health, greater clarity is needed about whether the topic is the health of the body or the health of the person.

1.7b. The purview of medicine includes the health of the body and the aspects of the health of the person that pertain to decisions about the health of the body.

1.7c. The purview of psychiatry is wholeness of the mind as it pertains to the proper functioning of the brain and to the aspects of flourishing that the patient and clinician together agree to address through dialogue; and the purview of counseling likewise consists of those aspects of flourishing that the patient and counselor together agree to address through dialogue.

1.7d. Given that flourishing will be understood differently across persons and communities, there ought to be room for tradition-specific practices of medicine, psychiatry, and counseling.

1.7e. The purview of public health and public policy ought to be the aspects of the health of persons, or human flourishing, around which societal consensus can be attained.

1.7f. In medical, public health, and public policy contexts, assessments should be made of human well-being and not only of physical health and financial circumstances.

1.7g. An exclusive focus on the health of the body leads to poor decision-making.

1.7h. Psychological theories of well-being are often impoverished by the absence of considerations of bodily health, virtue, and communal well-being and thus need to be supplemented with these other aspects of flourishing.

1.7i. Since the health of persons includes their social well-being, social and communal well-being should be assessed, and decisions made in clinical contexts and in public health and public policy should take relational considerations into account.

1.7j. Since the health of persons includes their spiritual well-being, attention should be given to tradition-specific understandings and assessments of spiritual well-being in discussions of public health, medicine, and public policy.

1.7k. Because the health of the body and the health of the person are ideals, health, in both senses, is thus a relative concept, and flourishing should be promoted in various ways even in the absence of bodily health.

Part II. Ill Health and Sin

"Our heart is restless"
(Augustine, *Confessions*, book 1, section 1)

Propositional Outline of Part II: The cause of ill health is sin.

II.0. Ill Health as the Absence of Wholeness

Proposition 2.0: Ill health is the absence of wholeness.

2.0a. Ill health is the absence of wholeness.

2.0b. Ill health of the body may arise from disease, injury, or infirmity.

2.0c. Ill health of the person, or brokenness, is constituted by lack of full flourishing.

2.0d. Ill health is lack of wholeness intended by God, and this has come about by free human action contrary to God's intent.

II.1. Agency, Sin, and Ill Health

Proposition 2.1: Ill health often follows from the wrongful action of ourselves or others.

2.1a. Wrong action toward others can bring about ill health.

2.1b. Wrong action toward others damages social relationships and community and can bring about ill health.

2.1c. Wrong action can bring about ill health for oneself.

2.1d. Poor habits can bring about ill health.

2.1e. Wrong action separates us from God, which constitutes and further brings about ill health.

2.1f. Wrong action impedes us from being who we were intended to be and produces guilt, which constitutes and results in ill health.

II.2. Injustice and Ill Health

Proposition 2.2: Wrongful actions can bring about unjust structures that may result in ill health over extended periods of time and even across generations.

2.2a. Wrongful human action can give rise to unjust structures.

2.2b. Unjust structures and communal relations can actively diminish human flourishing, give rise to lack of opportunities for flourishing, and impede each person from receiving what is his or her due.

2.2c. Unjust structures are contrary to God's intent and they constitute ill health of communities and contribute to ill health of individuals.

2.2d. Although unjust structures may have arisen from actions of individuals in the past, they may persist if left unaddressed and it is the responsibility of a community to alter unjust structures.

II.3. Fallenness and Ill Health

Proposition 2.3: Human nature is distorted by sin, and this fallenness of human nature has disrupted relations between human persons and the world, giving rise to external causes of ill health.

2.3a. Because of wrongful human actions, our nature and our relation to the world around us are fallen and are not as they should be.

2.3b. The body ages and deteriorates with time, bringing about ill health.

2.3c. The mental faculties and social interactions of human persons are not what they should be, and this is both constitutive of and brings about ill health.

2.3d. Because the human person's relation to creation is fallen, natural disasters, accidents, and pollution all bring about ill health.

2.3e. Corresponding to the free decisions of human persons to depart from God's intent are the free decisions of spiritual beings to depart from God's intent, which result in further ill health of persons.

2.3f. The trials of life lead to strain and distress, which constitute and result in ill health.

II.4. Sin and Death

Proposition 2.4: Sin has brought about and continues to bring about death.

> 2.4a. Death is the consequence of sin.
> 2.4b. Sin causes ill health that eventually results in death.
> 2.4c. Sin is separation from God and thus also constitutes spiritual death.
> 2.4d. Death, as the ending of life, is also a cessation of ill health in this life.

II.5. Incapacity and Sin

Proposition 2.5: Ill health cannot be prevented without addressing sin.

> 2.5a. Ill health cannot be prevented without addressing sin because sin brings about harmful actions for ourselves and others, unjust structures that perpetuate ill health, poor social relations, and poorly functioning communities.
> 2.5b. Ill health cannot be prevented without addressing sin because sin, as separation from God, is constitutive of ill health.
> 2.5c. Without God, we cannot address sin as a cause of ill health, and we are incapable of fully preserving or restoring the body, the mind, our relationships, and the world around us to be what God intended them to be.

II.6. Ill Health and Suffering

Proposition 2.6: The experience of distress over brokenness, or lack of wholeness, is suffering, whereby the need for healing and restoration is made clear.

> 2.6a. Suffering is the anguished experience of a negative physical or mental state of considerable duration or intensity.
> 2.6b. Our experience of suffering reflects the brokenness of the world and of the human person.
> 2.6c. Ill health of the body can bring about suffering.
> 2.6d. Ill health of the person can bring about suffering.
> 2.6e. Suffering can lead to a transformation in understanding, life orientation, relationships, and character and can thereby bring about a renewed health of the person.
> 2.6f. God allows suffering to help bring about the free conversion of the will to God's intent and thereby a fuller spiritual well-being.
> 2.6g. The impossibility of our fully alleviating suffering and ill health points to the need for final restoration by God.

II.7. The Implications of Ill Health and Sin

2.7a. Human wrongdoing should not be overlooked as a cause of ill health.
2.7b. Character ought to be emphasized as an important factor in maintaining health.
2.7c. Injustices, the social nature of wrongdoing, and unjust structures from past wrongdoing need to be addressed in order to maintain health.
2.7d. Respect for life and the averting of abortion and euthanasia is critical to maintaining health.
2.7e. Care for the environment is critical to maintaining health.
2.7f. The notion that we will ultimately overcome ill health and death in this life is a fiction that we should resist.
2.7g. Medicine, public health, and public policy should be attentive to questions of suffering and not just to mental disorders and physical diseases.
2.7h. Medicine, public health, and public policy should be attentive to and address the phenomenon of moral injury.

Part III. Healing and Salvation
". . . until it finds its rest in thee"
(Augustine, *Confessions*, book 1, section 1)

Propositional Outline of Part III: The restoration and fulfillment of health is salvation.

III.0. Healing as the Restoration of Wholeness

Proposition 3.0: Healing is the restoration of wholeness.

3.0a. Healing is the restoration of wholeness.
3.0b. Healing may pertain to the body or, more broadly, to the person.
3.0c. Numerous aspects of ill health can be addressed so that health is restored.
3.0d. God's intent is for health and thus for healing, a restoration to health.
3.0e. Healing of the person is constituted by a restoration to physical, mental, social, and spiritual well-being.
3.0f. God's intent now and in the life to come is the fulfillment of wholeness.

III.1. Healing of Persons and Healing from Sin

Proposition 3.1: Healing of the person cannot fully come about without a healing from sin.

3.1a. Complete healing of the person may seem like an ideal that is not possible to achieve.

3.1b. Restoration to wholeness cannot be achieved without addressing sin and the effects of sin.
3.1c. Complete health of the person requires communion with God and thus healing in relation to God so that sin no longer separates a person from God.
3.1d. Salvation is the deliverance from sin and its consequences and thereby a complete restoration and fulfillment of wholeness as God intended.

III.2. Healing and Love

Proposition 3.2: The principal ways that a restoration and fulfillment of wholeness are brought about are love of God and love of one's neighbor.

3.2a. Love of God is the foundation for healing.
3.2b. Loving one's neighbor brings healing to others.
3.2c. Loving one's neighbor brings healing to oneself.
3.2d. Loving God is integral to a full restoration to wholeness.
3.2e. Loving God empowers one to love one's neighbor.
3.2f. Communities are brought to wholeness by love.
3.2g. Love of enemies is a pathway to wholeness for all people and communities.
3.2h. Charity—the virtue of friendship with God, including love of one's neighbor—is brought about by God's grace.

III.3. Healing and Jesus Christ

Proposition 3.3: God has brought healing and salvation through Jesus Christ.

3.3a. God is the principal agent of healing.
3.3b. Sin cannot be fully dealt with through human efforts.
3.3c. God has dealt with the problem of sin in the person of Jesus Christ.
    3.3c.i. Jesus Christ restored human nature by uniting it to the divine.
    3.3c.ii. Jesus's life and teaching enables us to better know God.
    3.3c.iii. Jesus Christ demonstrated God's love, which can in turn prompt love in us.
    3.3c.iv. Jesus provided a model of a life lived in love for God and neighbor that we are to imitate.
    3.3c.v. Jesus did away with sin and guilt in uniting us to himself in his suffering and death.
    3.3c.vi. Jesus's resurrection empowers our life and guarantees we too will be raised from the dead and restored to complete wholeness.

3.3c.vii. Jesus's sending his Spirit and the formation of the Church enables our lives to conform to God's intent both here and now and in the life to come.

3.3d. The individual receives God's gift of salvation and is delivered from sin through faith in Jesus Christ.

III.4. The Church, Community, and Healing

Proposition 3.4: The Church and its members are both agents and recipients of healing and that healing comes about through communal life, forgiveness, prayer, fasting, the sacraments, growth in character, and the care of others, including the work of medicine.

3.4a. The Church is called to bring healing and the message of salvation to the world.

3.4b. The Christian is called to bring healing and the message of salvation to the world.

3.4c. Healing comes through community life.

3.4d. Healing comes through forgiveness.

3.4e. Healing comes through prayer.

3.4f. Healing comes through fasting.

3.4g. Healing comes through the sacraments.

    3.4g.i. Healing comes through the Eucharist.

    3.4g.ii. Healing comes through baptism.

    3.4g.iii. Healing comes through confirmation of faith.

    3.4g.iv. Healing comes through the sacrament of reconciliation.

    3.4g.v. Healing comes through the anointing of the sick.

    3.4g.vi. Healing comes through marriage.

    3.4g.vii. Healing comes through ordination to the priesthood.

3.4h. Healing comes through growth in character.

3.4i. Healing comes through the care of others.

    3.4i.i. The care of others can bring health and healing through the provision of material needs, the addressing of wounds and disease, the meeting of spiritual and emotional needs, and through the experience of love.

    3.4i.ii. Care and healing constitute acts of love and bring healing and wholeness to the person providing care.

    3.4i.iii. The Christian experiences Christ in the other when caring for those in need.

3.4j. Healing comes through the work of medicine.

    3.4j.i. Wounds and disease can be healed by the practice of medicine.

3.4j.ii. The practice of medicine is facilitated by God in his creating the body's natural capacity to heal and in granting human intellect and creativity endowed by God.
3.4j.iii. The Church is to empower and facilitate the practice of medicine.

III.5. The Limits of Healing

Proposition 3.5: There are limits to healing in this life, but healing in relation to God can come about in the midst of and sometimes even through ill health.

3.5a. Salvation does not, in this life, free the body from illness and death.
3.5b. Salvation in this life gradually, but not completely, frees the person from sin.
3.5c. Salvation does not, in this life, completely free the Church from sin.
3.5d. The Church, as an agent of healing, must seek to limit the presence and influence of sin.
3.5e. Even in the midst of ill health and suffering, there can be personal growth and healing.
3.5f. Even in the midst of ill health and sin, there can be a greater communion with God
3.5g. Those with faith in Jesus Christ are to hope for a fuller restoration and fulfillment of wholeness in the life to come.

III.6. God, Resurrection, and Salvation

Proposition 3.6: The fulfillment of wholeness, a communion with God and a completion of God's intent, comes only in the resurrection in the life to come and will be accomplished by God.

3.6a. God has promised a full healing of and restoration of creation.
3.6b. God's restoration of all creation will come about through Jesus Christ and is received by faith.
3.6c. God's restoration of all creation requires the establishing of justice and thus a judgment of good and evil.
3.6d. God will bring about a final and more perfect bodily health in the resurrection of the dead.
3.6e. God will bring about a fulfillment of healing of the person and complete freedom from sin.
3.6f. God will bring about a full restoration and transformation of all of creation.
3.6g. God will be fully present, and there will be full communion with God.

III.7. The Implications of Healing and Salvation

3.7a. Medicine and public health need to pay greater attention to psychological, social, and spiritual pathways to health and healing.

3.7b. Institutions of public health and medicine should partner with religious communities to promote health and healing.

3.7c. Participation in religious communities should be encouraged for those who already positively self-identify with a religious tradition to promote health and healing.

3.7d. Other forms of community participation should be supported and encouraged to promote health and healing.

3.7e. Character development should be promoted at local, national, and international scales to foster health and healing.

3.7f. Forgiveness should be promoted at local, national, and international scales to foster health and healing.

3.7g. Love should be promoted at local, national, and international scales to foster health and healing.

3.7h. Love needs to be promoted in order to ensure that the right to the highest attainable standard of health is upheld as best as possible.

3.7i. In the context of a pluralistic society, there should be open dialogue concerning how different communities understand health and what is ultimately most important.

3.7j. Religious individuals and communities should be free to pursue their ultimate goals and ends in promoting the health and the healing of persons.

A BRIEF GLOSSARY CONCERNING HEALTH AND ILLNESS

brain disease. *See* mental ill health (brain disease).

brain disorder. *See* mental ill health (brain disorder).

brokenness. *See* ill health (of the person; broad sense).

common good (multiple usages): the common shared end of a community, possibly including the broader flourishing of the community and its members and possibly including the means to attain the relevant end or ends.

common good, general: the flourishing of the community and its members together with the means to sustain such flourishing. *See also* flourishing, community (broad sense).

common good, particular: the shared ends, or aspects of flourishing, that are the particular focus of a community together with the means to attain that end. *See also* flourishing, community (narrow sense).

common good, political (or the common good in its primary sense): the particular common good of a nation; or "the sum of those conditions of social life which allow social groups and their individual members relatively thorough and ready access to their own fulfillment" (Catholic Church, 2004, 164).

common good, universal: the shared final end in God.

community flourishing. *See* flourishing, community (broad sense); flourishing, community (narrow sense).

complete human well-being. *See* well-being, complete human.

defect. *See* ill health (defect).

disability. *See* ill health (disability).

disease. *See* ill health (disease).

eternal flourishing. *See* flourishing, eternal.

frailty. *See* ill health (frailty).

flourishing: (n) complete human well-being; the state in which all aspects of a person's life are good (abstract noun); (gerund or present participle) living in a state in which all aspects of a person's life are good.

flourishing, community (broad sense): a state in which all aspects of a community's life are good; a state of flourishing of the community itself as a community and the flourishing of its members together with the means to sustain such flourishing. *See also* common good, general.

flourishing, community (narrow sense): a state in which the community has the relationships, leadership, practices, and unity needed for the fulfillment of the particular ends specific to that community. *See also* common good, particular.

flourishing, eternal: complete communion with God. *See also* well-being, spiritual.

flourishing, temporal: a state in which all aspects of a person's life are good as pertaining to the goods in this life.

general common good. *See* common good, general.

happiness: the experience of a desired state of quality.

happiness, perfect: the complete satisfaction of the will.

health: a state of wholeness; or (in a derivative sense) the condition of a thing with respect to an ideal state of wholeness.

health (of the body; narrow sense): the state of having the body's parts and systems being and functioning as normal so as to allow for the full range of activities characteristic of the human body.

health (of the person; broad sense): complete human well-being or flourishing, a state in which all aspects of a person's life are good; or (from a theological perspective) a state in which all aspects of a person's life are as intended by God. *See also* flourishing.

human well-being. *See* well-being, human.

ill health: a state involving lack of wholeness.

ill health (of the body; narrow sense): lack of wholeness of the body; the presence of disease, injury, defect, or frailty.

ill health (of the person; broad sense); brokenness, lack of wholeness of the person; any lack of human well-being or flourishing.

ill health (defect): a state of bodily anomaly.

ill health (disability): a lack of capacity to function, in some respect, as a person (as shaped in part by the accommodations and resources provided by others and by society). *See also* ill health (impairment).

ill health (disease): a bodily anomaly constituted by a process of a sequence of changes from normal or abnormal structure.

ill health (frailty): a bodily state of weakened or abnormal function accompanied by comparatively normal structure.

ill health (illness): the human experience of disease. *See also* mental ill health (mental illness).

ill health (impairment): a restriction on the normal range of activities characteristic of the human body.

ill health (injury): a bodily anomaly resulting from an extrinsic infliction.

ill health (sickness): the experience of physical symptoms suggestive of or similar to what is experienced in disease.

impairment. *See* ill health (impairment).

injury. *See* ill health (injury).

mental disorder. *See* mental ill health (mental disorder).

mental health (of the person; broad sense): the complete wholeness of the mind; a state in which all aspects of a person's mental life are good. *See also* well-being, mental.

mental health (as pertaining to the brain; narrow sense): no lack of wholeness of the mind arising from malfunction of the brain.

mental ill health (brain disease): abnormal function of the brain constituted by a process of a sequence of changes from normal or abnormal structure.

mental ill health (brain disorder): a particular abnormal function of the brain specified by the brain's physical processes.

mental ill health (mental disorder): a particular type of mental illness specified by the nature of the mental experience.

mental ill health (mental illness): lack of wholeness of the mind arising from malfunction of the brain of sufficiently severe quality.

mental ill health (of the person, broad sense): lack of wholeness of the mind.

mental ill health (as pertaining to the brain, narrow sense): lack of wholeness of the mind arising from malfunction of the brain.

particular common good. *See* common good, particular.

perfect happiness. *See* happiness, perfect.

physical health (of the body; narrow sense): a state of having the body's parts and systems being and functioning as normal so as to allow for the full range of activities characteristic of the human body.

physical health (of the person; broad sense): a state in which all aspects of a person's physical life are good. *See also* well-being, physical.

physical well-being. *See* well-being, physical.

political common good. *See* common good, political (or the common good in its primary sense).

sickness. *See* ill health (sickness).

social well-being. *See* well-being, social (as pertaining to the community; broad sense); well-being, social (as pertaining to the individual; narrow sense).

spiritual well-being. *See* well-being, spiritual.

temporal flourishing. *See* flourishing, temporal.

universal common good. *See* common good, universal.

well-being: a desirable state of quality; or (from a theological perspective) a state of goodness as intended by God. *See also* flourishing.

well-being, complete human: a state in which all aspects of a person's life are good. *See also* flourishing.

well-being, human: a state in which all aspects of a person's life are good as they pertain to that individual.

well-being, mental: a state in which all aspects of a person's mental life are good. *See also* mental health (of the person; broad sense).

well-being, physical: a state in which all aspects of a person's physical life are good.

well-being, social (as pertaining to the community; broad sense): a state in which all aspects of a person's social life are good, including the person's broader community. *See also* flourishing, community (broad sense).

well-being, social (as pertaining to the individual; narrow sense): a state in which all aspects of a person's social life are good as they pertain to that individual.

well-being, spiritual: a state in which all aspects of a person's spiritual life are good; or a state in which all aspects of a person's life are good with respect to his or her final end in God; or a state in which a person's life is oriented toward eternal flourishing. *See also* flourishing, eternal.

REFERENCES

Abbey, R., and Den Uyl, D. J., 2001. The Chief Inducement? The Idea of Marriage as Friendship. *Journal of Applied Philosophy* 18(1): 37–52.
Abu Raiya, H., and Pargament, K. I. (2010). Religiously Integrated Psychotherapy with Muslim Clients: From Research to Practice. *Professional Psychology: Research and Practice* 41(2): 181–188. DOI: 10.1037/a0017988.
Adams, M. M. (2000). *Horrendous Evils and the Goodness of God.* Ithaca, NY: Cornell University Press.
Adler, M. D., and Fleurbaey, M. (Eds.). (2016). *The Oxford Handbook of Well-Being and Public Policy.* Oxford: Oxford University Press.
Aftab, A., and Ryznar, E. (2021). Conceptual and Historical Evolution of Psychiatric Nosology. *International Review of Psychiatry* 33(5): 486–499.
Aksoy, O., Bann, D., Fluharty, M. E., and Nandi, A. (2022). Religiosity and Mental Wellbeing among Members of Majority and Minority Religions: Findings from Understanding Society, The UK Household Longitudinal Study. *American Journal of Epidemiology* 191: 20–30.
Alan, S., Boneva, T., and Ertac, S. (2019). Ever Failed, Try Again, Succeed Better: Results from a Randomized Educational Intervention on Grit. *Quarterly Journal of Economics* 134(3): 1121–1162.
Alan, S., and Ertac, S. (2018). Fostering Patience in the Classroom: Results from Randomized Educational Intervention. *Journal of Political Economy* 126(5): 1865–1911.
Alkire, S. (2005). *Valuing Freedoms: Sen's Capability Approach and Poverty Reduction.* Oxford: Oxford University Press.
Allen, J. D., Pérez, J. E., Tom, L., Leyva, B., Diaz, D., and Torres, M. I. (2014). A Pilot Test of a Church-Based Intervention to Promote Multiple Cancer-Screening Behaviors among Latinas. *Journal of Cancer Education* 29(1): 136–143.
Allen, S. (2018). The Science of Generosity. White paper prepared for the John Templeton Foundation by the Greater Good Science Center at UC Berkeley. Accessed January 4, 2024. https://ggsc.berkeley.edu/images/uploads/GGSC-JTF_White_Paper-Generosity-FINAL.pdf.
Amato, P. R., and Sobolewski, J. M. (2001). The Effects of Divorce and Marital Discord on Adult Children's Psychological Well-Being. *American Sociological Review* 66: 900–921.

American Psychiatric Association. (2013). *Diagnostic and Statistical Manual of Mental Disorders*. 5th ed. Arlington, VA: American Psychiatric Association.

Amundson, R. (2000). Against Normal Function. *Studies in History and Philosophy of Science Part C: Studies in History and Philosophy of Biological and Biomedical Sciences* 31(1): 33–53.

Aquinas, T. (1265/2014). *Summa contra Gentiles*. Translated by English Dominican Fathers. Frederick, MD: Aeterna Press.

Aquinas, T. (1270). *Super Evangelium S. Matthaei lectura (Commentary on Saint Matthew's Gospel)*. Chapters 1–12. Translated by R. F. Larcher. Accessed January 3, 2024. https://isidore.co/aquinas/SSMatthew.htm.

Aquinas, T. (1272a). *Sententia Libri Ethicorum* (Commentary on Aristotle's Nicomachean Ethics). Translated by C. I. Litzinger. Accessed January 3, 2024. https://isidore.co/aquinas/english/Ethics.htm

Aquinas, T. (1272b). *Commentary on Romans*. Accessed January 3, 2024. https://aquinas.cc/la/en/~Rom.

Aquinas, T. (1274/1920). *Summa Theologica*. Translated by the Fathers of the Dominican Province. Notre Dame, IN: Ave Maria Press.

Aquinas, Albert, and Philip the Chancelor. (2004). *The Cardinal Virtues: Aquinas, Albert, and Philip the Chancellor*. Translated by R. E. Houser. Toronto, ON: Pontifical Institute of Mediaeval Studies.

Aristotle. (4th C BCE/1980). *The Nicomachean Ethics*. Translated by W. D. Ross. Edited by J. L. Ackrill. Oxford: Oxford University Press.

Aristotle. (4th C BCE/1995). *The Politics of Aristotle*. Translated by E. Barker. Oxford: Oxford University Press.

Astin, J. A., Harkness, E., and Ernst, E. (2000). The Efficacy of "Distant Healing": A Systematic Review of Randomized Trials. *Annals of Internal Medicine* 2000(132): 903–910.

Augustine. (400/1991). *Confessions*. Translated by Henry Chadwick. Oxford: Oxford University Press.

Augustine. (417/2019). *On the Trinity*. Translated by Arthur W. Haddon. Philadelphia, PA: Dalcassian Publishing Company.

Augustine. (426/427). *On Rebuke and Grace*. Accessed January 3, 2024. Excerpts translated at https://www.newadvent.org/fathers/1513.htm.

Augustine. (426/1998). *Augustine: The City of God against the Pagans*. Cambridge: Cambridge University Press.

Avalos, H. (1999). *Health Care and the Rise of Christianity*. Peabody, MA: Hendrickson Publishers.

Baird, A., and Thompson, W. F. (2018). The Impact of Music on the Self in Dementia. *Journal of Alzheimer's Disease* 61(3): 827–841.

Balboni, M. J., and Balboni, T. A. (2018). *Hostility to Hospitality: Spirituality and Professional Socialization within Medicine*. Oxford: Oxford University Press.

Balboni, M. J., Sullivan, A., Amobi, A., Phelps, A. C., Gorman, D. P., Zollfrank, A., Peteet, J. R., Prigerson, H. G., VanderWeele, T. J., and Balboni, T. A. (2013). Why Is Spiritual Care Infrequent at the End of Life? Spiritual Care Perceptions among Patients, Nurses, and Physicians and the Role of Training. *Journal of Clinical Oncology* 30: 2538–2544.

Balboni, T. A., VanderWeele, T. J., Doan-Soares, S. D., Long, K. N. G., Ferrell, B. R., Fitchett, G., Koenig, H. G., Bain, P. A., Puchalski, C., Steinhauser, K. E., Sulmasy, D. P., and Koh, H. K. (2022). Spirituality in Serious Illness and Health. *Journal of the American Medical Association* 328(2): 184–197.

Barbieri, W. A. (2001). Beyond the Nations: The Expansion of the Common Good in Catholic Social Thought. *Review of Politics* 63(4): 723–754.

Barth, K. (1961). *Church Dogmatics*. Vol. III, Part 4. *The Doctrine of Creation*. Edited by G. W. Bromiley and T. F. Torrance. Edinburgh: T & T Clark.

St. Basil the Great. (1962). *St. Basil: Ascetical Works*. Translated by M. Monica Wagner. Washington, DC: Catholic University of America Press.

Benedict XVI. (2007). *Spe salvi: On Christian hope*. Libreria Editrice Vaticana. https://www.vatican.va/content/benedict-xvi/en/encyclicals/documents/hf_ben-xvi_enc_20071130_spe-salvi.html.

Benedict XVI. (2009). *Caritas in veritate: On integral human development*. Libreria Editrice Vaticana. https://www.vatican.va/content/benedict-xvi/en/encyclicals/documents/hf_ben-xvi_enc_20090629_caritas-in-veritate.html.

Berkman, L. F., Kawachi, I., and Glymour, M. M. (Eds.). (2014). *Social Epidemiology*. Oxford: Oxford University Press.

Bice, T. W. (1976). Comments on Health Indicators: Methodological Perspectives. *International Journal of Health Services* 6(3): 509–520.

Bickenbach, J. (2017). WHO's Definition of Health: Philosophical Analysis. In *Handbook of the Philosophy of Medicine*, edited by T. Schramme and S. Edwards, 961–974. Dordrecht: Springer.

Biggar, N. (2011). *Behaving in Public: How to do Christian Ethics*. Grand Rapids, MI: William B. Eerdmans Publishing.

Bishop, J. P. (2009). Biopsychosociospiritual Medicine and Other Political Schemes. *Christian Bioethics* 15: 254–276.

Bishop, S. R., Lau, M., Shapiro, S., Carlson, L., Anderson, N. D., Carmody, J., Segal, Z. V., Abbey, S., Speca, M., Velting, D., and Devins, G. (2004). Mindfulness: A Proposed Operational Definition. *Clinical Psychology: Science and Practice* 11(3): 230–231.

Blythe, J. A., and Curlin, F. A. (2019). How Should Physicians Respond to Patient Requests for Religious Concordance? *AMA Journal of Ethics* 21(6): 485–492.

Bolier, L., Haverman, M., Westerhof, G. J., Riper, H., Smit, F., and Bohlmeijer, E. (2013). Positive Psychology Interventions: A Meta-Analysis of Randomized Controlled Studies. *BMC Public Health* 13(119). DOI: 10.1186/1471-2458-13-119.

Boorse, C. (1975). On the Distinction between Disease and Illness. *Philosophy & Public Affairs* 5(1): 49–68.

Bowling, N. A., Eschleman, K. J., and Wang, Q. (2010). A Meta-Analytic Examination of the Relationship between Job Satisfaction and Subjective Well-Being. *Journal of Occupational and Psychology* 83(4): 915–934.

Brady, M. S. (2018). *Suffering and Virtue*. Oxford: Oxford University Press.

Brandt, B. (1979). *A Theory of the Good and the Right*. Oxford: Clarendon Press.

Breslow, L. (1972). A Quantitative Approach to the World Health Organization Definition of Health: Physical, Mental and Social Well-Being. *International Journal of Epidemiology* 1(4): 347–355.

Brinkman, S. (2017). *A Catholic Guide to Mindfulness*. Bessemer, AL: Avila Institute for Spiritual Formation.

Brooks, A. C. (2019). *Love Your Enemies*. New York: HarperCollins.

Brown, C. G. (2012). *Testing Prayer*. Cambridge, MA: Harvard University Press.

Brown, P. J. (2014). Religion and Global Health. In *Religion as a Social Determinant of Public Health*, edited by Ellen Idler. New York: Oxford University Press.

Bryan, C. J., Bryan, A. O., Roberge, E., Leifker, F. R., and Rozek, D. C. (2018). Moral Injury, Posttraumatic Stress Disorder, and Suicidal Behavior among National Guard Personnel. *Psychological Trauma: Theory, Research, Practice, and Policy* 10(1): 36.

Bulzacchelli, R. H. (2012). Developing the Seminal Theology of Pope Paul VI: Toward a Civilization of Love in the Confident Hope of the Gospel of Life. *Ave Maria Law Review*, 11: 49–64.

Burgos, J. M. (2018). *An Introduction to Personalism*. Washington, DC: Catholic University of America Press.

Cadge, W., Freese, J., and Christakis, N. A. (2008). The Provision of Hospital Chaplaincy in the United States: A National Overview. *Southern Medical Journal* 101: 626–630.

Callahan, D. (1973). The WHO Definition of "Health." *Hastings Center Studies* 1(3): 77–87.

Campaign to End Loneliness. (2015). Measuring Your Impact on Loneliness in Later Life. https://www.campaigntoendloneliness.org/wp-content/uploads/Loneliness-Measurement-Guidance1.pdf.

Campbell, M. K., Hudson, M. A., Resnicow, K., Blakeney, N., Paxton, A., and Baskin. M. (2007). Church-Based Health Promotion Interventions: Evidence and Lessons Learned. *Annual Review of Public Health* 28: 213–234.

Cantril, H. (1965). *The Pattern of Human Concerns*. New Brunswick, NJ: Rutgers University Press.

Cary, P. (2008). *Outward Signs: The Powerlessness of External Things in Augustine's Thought*. Oxford: Oxford University Press.

Case, B. (2021). *The Accountable Animal: Justice, Justification, and Judgment*. New York: Bloomsbury Publishing.

Caspary, A. (2010). *In Good Health: Philosophical-Theological Analysis of the Concept of Health in Contemporary Medical Ethics*. Franz Steiner Verlag Stuttgart.

Cassell, E. J. (1982). The Nature of Suffering and the Goals of Medicine. *New England Journal of Medicine*. 306 (11): 639–645.

Cassell, E. J. (1991). *The Nature of Suffering and the Goals of Medicine*. New York: Oxford University Press.

Catholic Church. (2000). *Catechism of the Catholic Church*. 2nd ed. Vatican City: Libreria Editrice Vaticana.

Catholic Church. (2004). *Compendium of the Social Doctrine of the Church.* Cittá del Vaticano: Libreria Editrice Vaticana.

Cavanaugh, W. T., and Smith, J. K. (2017). *Evolution and the Fall.* Grand Rapids, MI: William B. Eerdmans.

Chancellor, J., Margolis, S., and Lyubomirsky, S. (2018). The Propagation of Everyday Prosociality in the Workplace. *Journal of Positive Psychology* 13(3): 271–283.

Chang, E. H., Milkman, K. L., Gromet, D. M., Rebele, R. W., Massey, C., Duckworth, A. L., and Grant, A. M. (2019). The Mixed Effects of Online Diversity Training. *Proceedings of the National Academy of Sciences* 116: 7778–7783.

Chang, S. C., Glymour, M., Cornelis, M., Walter, S., Rimm, E. B., Tchetgen, E., Kawachi, I., and Kubzansky, L. D. (2017). Social Integration and Reduced Risk of Coronary Heart Disease in Women: The Role of Lifestyle Behaviors. *Circulation Research* 120(12): 1927–1937.

Chatters, L. M. (2000). Religion and Health: Public Health Research and Practice. *Annual Review of Public Health* 21: 335–367.

Chen, Y., Haines, J., Charlton, B. M., and VanderWeele, T. J. (2019). Positive Parenting Improves Multiple Aspects of Health and Well-Being in Young Adulthood. *Nature Human Behavior* 3: 684–691.

Chen, Y., Harris, S. K, Worthington, E. L., and VanderWeele, T. J. (2019). Religiously or Spiritually-Motivated Forgiveness and Subsequent Health and Well-Being among Young Adults: An Outcome-Wide Analysis. *Journal of Positive Psychology* 187: 2355–2364.

Chen, Y., Kim, E. S., Koh, H. K., Frazier, A. L., and VanderWeele, T. J. (2019). Sense of Mission and Subsequent Health and Well-Being among Young Adults: An Outcome-Wide Analysis. *American Journal of Epidemiology* 188(4): 664–673.

Chen, Y., Kim, E. S., and VanderWeele, T. J. (2020). Religious-Service Attendance and Subsequent Health and Well-Being throughout Adulthood: Evidence from Three Prospective Cohorts. *International Journal of Epidemiology* 49(6): 2030–2040.

Chen, Y., Kubzansky, L. D., and VanderWeele, T. J. (2019). Parental Warmth and Flourishing in Mid-Life. *Social Science & Medicine* 220: 65–72.

Chen, Y., Mathur, M. B., Case, B. W., and VanderWeele, T. J. (2023). Marital Transitions during Earlier Adulthood and Subsequent Health and Well-Being in Mid- to Late-Life among Female Nurses: An Outcome-Wide Analysis. *Global Epidemiology* 5: 100099.

Chen, Y., and VanderWeele, T. J. (2018). Associations of Religious Upbringing with Subsequent Health and Well-Being from Adolescence to Young Adulthood: An Outcome-Wide Analysis. *American Journal of Epidemiology* 187(11): 2355–2364.

Chetty, R., Friedman, J., and Rockoff, J. (2014a). Measuring the Impacts of Teachers II: Teacher Value-Added and Student Outcomes in Adulthood. *American Economic Review* 104(9): 2633–2679.

Chetty, R., Hendren, N., Kline, P., Saez, E., and Turner, N. (2014b). Is the United States Still a Land of Opportunity? Recent Trends in Intergenerational Mobility. *American Economic Review* 104(5): 141–147.

Chida, Y., Steptoe, A., and Powell, L. H. (2009). Religiosity/Spirituality and Mortality. *Psychotherapy and Psychosomatics* 78(2): 81–90.

Cloninger, C. R., Zohar, A. H., and Cloninger, K. M. (2010). Promotion of Well-Being in Person-Centered Mental Health Care. *Focus* 8(2): 165–179.

Cohen, R., Bavishi, C., and Rozanski, A. (2016). Purpose in Life and Its Relationship to All-Cause Mortality and Cardiovascular Events: A Meta-Analysis. *Psychosomatic Medicine* 78: 122–133.

Coleman, P. K. (2011). Abortion and Mental Health: Quantitative Synthesis and Analysis of Research Published 1995–2009. *British Journal of Psychiatry* 199: 180–186.

Craig, W. L. (2000). *The Son Rises: Historical Evidence for the Resurrection of Jesus*. Wipf and Stock Publishers.

Cregg, D. R., and Cheavens, J. S. (2020). Gratitude Interventions: Effective Self-Help? A Meta-Analysis of the Impact on Symptoms of Depression and Anxiety. *Journal of Happiness Studies* 22: 1–33.

Crislip, A. T. (2005). *From Monastery to Hospital: Christian Monasticism and the Transformation of Health Care in Late Antiquity*. Ann Arbor, MI: University of Michigan Press.

Crofts, R. A. (1973). The Common Good in the Political Theory of Thomas Aquinas. *The Thomist: A Speculative Quarterly Review* 37(1): 155–173.

Cuñado, J., and de Gracia, F. P. (2012). Does Education Affect Happiness? Evidence for Spain. *Social Indicators Research* 108(1): 185–196.

Curlin, F., and Tollefsen, C. (2021). *The Way of Medicine: Ethics and the Healing Profession*. Notre Dame, IN: University of Notre Dame Press.

Curlin, F. A. (2018). Palliative Sedation: Clinical Context and Ethical Questions. *Theoretical Medicine and Bioethics* 39(3): 197–209.

Curlin, F. A., and Hall, D. E. (2005). Strangers or Friends? A Proposal for a New Spirituality-in-Medicine Ethic. *Journal of General Internal Medicine* 20: 370–374.

Curry, O. S., Rowland, L. A., Van Lissa, C. J., Zlotowitz, S., McAlaney, J., and Whitehouse, H. (2018). Happy to Help? A Systematic Review and Meta-Analysis of the Effects of Performing Acts of Kindness on the Well-Being of the Actor. *Journal of Experimental Social Psychology* 76: 320–329.

Dahlsgaard, K., Peterson, C., and Seligman, M. E. (2005). Shared Virtue: The Convergence of Valued Human Strengths across Culture and History. *Review of General Psychology* 9(3): 203–213.

Dalmida, S. G., and Thurman, S. (2014). HIV/AIDS. In *Religion as a Social Determinant of Health*, edited by E. Idler, 369–381. New York: Oxford University Press.

Daly, D. J. (2011). Structures of Virtue and Vice. *New Blackfriars* 92(1039): 341–357.

Daniels, N. (2008). *Just Health: Meeting Health Needs Fairly.* New York: Cambridge University Press.

Davis, D. E., Choe, E., Meyers, J., Wade, N., Varjas, K., Gifford, A., and Worthington, Jr., E. L. (2016). Thankful for the Little Things: A Meta-Analysis of Gratitude Interventions. *Journal of Counseling Psychology* 63(1): 20.

Dayrit, M. M., and Ambegaokar, M. (2015). Leadership in Public Health. In *The Oxford Textbook of Global Public Health*, 6th ed., edited by Roger Detels, Martin Gulliford, Quarraisha Abdool Karim, and Chorh Chuan Tan. Oxford: Oxford University Press.

De Cabo, R., and Mattson, M. P. (2019). Effects of Intermittent Fasting on Health, Aging, and Disease. *New England Journal of Medicine* 381: 2541–2551.

DeHaven, M. J., Hunter, I. B., Wilder, L., Walton, J. W., and Berry, J. (2004). Health Programs in Faith-Based Organizations: Are They Effective? *American Journal of Public Health* 94(6): 1030–1036.

Derose, K. P., Mendel, P. J., Palar, K., Kanouse, D. E., Bluthenthal, R. N., Castaneda, L. W., Corbin, D. E., Domínguez, B. X., Hawes-Dawson, J., Mata, M. A., and Oden, C. W. (2011). Religious Congregations' Involvement in HIV: A Case Study Approach. *AIDS and Behavior* 15: 1220–1232.

Detels, R., Gulliford, M., Karim, Q. A., and Tan, C. C. (Eds.). (2015). *Oxford Textbook of Global Public Health.* 6th ed. Oxford: Oxford University Press.

Devakumar, D., Selvarajah, S., Shannon, G., Muraya, K., Lasoye, S., Corona, S., Paradies, Y., Abubakar, I., and Achiume, E. T. (2020). Racism, The Public Health Crisis We Can No Longer Ignore. *The Lancet* 395(10242): e112–e113.

Diener, E., Lucas, R., Helliwell, J. F., Schimmack, U., and Helliwell, J. (2009). *Well-Being for Public Policy.* Series in Positive Psychology. Oxford: Oxford University Press.

Diener, E., Tay, L., and Myers, D. G. (2011). The Religion Paradox: If Religion Makes People Happy, Why Are So Many Dropping Out? *Journal of Personality and Social Psychology* 101(6): 1278–1290.

Diener, E. D., Emmons, R. A., Larsen, R. J., and Griffin, S. (1985). The Satisfaction with Life Scale. *Journal of Personality Assessment* 49(1): 71–75.

DiLoreto, R., and Murphy, C. T. (2015). The Cell Biology of Aging. *Molecular Biology of the Cell* 26(25): 4524–4531.

Dobbin, F., and Kalev, A. (2016). Why Diversity Programs Fail. *Harvard Business Review* 94(7): 14.

Dobson, M. L. (2014). *Health as a Virtue: Thomas Aquinas and the Practice of Habits of Health.* N.p.: Wipf and Stock Publishers.

Doss, B. D., Cicila, L. N., Georgia, E. J., Roddy, M. K., Nowlan, K. M., Benson, L. A., and Christensen, A. (2016). A Randomized Controlled Trial of the Web-Based OurRelationship Program: Effects on Relationship and Individual Functioning. *Journal of Consulting and Clinical Psychology* 84: 285–296.

Duffee, C. (2023). Existential Spectrum of Suffering: Concepts and Moral Valuations for Assessing Intensity and Tolerability. *Journal of Medical Ethics.* doi: 10.1136/jme-2023-109183

Duffin, J. (2009). *Medical Miracles: Doctors, Saints, and Healing in the Modern World*. Oxford: Oxford University Press.
Dugdale, L. S. (Ed.). (2017). *Dying in the Twenty-First Century: Toward a New Ethical Framework for the Art of Dying Well*. Cambridge, MA: MIT Press.
Dugdale, L. S. (2021). *The Lost Art of Dying: Reviving Forgotten Wisdom*. New York: HarperCollins.
Emanuel, E. (2017). Euthanasia and Physician-Assisted Suicide: Focus on the Data. *Medical Journal of Australia* 206(8): 339–340.
Emmons, R. A., and Mccullough, M. E. (2003). Counting Blessings versus Burdens: An Experimental Investigation of Gratitude and Subjective Well-Being in Daily Life. *Journal of Personality and Social Psychology* 84(2): 377–389.
Engelhardt, H. T. (1974). The Disease of Masturbation: Values and the Concept of Disease. *Bulletin of the History of Medicine* 48(2): 234–248.
Enright, R. D., and Fitzgibbons, R. P. (2000). *Helping Clients Forgive: An Empirical Guide for Resolving Anger and Restoring Hope*. Washington, DC: American Psychological Association.
Evans, A. R. (1999). *Healing Church: Practical Programs for Health Ministries*. Cleveland, OH: United Church Press.
Fagerlind, H., Ring, L., Brülde, B., Feltelius, N., and Lindblad, Å. K. (2010). Patients' Understanding of the Concepts of Health and Quality of Life. *Patient Education and Counseling* 78(1): 104–110.
Fancourt, D., and Finn, S. (2019). *What Is the Evidence on the Role of the Arts in Improving Health and Well-Being? A Scoping Review*. Copenhagen: World Health Organization. Regional Office for Europe.
Fancourt, D., and Steptoe, A. (2018). Community Group Membership and Multidimensional Subjective Well-Being in Older Age. *Journal of Epidemiology and Community Health* 72(5): 376–382.
Fedoryka, K. (1997). Health as a Normative Concept: Towards a New Conceptual Framework. *Journal of Medicine and Philosophy* 22(2): 143–160.
Ferngren, G. B. (2016). *Medicine and Health Care in Early Christianity*. Baltimore, MD: Johns Hopkins University Press.
Finn, D. K. (2016). What Is a Sinful Social Structure? *Theological Studies* 77(1): 136–164.
Finnis, J. (1998). *Aquinas: Moral, Political, and Legal Theory*. Oxford: Oxford University Press.
Finnis, J. (2011). *Natural Law and Natural Rights*. Oxford: Oxford University Press.
First, M. B., and Wakefield, J. C. (2013). Diagnostic Criteria as Dysfunction Indicators: Bridging the Chasm between the Definition of Mental Disorder and Diagnostic Criteria for Specific Disorders. *Canadian Journal of Psychiatry* 58(12): 663–669.
Fischer, C. S. (2009). The 2004 GSS Finding of Shrunken Social Networks: An Artifact? *American Sociological Review* 74(4): 657–669.
Fisher, J. (2010). Development and Application of a Spiritual Well-Being Questionnaire Called SHALOM. *Religions* 1(1): 105–121.

Fletcher, G. (2013). A Fresh Start for the Objective-List Theory of Well-Being. *Utilitas* 25(2): 206.
Fletcher, G. (2015). Objective List Theories. In *The Routledge Handbook of Philosophy of Well-Being*, edited by G. Fletcher, 164–176. London: Routledge.
Fletcher, G. (2016). *The Philosophy of Well-Being: An Introduction*. London: Routledge.
Fowers, B. J. (2014). Toward Programmatic Research on Virtue Assessment: Challenges and Prospects. *Theory and Research in Education* 12(3): 309–328.
Fowler, J. H., and Christakis, N. A. (2010). Cooperative Behavior Cascades in Human Social Networks. *Proceedings of the National Academy of Sciences* 107(12): 5334–5338.
Fox, K. E., Johnson, S. T., Berkman, L. F., Sianoja, M., Soh, Y., Kubzansky, L. D., and Kelly, E. L. (2021). Organisational- and Group-Level Workplace Interventions and Their Effect on Multiple Domains of Worker Well-Being: A Systematic Review. *Work & Stress* 36(1): 30–59.
Francis. (2015). *Laudato si': On Care for Our Common Home*. https://www.vatican.va/content/francesco/en/encyclicals/documents/papa-francesco_20150524_enciclica-laudato-si.html.
Francis. (2017). Address to Participants in the Meeting Promoted by the Pontifical Council for Promoting the New Evangelization. https://www.vatican.va/content/francesco/en/speeches/2017/october/documents/papa-francesco_20171011_convegno-nuova-evangelizzazione.html.
Francis. (2020). *Fratelli tutti: On Fraternity and Social Friendship*. Libreria Editrice Vaticana. https://www.vatican.va/content/francesco/en/encyclicals/documents/papa-francesco_20201003_enciclica-fratelli-tutti.html.
Frederick, D. E., and VanderWeele, T. J. (2020). Longitudinal Meta-Analysis of Job Crafting Shows Positive Association with Work Engagement. *Cogent Psychology* 7(1): 1746733.
Frey, J. A. (2018). Aquinas on Sin, Self-Love, and Self-Transcendence. In *Self-Transcendence and Virtue: Perspectives from Philosophy, Psychology, and Theology*, edited by J. A. Frey and C. Vogler. London: Routledge.
Fruehwirth, J. C., Iyer, S., and Zhang, A. (2019). Religion and Depression in Adolescence. *Journal of Political Economy* 127(3): 1178–1209.
Fulford, K. W. (1993). Praxis Makes Perfect: Illness as a Bridge between Biological Concepts of Disease and Social Conceptions of Health. *Theoretical Medicine* 14(4): 305–320.
Fulford, K. W. M., Thornton, T., and Graham, G. (2006). *Oxford Textbook of Philosophy and Psychiatry*. Oxford: Oxford University Press.
Gadamer, H. G. (1996). *The Enigma of Health*. Translated by J. Gaiger and N. Walker. Stanford, CA: Stanford University Press.
Galante, J., Galante, I., Bekkers, M. J., and Gallacher, J. (2014). Effect of Kindness-Based Meditation on Health and Well-Being: A Systematic Review and Meta-Analysis. *Journal of Consulting and Clinical Psychology* 82(6): 1101–1114.

Gammelgaard, A. (2000). Evolutionary Biology and the Concept of Disease. *Medicine, Health Care and Philosophy* 3(2): 109–116.

Garner, L. (1979). *The NHS: Your Money or Your Life.* New York: Penguin.

Garrigou-Lagrange, R. (1937). *Christian Perfection and Contemplation.* St. Louis, MO: B. Herder Book Co.

Garrigou-Lagrange, R. (1999). *Three Ages of the Interior Life.* Rockford, IL: Tan Books & Publishers.

Garssen, B., Visser, A., and Pool, G. (2021). Does Spirituality or Religion Positively Affect Mental Health? Meta-Analysis of Longitudinal Studies. *International Journal for the Psychology of Religion* 31(1): 4–20.

George, L. S., and Park, C. L. (2016). Meaning in Life as Comprehension, Purpose, and Mattering: Toward Integration and New Research Questions. *Review of General Psychology* 20(3): 205–220.

George, R. P. (1995). *Making Men Moral: Civil Liberties and Public Morality.* Oxford: Clarendon Press.

Gilby, T. (1958). *The Political Thought of Thomas Aquinas.* Chicago: University of Chicago Press.

Girgis, S., Anderson, R. T., and George, R. P. (2012). *What Is Marriage? Man and Woman: A Defense.* Encounter Books.

Goodman, F. R., Disabato, D. J., Kashdan, T. B., and Kauffman, S. B. (2018). Measuring Well-Being: A Comparison of Subjective Well-Being and PERMA. *Journal of Positive Psychology* 13(4): 321–332.

Griffin, B. J., Purcell, N., Burkman, K., Litz, B. T., Bryan, C. J., Schmitz, M., . . . and Maguen, S. (2019). Moral Injury: An Integrative Review. *Journal of Traumatic Stress* 32(3): 350–362.

Grim, B. J., and Finke, R. (2011). *The Price of Freedom Denied: Religious Persecution and Conflict in the Twenty-First Century.* Cambridge: Cambridge University Press.

Gunderson, G., and Cochrane, J. (2012). *Religion and the Health of the Public: Shifting the Paradigm.* New York: Palgrave Macmillan.

Hacker, P. M. S. (1996). *Wittgenstein: Mind and Will.* Vol. 4 of *An Analytical Commentary on the Philosophical Investigations.* Oxford: Blackwell.

Hall, J., and Rickard, L. (2013). *People, Progress and Participation: How Initiatives Measuring Social Progress Yield Benefits beyond Better Metrics.* Gütersloh, Germany: Bertelsmann Stiftung.

Handzo, G., Flannelly, K. J., and Hughes, B. P. (2017). Hospital Characteristics Affecting Healthcare Chaplaincy and the Provision of Chaplaincy Care in the United States: 2004 vs. 2016. *Journal of Pastoral Care & Counseling* 71(3): 156–162.

Hanson, J. A. (2022a). *Philosophies of Work in the Platonic Tradition: A History of Labor and Human Flourishing.* New York: Bloomsbury.

Hanson, J. A. (2022b). "That is giving a banquet": Neighbor-Love as Spiritualization of Romantic Love in Works of Love. *Journal of Religious Ethics* 50(2): 196–218.

Hanson, J. A., and VanderWeele, T. J. (2021). The Comprehensive Measure of Meaning: Psychological and Philosophical Foundations. In *Measuring*

Well-Being: Interdisciplinary Perspectives from the Social Sciences and the Humanities, edited by M. Lee, L. D. Kubzansky, and T. J. Vander-Weele, 339–376. New York: Oxford University Press.

Harper, Q., Worthington Jr., E. L., Griffin, B. J., Lavelock, C. R., Hook, J. N., Vrana, S. R., and Greer, C. L. (2014). Efficacy of a Workbook to Promote Forgiveness: A Randomized Controlled Trial with University Students. *Journal of Clinical Psychology* 70(12): 1158–1169.

Harr, J. (1996). *A Civil Action*. New York: Random House.

Heinrich, G., Leege, D., and Miller, C. (2009). *A User's Guide to Integral Human Development (IHD): Practical Guidance for CRS Staff and Partners*. Catholic Relief Services. https://www.crs.org/sites/default/files/tools-research/users-guide-to-integral-human-development.pdf.

Helliwell, J. F., Layard, R., Sachs, J. D., and De Neve, J.-E. (2021). *World Happiness Report 2021*. New York: Sustainable Development Solutions Network.

Hendriks, T., Schotanus-Dijkstra, M., Hassankhan, A., de Jong, J., and Bohlmeijer, E. (2019). The Efficacy of Multi-Component Positive Psychology Interventions: A Systematic Review and Meta-Analysis of Randomized Controlled Trials. *Journal of Happiness Studies* 21: 1–34.

Hernandez, R., Bassett, S. M., Boughton, S. W., Schuette, S. A., Shiu, E. W., and Moskowitz, J. T. (2018). Psychological Well-Being and Physical Health: Associations, Mechanisms, and Future Directions. *Emotion Review* 10(1): 18–29.

Ho, M. Y., Worthington, E., Cowden, R., Bechara, A. O., Chen, Z. J., Gunatirin, E. Y., Joynt, S., Khalanskyi, V. V., Korzhov, H., Kurniati, N. M. T., Rodriguez, N., Salnykova, A., Shtanko, L., Tymchenko, S., Voytenko, V. L., Zulkaida, A., Mathur, M., and VanderWeele, T. (2024, March 3). International REACH Forgiveness Intervention: A Multi-Site Randomised Controlled Trial. *BMJ Public Health*, 2:e000072.

Hoad, T. F. (Ed.). (1986). *The Concise Oxford Dictionary of English Etymology*. Oxford: Clarendon Press.

Hogan, R. M. (2006). *The Theology of the Body in John Paul II: What It Means, Why It Matters*. Frederick, MD: Word Among Us Press.

Holmgren, M. R. (1993). Forgiveness and the Intrinsic Value of Persons. *American Philosophical Quarterly* 30: 341–352.

Höltge, J., Cowden, R., Lee, M., Bechara, A., Joynt, S., Kamble, S., Khalanskyi, V., Shtanko, L., Kurniati, N., Tymchenko, S., Voytenko, V., McNeely, E., and VanderWeele, T. J. (2023). A Systems Perspective on Human Flourishing: Exploring Cross-Country Similarities and Differences of a Multisystemic Flourishing Network. *Journal of Positive Psychology* 18: 695–710.

Holt-Lunstad, J. (2022). Social Connection as a Public Health Issue: The Evidence and a Systemic Framework for Prioritizing the "Social" in Social Determinants of Health. *Annual Review of Public Health* 43: 193–213.

Holt-Lunstad, J., Smith, T. B., Baker, M., Harris, T., and Stephenson, D. (2015). Loneliness and Social Isolation as Risk Factors for Mortality: A Meta-Analytic Review. *Perspectives on Psychological Science* 10(2): 227–237.

Hone, L. C., Jarden, A., Schofield, G. M., and Duncan, S. (2014). Measuring Flourishing: The Impact of Operational Definitions on the Prevalence of High Levels of Wellbeing. *International Journal of Wellbeing* 4(1): 62–90.

Hong, J. H., Berkman, L. F., Chen, F. S., Shiba, K., Chen, Y., Kim, E. S., and VanderWeele, T. J. (2023). Are Loneliness and Social Isolation Equal Threats to Health and Well-Being? An Outcome-Wide Longitudinal Approach. *Social Science & Medicine—Population Health* 23: 101459.

Hordern, J. (2020). *Compassion in Healthcare: Pilgrimage, Practice, and Civic Life*. Oxford: Oxford University Press.

Houck, D. W. (2020). *Aquinas, Original Sin, and the Challenge of Evolution*. Cambridge: Cambridge University Press.

Huber, M., Knottnerus, J. A., Green, L., van der Horst, H., Jadad, A. R., Kromhout, D., Leonard, B., Lorig, K., Loureiro, M. I., van der Meer, J. W. M., Schnabel, P., Smith, R., van Weel, C., and Smid, H. (2011). How Should We Define Health? *British Medical Journal* 343: d4163.

Hunt, P., Backman, G., de Mesquita, J. B., Finer, L., Khosla, R., Korljan, D., and Oldring, L. (2015). The Right to the Highest Attainable Standard of Health. In *The Oxford Textbook of Global Public Health*, 6th ed., edited by Roger Detels, Martin Gulliford, Quarraisha Abdool Karim, and Chorh Chuan Tan. Oxford: Oxford University Press.

Huppert, F. A., Abbott, R. A., Ploubidis, G. B., Richards, M., and Kuh, D. (2010). Parental Practices Predict Psychological Well-Being in Midlife: Life-Course Associations among Women in the 1946 British Birth Cohort. *Psychological Medicine* 40(9): 1507–1518.

Huppert, F. A., and So, T. T. (2013). Flourishing across Europe: Application of a New Conceptual Framework for Defining Well-Being. *Social Indicators Research* 110(3): 837–861.

Hurka, T. (1993). *Perfectionism*. Oxford: Clarendon Press.

Idler, E. L. (2014a). Ingenious Institutions: Religious Origins of Health and Development Organization. In *Religion as a Social Determinant of Public Health*, edited by Ellen Idler. New York: Oxford University Press.

Idler, E. L. (2014b). *Religion as a Social Determinant of Public Health*. New York: Oxford University Press.

Idler, E., Levin, J., VanderWeele, T. J., and Khan, A. (2019). Partnerships between Public Health Agencies and Faith Communities. *American Journal of Public Health* 109(3): 346–347.

International Theological Commission. (2009, May 20). In Search of a Universal Ethic: A New Look at the Natural Law. Accessed May 24, 2003. https://www.vatican.va/roman_curia/congregations/cfaith/cti_documents/rc_con_cfaith_doc_20090520_legge-naturale_en.html.

Jankowski, P. J., Sandage, S. J., Bell, C. A., Davis, D. E., Porter, E., Jessen, M., Motzny, C. L., Ross, K. V., and Owen, J. (2020). Virtue, Flourishing, and Positive Psychology in Psychotherapy: An Overview and Research Prospectus. *Psychotherapy* 57(3): 291.

Jazaieri, H., Jinpa, G. T., McGonigal, K., Rosenberg, E. L., Finkelstein, J., Simon-Thomas, E., Cullen, M., Doty, J. R., Gross, J. J., and Goldin, P. R. (2013). Enhancing Compassion: A Randomized Controlled Trial of a Compassion Cultivation Training Program. *Journal of Happiness Studies* 14(4): 1113–1126.

Jazaieri, H., McGonigal, K., Jinpa, T., Doty, J. R., Gross, J. J., and Goldin, P. R. (2014). A Randomized Controlled Trial of Compassion Cultivation Training: Effects on Mindfulness, Affect, and Emotion Regulation. *Motivation and Emotion* 38(1): 23–35.

Jeffrey, D. L., and Levin, J. (2020). Are the Wages of Sin Really Death? Moral and Epidemiologic Observations. *Christian Scholar's Review* 49(3): 263–279.

Jeste, D. V., Palmer, B. W., Rettew, D. C., and Boardman, S. (2015). Positive Psychiatry: Its Time Has Come. *Journal of Clinical Psychiatry* 76(6): 675–683.

John Paul II. (1980). *Dives in misericordia*. Libreria Editrice Vaticana. https://www.vatican.va/content/john-paul-ii/en/encyclicals/documents/hf_jp-ii_enc_30111980_dives-in-misericordia.html.

John Paul II. (1981). *Laborem exercens*. Libreria Editrice Vaticana. https://www.vatican.va/content/john-paul-ii/en/encyclicals/documents/hf_jp-ii_enc_14091981_laborem-exercens.html.

John Paul II. (1984). *Salvifici doloris*. https://www.vatican.va/content/john-paul-ii/en/apost_letters/1984/documents/hf_jp-ii_apl_11021984_salvifici-doloris.html.

John Paul II. (1987). *Sollicitudo rei socialis*. Libreria Editrice Vaticana. https://www.vatican.va/content/john-paul-ii/en/en16cyclicals/documents/hf_jp-ii_enc_30121987_sollicitudo-rei-socialis.html.

John Paul II. (1991). *Centesimus annus*. Libreria Editrice Vaticana. https://www.vatican.va/content/john-paul-ii/en/encyclicals/documents/hf_jp-ii_enc_01051991_centesimus-annus.html.

John Paul II. (1995). *Evangelium vitae: On the Value and Inviolability of Human Life*. Libreria Editrice Vaticana. https://www.vatican.va/content/john-paul-ii/en/encyclicals/documents/hf_jp-ii_enc_25031995_evangelium-vitae.html.

John Paul II. (2006). *Man and Woman He Created Them: A Theology of the Body*. Boston, MA: Pauline Books & Media.

John XXIII. (1961). *Mater and magistra*. Libreria Editrice Vaticana. https://www.vatican.va/content/john-xxiii/en/encyclicals/documents/hf_j-xxiii_enc_15051961_mater.html.

John XXIII. (1963). *Pacem in terries: On Establishing Universal Peace in Truth*. Libreria Editrice Vaticana. https://www.vatican.va/content/john-xxiii/en/encyclicals/documents/hf_j-xxiii_enc_11041963_pacem.html.

Jordan, J. J., Rand, D. G., Arbesman, S., Fowler, J. H., and Christakis, N. A. (2013). Contagion of Cooperation in Static and Fluid Social Networks. *PLOS One* 8(6): e66199.

Justinian. (533/1985). *The Digest of Justinian*. Edited by T. Mommsen, P. Krueger, and A. Watson. Philadelphia: University of Pennsylvania Press. Accessed January 4, 2023. https://www.vatican.va/content/john-xxiii/en/encyclicals/documents/hf_j-xxiii_enc_11041963_pacem.html.

Kass, L. R. (1975). Regarding the End of Medicine and the Pursuit of Health. *The Public Interest* 40: 11.

Kass, N. E. (2001). An Ethics Framework for Public Health. *American Journal of Public Health* 91(11): 1776–1782.

Kee, H. C. (1992). Medicine and Healing. In *The Anchor Bible Dictionary*, edited by D. N. Freedman. New York: Doubleday.

Keenan, J. F. (1993). The Function of the Principle of Double Effect. *Theological Studies* 54(2): 294–315.

Kelly, G. (1955). Pope Pius XII and the Principle of Totality. *Theological Studies* 16: 373–396.

Kendler, K. S. (2009). An Historical Framework for Psychiatric Nosology. *Psychological Medicine* 39(12): 1935–1941.

Kendler, K. S. (2016). The Nature of Psychiatric Disorders. *World Psychiatry* 15(1): 5–12.

Kendler, K. S., and Parnas, J. (2012). *Philosophical Issues in Psychiatry II: Nosology*. Oxford: Oxford University Press.

Kenny, A. J. P. (1976). *Will, Freedom, and Power*. Oxford: Blackwell Publishers.

Kern, M. L., Allen, K. A., Furlong, M., Vella-Brodrick, S., and Suldo, S. (2021). PERMAH: A Useful Model for Focusing on Wellbeing in Schools. In *Handbook of Positive Psychology in Schools*, 3rd ed., edited by M. J. Furlong, R. Gilman, and E. S. Huebner. London: Routledge.

Keyes, C. L. (2002). The Mental Health Continuum: From Languishing to Flourishing in Life. *Journal of Health and Social Behavior* 43(2): 207–222.

Keys, M. M. (1995). Personal Dignity and the Common Good: A Twentieth-Century Thomistic Dialogue. In *Catholicism, Liberalism, and Communitarianism: The Catholic Intellectual Tradition and the Moral Foundations of Democracy*, edited by Kenneth L. Grasso, Gerard Y. Bradley, and Robert P. Hunt. Lanham, MD: Rowman and Littlefield, 1995.

Kheriaty, A. D. (2012). *A Catholic Guide to Depression*. Manchester, NJ: Sophia Institute Press.

Kierkegaard, S. (1847/1995). *Works of Love*. Edited and translated by H. V. Hong and E. H. Hong. Princeton, NJ: Princeton University Press.

Kim, E. S., Nakamura, J. S., Chen, Y., Ryff, C. D., and VanderWeele, T. J. (2022). Sense of Purpose in Life and Subsequent Health and Well-Being in Older Adults: An Outcome-Wide Analysis. *American Journal of Health Promotion* 36: 137–147.

Kim, E. S., and VanderWeele, T. J. (2019). Mediators of the Association between Religious Service Attendance and Mortality. *American Journal of Epidemiology* 188(1): 96–101.

Kim, E. S., Whillans, A. V., Lee, M. T., Chen, Y., and VanderWeele, T. J. (2020). Volunteering and Subsequent Health and Well-Being in Older Adults: An Outcome-Wide Longitudinal Approach. *American Journal of Preventive Medicine* 59: 176–186.

Kinghorn, W. (2013). "Hope that is seen is no hope at all": Theological Constructions of Hope in Psychotherapy. *Bulletin of the Menninger Clinic* 77(4): 369–394.

Kirby, J. N., Tellegen, C. L., and Steindl, S. R. (2017). A Meta-Analysis of Compassion-Based Interventions: Current State of Knowledge and Future Directions. *Behavior Therapy* 48(6): 778–792.

Kirkman, M., Rowe, H., Hardiman, A., Mallett, S., and Rosenthal, D. (2009). Reasons Women Give for Abortion: A Review of the Literature. *Archives of Women's Mental Health* 12: 365–378.

Koenig, H. G. (2000a). Medicine and Religion. *New England Journal of Medicine* 343: 1339.

Koenig, H. G. (2000b). Religion, Spirituality, and Medicine: Application to clinical practice. *Journal of the American Medical Association* 284(13): 1708.

Koenig, H. G., and Al Zaben, F. (2021). Moral Injury: An Increasingly Recognized and Widespread Syndrome. *Journal of Religion and Health* 60(5): 2989–3011.

Koenig, H. G., Hooten, E. G., Lindsay-Calkins, E., Meador, K. G. (2010). Spirituality in Medical School Curricula: Findings from a National Survey. *International Journal of Psychiatry in Medicine* 40(4): 391–398.

Koenig, H. G., VanderWeele, T. J., and Peteet, J. (2023). *Handbook of Religion and Health*. 3rd ed. Oxford: Oxford University Press.

Koritansky, P. K. (2012). *Thomas Aquinas and the Philosophy of Punishment*. Washington, DC: Catholic University of America Press.

Kovács, J. (1998). The Concept of Health and Disease. *Medicine, Health Care and Philosophy* 1(1): 31–39.

Krieger, N. (2017). Religious Service Attendance and Suicide Rates. *Journal of the American Medical Association Psychiatry* 74(2): 197.

Krieger, N., Chen, J. T., Coull, B. A., Beckfield, J., Kiang, M. V., and Waterman, P. D. (2014). Jim Crow and Premature Mortality among the US Black and White Population, 1960–2009: An Age-Period-Cohort Analysis. *Epidemiology* 25(4): 494.

Krom, M. P. (2020). *Justice and Charity: An Introduction to Aquinas's Moral, Economic, and Political Thought*. Grand Rapids, MI: Baker Academic.

Larchet, J.-C. (2002). *The Theology of Illness*. Crestwood, NY: St. Vladimir's Seminary Press.

Larrimore, M. (2000). *The Problem of Evil: A Reader*. New York: Wiley-Blackwell.

Larson, J. S. (1996). The World Health Organization's Definition of Health: Social versus Spiritual Health. *Social Indicators Research* 38(2): 181–192.

Lasater, T. M., Becker, D. M., Hill, M. N., and Gans, K. M. 1997. Synthesis of Findings and Issues from Religious-Based Cardiovascular Disease Prevention Trials. *Annals of Epidemiology* 7(57): s47–53.

Lauinger, W. (2013). The Missing-Desires Objection to Hybrid Theories of Well-Being. *Southern Journal of Philosophy* 51(2): 270–295.

Law, I., and Widdows, H. (2008). Conceptualising Health: Insights from the Capability Approach. *Health Care Analysis* 16(4): 303–314.

Lee, M., Kubzansky, L. D., and VanderWeele, T. J. (2021). *Measuring Well-Being: Interdisciplinary Perspectives from the Social Sciences and the Humanities*. Oxford: Oxford University Press.

Leo XIII. (1891). *Rerum Novarum: On Capital and Labour.* Accessed January 5, 2024. https://www.vatican.va/content/leo-xiii/en/encyclicals/documents/hf_l-xiii_enc_15051891_rerum-novarum.html.
Letourneau, B. (2019, November 14). Attempts in Reconciliation. *North American Anglican.* https://northamanglican.com/attempts-in-reconciliation/.
Levin, J. (2014). Faith-Based Initiatives in Health Promotion: History, Challenges, and Current Partnerships. *American Journal of Health Promotion* 28: 139–141.
Levin, J. (2016). Partnerships between the Faith-Based and Medical Sectors: Implications for Preventive Medicine and Public Health. *Preventive Medicine Reports* 4: 344–350.
Levin, J., Idler, E. L., and VanderWeele, T. J. (2021). Faith-Based Organizations and SARS-CoV-2 Vaccination: Challenges and Recommendations. *Public Health Reports* 137(1): 11–16.
Levin, J., and Meador, K. (Eds.). (2012). *Healing to All Their Flesh: Jewish and Christian Perspectives on Spirituality, Theology, and Health.* West Conshohocken, PA: Templeton Foundation Press.
Li, S., Stamfer, M., Williams, D. R., and VanderWeele, T. J. (2016). Association between Religious Service Attendance and Mortality among Women. *Journal of the American Medical Association Internal Medicine* 176(6): 777–785.
Litwin, H. (2007). What Really Matters in the Social Network-Mortality Association? A Multivariate Examination among Older Jewish-Israelis. *European Journal of Ageing* 4(2): 71–82.
Litz, B. T., and Kerig, P. K. (2019). Introduction to the Special Issue on Moral Injury: Conceptual Challenges, Methodological Issues, and Clinical Applications. *Journal of Traumatic Stress* 32(3): 341–349.
Litz, B. T., Lebowitz, L., Gray, M. J., and Nash, W. P. (2016). *Adaptive Disclosure: A New Treatment for Military Trauma, Loss, and Moral Injury.* New York: The Guilford Press.
Litz, B. T., Stein, N., Delaney, E., Lebowitz, L., Nash, W. P., Silva, C., and Maguen, S. (2009). Moral Injury and Moral Repair in War Veterans: A Preliminary Model and Intervention Strategy. *Clinical Psychology Review* 29(8): 695–706.
Lomas, T., and VanderWeele, T. J. (2023). Toward an Expanded Taxonomy of Happiness: A Conceptual Analysis of 16 Distinct Forms of Mental Wellbeing. *Journal of Humanistic Psychology* 0(0). DOI: 10.1177/00221678231155512.
Lomas, T., and VanderWeele, T. J. (N.d.). A Flexible Map of Flourishing: The Dynamics and Drivers of Flourishing, Wellbeing, Health, and Happiness. Unpublished paper.
Long, K. N., Chen, Y., Potts, M., Hanson, J., and VanderWeele, T. J. (2020). Spiritually Motivated Self-Forgiveness and Divine Forgiveness, and Subsequent Health and Well-Being among Middle-Aged Female Nurses: An Outcome-Wide Longitudinal Approach. *Frontiers in Psychology* 11: 1337.

Long, K. N., Kim, E. S., Chen, Y., Wilson, M. F., Worthington Jr., E. L., and VanderWeele, T. J. (2020). The Role of Hope in Subsequent Health and Well-Being for Older Adults: An Outcome-Wide Longitudinal Approach. *Global Epidemiology* 2: 100018.

Long, K., Worthington, E. L., VanderWeele, T. J., and Chen, Y. (2020). Forgiveness of Others and Subsequent Health and Well-Being in Mid-Life: A Longitudinal Study on Female Nurses. *BMC Psychology* 8: 104.

Lyubomirsky, S., King, L., and Diener, E. (2005). The Benefits of Frequent Positive Affect: Does Happiness Lead to Success? *Psychological Bulletin* 131(6): 803–855.

Mafico, T. L. J. Just, Justice. (1992). In *The Anchor Bible Dictionary*, edited by D. N. Freedman. New York: Doubleday.

Manzoli, L., Villari, P. M., Pirone, G., and Boccia, A. (2007). Marital Status and Mortality in the Elderly: A Systematic Review and Meta-Analysis. *Social Science & Medicine* 64: 77–94.

Maritain, J. (1936/1996). *Integral Humanism, Freedom in the Modern World, and A Letter on Independence*. Translated by Otto Bird. Notre Dame, IN: University of Notre Dame Press.

Maritain, J. (1947). *The Person and the Common Good*. Translated by John J. Fitzgerald. New York: Charles Scribner's Sons.

Marks, N. F., and Lambert, J. D. (1998). Marital Status Continuity and Change among Young and Midlife Adults: Longitudinal Effects on Psychological Well-Being. *Journal of Family Issues* 19: 652–686.

Martela, F., and Steger, M. F. (2016). The Three Meanings of Meaning in Life: Distinguishing Coherence, Purpose, and Significance. *Journal of Positive Psychology* 11(5): 531–545.

Martín-María, N., Miret, M., Caballero, F. F., Rico-Uribe, L. A., Steptoe, A., Chatterji, S., and Ayuso-Mateos, J. L. (2017). The Impact of Subjective Well-Being on Mortality: A Meta-Analysis of Longitudinal Studies in the General Population. *Psychosomatic Medicine* 79(5): 565–575.

Massingale, B. N. (2014). *Racial Justice and the Catholic Church*. Maryknoll, NY: Orbis Books.

Maves, P. B. (1960). Aging, Religion, and the Church. In *Handbook of Social Gerontology*, edited by Clark Tibbits. Chicago, IL: University of Chicago Press.

Max-Neef, M. A. (1992). *Human Scale Development: Conception, Application and Further Reflections*. New York: Apex.

May, G. G. (2009). *The Dark Night of the Soul: A Psychiatrist Explores the Connection Between Darkness and Spiritual Growth*. Grand Rapids, MI: Zondervan.

May, W. (2008). *Catholic Bioethics and the Gift of Human Life*. Huntington, IN: Our Sunday Visitor.

McCormick, R. (1987). *Health and Medicine in the Catholic Tradition*. New York: Crossroad.

McHugh, P. R., and Slavney, P. R. (1998). *The Perspectives of Psychiatry*. Baltimore, MD: Johns Hopkins University Press.

McKee-Ryan, F., Song, Z., Wanberg, C. R., and Kinicki, A. J. (2005). Psychological and Physical Well-Being during Unemployment: A Meta-Analytic Study. *Journal of Applied Psychology* 90(1): 53.

McMinn, M. R., and Campbell, C. D. (2007). *Integrative Psychotherapy: Toward a Comprehensive Christian Approach.* Downers Grove, IL: InterVarsity Press.

McPherson, M., Smith-Lovin, L., and Brashears, M. E. (2006). Social Isolation in America: Changes in Core Discussion Networks over Two Decades. *American Sociological Review* 71(3): 353–375.

Megone, C. (1998). Aristotle's Function Argument and the Concept of Mental Illness. *Philosophy, Psychiatry, & Psychology* 5(3): 187–201.

Meister, C., and Dew Jr, J. K. (Eds.). (2017). *God and the Problem of Evil: Five Views.* Downer's Grove, IL: InterVarsity Press.

Merriam, G. (2009). Rehabilitating Aristotle: A Virtue Ethics Approach to Disability and Human Flourishing. In *Philosophical Reflections on Disability*, edited by D. Christopher Ralston and Justin Ho, 133–151. Dordrecht: Springer.

Messer, N. (2013). *Flourishing: Health, Disease, and Bioethics in Theological Perspective.* Grand Rapids, MI: William B. Eerdmans Publishing.

Michels, R., and Frances, A. (2013). Should Psychiatry Be Expanding Its Boundaries? *Canadian Journal of Psychiatry* 58(10): 566–569.

Miettinen, O. S. (2011). *Epidemiological Research: Terms and Concepts.* Dordrecht: Springer Science & Business Media.

Miller, T. S. (1997). *The Birth of the Hospital in the Byzantine Empire.* Baltimore, MD: Johns Hopkins University Press.

Mordacci, R. (1995). Health as an Analogical Concept. *Journal of Medicine and Philosophy* 20(5): 475–497.

Moreira-Almeida, A., Araujo, S. D. F., and Cloninger, C. R. (2018). The Presentation of the Mind-Brain Problem in Leading Psychiatry Journals. *Brazilian Journal of Psychiatry* 40: 335–342.

Morgan, J., and Sandage, S. J. (2016). A Developmental Model of Interreligious Competence. *Archive for the Psychology of Religion* 38(2): 129–158.

Morris, A. D. (1986). *The Origins of the Civil Rights Movements.* The Free Press.

Moyse, A. J., and Hordern, J. (2021). Illuminating the Darker Side of Ageing: A Special Issue of the Journal of Population Ageing. *Journal of Population Ageing* 14(3): 317–322.

Murphy, M. C. (1999). The Simple Desire-Fulfillment Theory. *Noûs* 33(2): 247–272.

Murphy, M. C. (2001). *Natural Law and Practical Rationality.* Cambridge: Cambridge University Press.

Murray, L. R., Garcia, J., Munoz-Laboy, M., and Parker, R. G. (2011). Strange Bedfellows: The Catholic Church and Brazilian National AIDS Program in the Response to HIV/AIDS in Brazil. *Social Science & Medicine* 72: 945–952.

Murthy, V. (2023). *Our Epidemic of Loneliness and Isolation: The U.S. Surgeon General's Advisory on the Healing Effects of Social Connection and Com-*

munity. Washington, DC: Office of the Surgeon General. https://www.hhs.gov/sites/default/files/surgeon-general-social-connection-advisory.pdf.

Mwenda, S. (2011). The African Christian Health Association Platform: Showcasing the Contributions of CHAs. *Contact* 190: 2.

Narayan, D. (2000). *Voices of the Poor: Can Anyone Hear Us?* Oxford: Oxford University Press for the World Bank.

National Collaborating Centre for Mental Health at the Royal College of Psychiatrists. (2011). *Induced Abortion and Mental Health: A Systematic Review of the Mental Health Outcomes of Induced Abortion, Including Their Prevalence and Associated Factors*. London: Royal College of Psychiatrists.

National Research Council. (2013). *Subjective Well-Being*. Washington, DC: National Academies Press.

NHS England. (2019, June). *Social Prescribing and Community-Based Support: Summary Guide*. Accessed April 5, 2021. https://www.england.nhs.uk/wp-content/uploads/2020/06/social-prescribing-summary-guide-updated-june-20.pdf.

Nicklin, D. E. (2000). Medicine and Religion. *New England Journal of Medicine* 343(18): 1340.

Nordenfelt, L. (2001). *Health, Science, and Ordinary Language*. New York: Rodopi.

Nordenfelt, L. Y. (1995). *On the Nature of Health: An Action-Theoretic Approach*. Dordrecht: Springer Netherlands.

North, J. (1987). Wrongdoing and Forgiveness. *Philosophy* 62: 499–508.

Nussbaum, M. C. (2001). *Women and Human Development: The Capabilities Approach*. Cambridge: Cambridge University Press.

Oderberg, D. S. (2004). The Structure and Content of the Good. In *Human Values*, edited by D. S. Oderberg and T. Chappell, 127–165. London: Palgrave Macmillan.

Okun, M. A., Yeung, E. W., and Brown, S. (2013). Volunteering by Older Adults and Risk of Mortality: A Meta-Analysis. *Psychology and Aging* 28(2): 564–577.

Olivier, J., Cochrane, J. R., and Schmid, B., with Graham, L. (2006). *ARHAP Literature Review: Working in a Bounded Field of Unknowing*. African Religious Health Assets Programme. https://jliflc.com/wp-content/uploads/2014/05/arhaplitreview_oct2006.pdf.

Olivier, J., Tsimpo, C., Gemignani, R., Shojo, M., Coulombe, H., Dimmock, F., Nguyen, M. C., Hines, H., Mills, E. J., Dieleman, J. L., and Haakenstad, A. (2015). Understanding the Roles of Faith-Based Health-Care Providers in Africa: Review of the Evidence with a Focus on Magnitude, Reach, Cost, and Satisfaction. *The Lancet* 386(10005): 1765–1775.

Osewska, E., and Simonič, B. (2019). A Civilization of Love According to John Paul II. The Person and the Challenges. *Journal of Theology, Education, Canon Law and Social Studies Inspired by Pope John Paul II* 9(1): 23–32.

Otolok-Tanga, E., Atuyambe, L., Murphy, C. K., Ringheim, K. E., and Woldehanna, S. (2007). Examining the Actions of Faith-Based Organizations and Their Influence on HIV/AIDS-Related Stigma: A Case Study of Uganda. *African Health Sciences* 7(1): 55–60.

Paloutzian, R. F., and Ellison, C. W. (1982). Loneliness, Spiritual Well-Being, and the Quality of Life. In *Loneliness: A Sourcebook of Current Theory, Research and Therapy*, edited by L. A. Peplau and D. Perlman, 224–237. New York: John Wiley & Sons.

Paluck, E. L., Porat, R., Clark, C. S., and Green, D. P. (2021). Prejudice Reduction: Progress and Challenges. *Annual Review of Psychology* 72: 533–560.

Pannenberg, W. (2013). *Jesus God and man*. Scm Press.

Parfit, D. (1984). *Reasons and Persons*. Oxford: Clarendon Press.

Pargament, K. I., Feuille, M., and Burdzy, D. (2011). The Brief RCOPE: Current Psychometric Status of a Short Measure of Religious Coping. *Religions* 2: 51–76.

Pargament, K. I., Koenig, H. G., and Perez, L. M. (2000). The Many Methods of Religious Coping: Development and Initial Validation of the RCOPE. *Journal of Clinical Psychology* 56(4): 519–543.

Pargament, K. I., Wong, S., and Exline, J. J. (2022). The Holiness of Wholeness: Religious Contributions to Human Flourishing. In *The Oxford Handbook of Humanities and Human Flourishing*, edited by J. O. Pawelski, and L. Tay. New York: Oxford Press.

Paul, K. I., and Moser, K. (2009). Unemployment Impairs Mental Health: Meta-Analyses. *Journal of Vocational Behavior* 74(3): 264–282.

Paul VI. (1964a). *Lumen gentium*. Libreria Editrice Vaticana. https://www.vatican.va/archive/hist_councils/ii_vatican_council/documents/vat-ii_decree_19641121_unitatis-redintegratio_en.html.

Paul VI. (1964b). *Unitatis redintegratio*. Libreria Editrice Vaticana. https://www.vatican.va/archive/hist_councils/ii_vatican_council/documents/vat-ii_decree_19641121_unitatis-redintegratio_en.html.

Paul VI. (1965). *Gaudium et spes: Pastoral Constitution on the Church in the Modern World*. Boston, MA: Pauline Books & Media.

Paul VI. (1967). *Populorum progressio: On the Development of Peoples*. Libreria Editrice Vaticana. https://www.vatican.va/content/paul-vi/en/encyclicals/documents/hf_p-vi_enc_26031967_populorum.html.

Paul VI. (1968). *Humanae vitae: On the Regulation of Birth*. Libreria Editrice Vaticana. https://www.vatican.va/content/paul-vi/en/encyclicals/documents/hf_p-vi_enc_25071968_humanae-vitae.html.

Peng-Keller, S., Winiger, F., and Rauch, R. (Eds.). (2022). *The Spirit of Global Health: The World Health Organization and the "Spiritual Dimension" of Health, 1946–2021*. Oxford: Oxford University Press.

Peteet, J. R. (2018). A Fourth Wave of Psychotherapies: Moving beyond Recovery toward Well-Being. *Harvard Review of Psychiatry* 26(2): 90–95.

Peteet, J. R. (Ed.). (2022). *The Virtues in Psychiatric Practice.* New York: Oxford University Press.
Peterson, C., and Seligman, M. E. (2004). *Character Strengths and Virtues: A Handbook and Classification.* New York: Oxford University Press.
Pew Research Center. (2012). *The Global Religious Landscape: A Report on the Size and Distribution of the World's Major Religious Groups as of 2010.* https://assets.pewresearch.org/wp-content/uploads/sites/11/2014/01/global-religion-full.pdf.
Pfeil, M. (2018). Fifty Years after Populorum Progressio: Understanding Integral Human Development in Light of Integral Ecology. *Journal of Catholic Social Thought* 15(1): 5–17.
Phelps, A. C., Lauderdale, K. E., Alcorn, S., Dillinger, J., Balboni, M. T., Van Wert, M., Vanderweele, T. J., and Balboni, T. A. (2012). Addressing Spirituality within the Care of Patients at the End of Life: Perspectives of Advanced Cancer Patients, Oncologists, and Oncology Nurses. *Journal of Clinical Oncology* 30: 2538–2544.
Philippe, J. (2005). *Time for God: A Guide to Prayer.* New York: Pauline Books & Media.
Phillips, R., and Wong, C. (2017). *Handbook of Community Well-being Research.* Dordrecht: Springer.
Pieper, J. (1974). *About Love.* Translated by R. Winston and C. Winston. Chicago: Franciscan Herald Press.
Pieper, J. (1990). *The Four Cardinal Virtues: Human Agency, Intellectual Traditions, and Responsible Knowledge.* Notre Dame, IN: University of Notre Dame Press.
Pieper, J. (1986). *On Hope.* San Francisco, CA: Ignatius Press.
Pieper, J. (1998). *Happiness and Contemplation.* South Bend, IN: St. Augustine's Press.
Pieper, J. (2009). *Leisure: The Basis of Culture.* San Francisco, CA: Ignatius Press.
Pies, R. (2014). The Bereavement Exclusion and DSM-5: An Update and Commentary. *Innovations in Clinical Neuroscience* 11(7–8): 19.
Pilch, J. J. (2000). *Healing in the New Testament.* Minneapolis, MN: Fortress Press.
Pius XI. (1931). *Quadragesimo anno: On the Reconstruction of the Social Order.* Accessed January 5, 2024. https://www.vatican.va/content/pius-xi/en/encyclicals/documents/hf_p-xi_enc_19310515_quadragesimo-anno.html.
Pius XII. (1952). Address to the First International Congress on the Histopathology of the Nervous System. *Acta Apostolicae Sedis* 44 (1952): 779–789.
Pius XII. (1957). The Prolongation of Life: An Address of Pope Pius XII to an International Congress of Anesthesiologists. November 24, 1957. Accessed January 5, 2024. https://www.pdcnet.org/C1257D43006C9AB1/file/ADFD88433FCE0B7EC1257D660057B7AD/$FILE/ncbq_2009_0009_0002_0119_0124.pdf.

Plato. (4th C BCE/2004). *The Republic*. Indianapolis, IN: Hackett.
Plough, A. L. (Ed.). (2020). *Well-Being: Expanding the Definition of Progress: Insights from Practitioners, Researchers, and Innovators from Around the Globe*. Oxford: Oxford University Press.
Porterfield, A. (2005). *Healing in the History of Christianity*. Oxford: Oxford University Press.
Post, S. G. (2017). Rx It's Good to Be Good (G2BG) 2017 Commentary: Prescribing Volunteerism for Health, Happiness, Resilience, and Longevity. *American Journal of Health Promotion* 31: 164–172.
Potts, M. I. (2022). *Forgiveness: An Alternative Account*. New Haven, CT: Yale University Press.
Powdthavee, N., Lekfuangfu, W. N., and Wooden, M. (2015). What's the Good of Education on Our Overall Quality of Life? A Simultaneous Equation Model of Education and Life Satisfaction for Australia. *Journal of Behavioral and Experimental Economics* 54: 10–21.
Puchalski, C. M., and Romer, A. L. (2000). Taking a Spiritual History Allows Clinicians to Understand Patients More Fully. *Journal of Palliative Medicine* 3: 129–137.
Railton, P. (1986). Facts and Values. *Philosophical Topics* 14(2): 5–31.
Ramos, C., and Leal, I. (2013). Posttraumatic Growth in the Aftermath of Trauma: A Literature Review about Related Factors and Application Contexts. *Psychology, Community, & Health* 2: 43–54.
Rand, S. (2015). The Real Marriage Penalty: How Welfare Law Discourages Marriage Despite Public Policy Statements to the Contrary—and What Can Be Done about It. *The University of the District of Columbia Law Review* 18(1): 93–143.
Regnerus, M. (2017). *Cheap Sex: The Transformation of Men, Marriage, and Monogamy*. Oxford: Oxford University Press.
Roberts, L., Ahmed, I., and Hall, S. (2000). Intercessory Prayer for the Alleviation of Ill Health. *Cochrane Database of Systematic Reviews* 2.
Roberts, L., Ahmed, I., and Hall, S. (2007). Intercessory Prayer for the Alleviation of Ill Health. *Cochrane Database of Systematic Reviews* 1.
Roberts, L., Ahmed, I., Hall, S., and Davison, A. (2009). Intercessory Prayer for the Alleviation of Ill Health. *Cochrane Database of Systematic Reviews* 2: CD000368.
Roelfs, D. J., Shor, E., Davidson, K. W., and Schwartz, J. E. (2011). Losing Life and Livelihood: A Systematic Review and Meta-Analysis of Unemployment and All-Cause Mortality. *Social Science & Medicine* 72(6): 840–854.
Roest, A. M., Martens, E. J., Denollet, J., and De Jonge, P. (2010). Prognostic Association of Anxiety Post Myocardial Infarction with Mortality and New Cardiac Events: A Meta-Analysis. *Psychosomatic Medicine* 72(6): 563–569.
Rose, N. (2006). Disorders without Borders? The Expanding Scope of Psychiatric Practice. *BioSocieties* 1(4): 465–484.
Rosmarin, D. H., and Koenig, H. G. (Eds.). (2020). *Handbook of Spirituality, Religion, and Mental Health*. Cambridge, MA: Academic Press.

Rosmarin, D. H., Pirutinsky, S., Pargament, K. I., and Krumrei, E. J. (2009). Are Religious Beliefs Relevant to Mental Health among Jews? *Psychology of Religion and Spirituality*, 1(3): 180–190.

Rothman, E. F. (2021). *Pornography and Public Health*. Oxford: Oxford University Press.

Rozier, M. D. (2016). Structures of Virtue as a Framework for Public Health Ethics. *Public Health Ethics* 9(1): 37–45.

Rozier, M. (2017). Religion and Public Health: Moral Tradition as Both Problem and Solution. *Journal of Religion and Health* 56(3): 1052–1063.

Rozier, M. (2020). A Catholic Contribution to Global Public Health. *Annals of Global Health* 86: 1–5.

Russell, D. W. (1996). UCLA Loneliness Scale (Version 3): Reliability, Validity, and Factor Structure. *Journal of Personality Assessment* 66(1): 20–40.

Ryff, C. D. (1989). Happiness Is Everything, or Is It? Explorations on the Meaning of Psychological Well-Being. *Journal of Personality and Social Psychology* 57(6): 1069–1081.

Sachs, J. D., Kroll, C., Lafortune, G., Fuller, G., and Woelm F. (2021). *Sustainable Development Report 2021*. Cambridge: Cambridge University Press.

Sadler, J. Z. (2005). *Values and Psychiatric Diagnosis*. New York: Oxford.

Sajeev, G., Weuve, J., Jackson, J. W., VanderWeele, T. J., Bennett, D. A., Grodstein, F., and Blacker, D. (2016). Late-Life Cognitive Activity and Dementia: A Systematic Review and Bias Analysis. *Epidemiology* 27: 732–742.

Saracci, R. (1997). The World Health Organisation Needs to Reconsider Its Definition of Health. *British Medical Journal* 314(7091): 1409.

Sarah, R. (2011). Caritas: The Practice of Love by the Church as a "Community of Love." Catholic Culture. https://www.catholicculture.org/culture/library/view.cfm?recnum=9628.

Sayer, L. C., England, P., Allison, P. D., Kangas, N. (2011). She Left, He Left: How Employment and Satisfaction Affect Women's and Men's Decisions to Leave Marriages. *American Journal of Sociology* 116: 1982–2018.

Scheinman, S. J., Fleming, P., and Niotis, K. (2018). Oath Taking at US and Canadian Medical School Ceremonies: Historical Perspectives, Current Practices, and Future Considerations. *Academic Medicine* 93(9): 1301–1306.

Scheler, M. (1992). The Meaning of Suffering. In *On Feeling, Knowing, and Valuing: Selected Writings*, edited by Harold J. Bershady, 82–115. Chicago, IL: University of Chicago Press.

Schramme, T. (2007). A Qualified Defence of a Naturalist Theory of Health. *Medicine, Health Care and Philosophy* 10(1): 11–17.

Schulz, J. (2015). The Principle of Totality and the Limits of Enhancement. *Ethics and Medicine* 31: 143–157.

Schutte, N. S., and Malouff, J. M. (2019). The Impact of Signature Character Strengths Interventions: A Meta-Analysis. *Journal of Happiness Studies* 20(4): 1179–1196.

Schwartz, S. H. (1994). Are There Universal Aspects in the Structure and Contents of Human Values? *Journal of Social Issues* 50(4): 19–45.

Seligman, M. E. (2011). *Flourish: A Visionary New Understanding of Happiness and Well-Being.* New York: Simon and Schuster.

Seligman, M. E., Steen, T. A., Park, N., and Peterson, C. (2005). Positive Psychology Progress: Empirical Validation of Interventions. *American Psychologist* 60(5): 410.

Shor, E., and Roelfs, D. J. (2013). The Longevity Effects of Religious and Non-Religious Participation: A Meta-Analysis and Meta-Regression. *Journal of the Scientific Study of Religion* 52(1): 120–145.

Sidgwick, H. (1981). *The Methods of Ethics.* 7th ed. Indianapolis, IN: Hackett.

Silvestri, G. A., Knittig, S., Zoller, J. S., and Nietert, P. J. (2003). Importance of Faith on Medical Decisions Regarding Cancer Care. *Journal of Clinical Oncology* 21(7): 1379–1382.

Simundson, D. J. (1992). Suffering. In *The Anchor Bible Dictionary*, edited by D. N. Freedman. New York: Doubleday.

Sin, N. L., and Lyubomirsky, S. (2009). Enhancing Well-Being and Alleviating Depressive Symptoms with Positive Psychology Interventions: A Practice-Friendly Meta-Analysis. *Journal of Clinical Psychology: In Session* 65(5): 467–487.

Sloan, R. P. (2011). Virtue and Vice in Health and Illness: The Idea that Wouldn't Die. *Lancet* 377(9769): 896–897.

Sloan, R. P., Bagiella, E., VandeCreek, L., Hover, M., Casalone, C., Hirsch, T. J., Hasan, Y., Kreger, R., and Poulos, P. (2000). Should Physicians Prescribe Religious Activities? *New England Journal of Medicine* 342: 1913–1916.

Smith, C. (2015). *To Flourish or Destruct: A Personalist Theory of Human Goods, Motivations, Failure, and Evil.* Chicago, IL: University of Chicago Press.

Snyder, C. R. (Ed.). (2000). *Handbook of Hope: Theory, Measures, and Applications.* Cambridge, MA: Academic Press.

St. John of the Cross. (1585/1959). *Dark Night of the Soul.* Translated by E. A. Peers. New York: Image Books.

Stein, D. J. (2021). *Problems of Living: Perspectives from Philosophy, Psychiatry, and Cognitive-Affective Science.* Cambridge, MA: Academic Press.

Stein, D. J., Palk, A. C., and Kendler, K. S. (2021). What Is a Mental Disorder? An Exemplar-Focused Approach. *Psychological Medicine* 51(6): 894–901.

Steinberg, J. R., Trussell, J., Hall, K. S., and Guthrie, K. (2012). Fatal Flaws in a Recent Meta-Analysis on Abortion and Mental Health. *Contraception* 86(5): 430–437.

Steinhauser, K. E., Christakis, E. C., Clipp, E. C., McNeilly, M., McIntyre, I., and Tulsky, J. A. (2000). Factors Considered Important at the End of Life by Patients, Family, Physicians, and Other Care Providers. *Journal of the American Medical Association* 284: 2476–2482.

Steptoe, A. (2019). Happiness and Health. *Annual Review of Public Health* 40: 339–359.

Stevenson, D. H., Eck, B. E., and Hill, P. C. (Eds.). (2007). *Psychology & Christianity Integration: Seminal Works that Shaped the Movement.* Batavia, IL: Christian Association for Psychological Studies.

Stiglitz, J., Sen, A., and Fitoussi, J.-P. (2009). *Report by the Commission on the Measurement of Economic Performance and Social Progress*. Paris: CMEPS.
Stiglitz, J. E., Sen, S., and Fitoussi, J.-P. (2010). *Mismeasuring Our Lives: Why GDP Doesn't Add Up*. New York: New Press.
Stiglitz, J. E., Fitoussi, J.-P., and Durand, M. (2019). *Measuring What Counts: The Global Movement for Well-Being*. New York: New Press.
Strawbridge, W. J., Shema, S. J., Cohen, R. D., and Kaplan, G. A. (2001). Religious Attendance Increases Survival by Improving and Maintaining Good Health Behaviors, Mental Health, and Social Relationships. *Annals of Behavioral Medicine* 23(1): 68–74.
Stump, E. (1996). *Aquinas on the Sufferings of Job. The Evidential Argument from Evil*. Edited by D. Howard-Snyder. Bloomington, IN: Indiana University Press, 49–68.
Stump, E. (2006). Love, by All Accounts. In *Proceedings and Addresses of the American Philosophical Association* 80(2): 25–43.
Stump, E. (2010). *Wandering in Darkness: Narrative and the Problem of Suffering*. Oxford: Oxford University Press.
Stump, J. B., and Meister, C. (2020). *Original Sin and the Fall: Five Views*. Downers Grove, IL: Intervarsity Press.
Su, R., Tay, L., and Diener, E. (2014). The Development and Validation of the Comprehensive Inventory of Thriving (CIT) and the Brief Inventory of Thriving (BIT). *Applied Psychology: Health and Well-Being* 6(3): 251–279.
Sulmasy, D. P. (2009). Dignity, Disability, Difference, and Rights. In *Philosophical Reflections on Disability*, edited by D. Christopher Ralston and Justin Ho, 183–198. Dordrecht: Springer.
Swinburne, R. (1998). *Providence and the Problem of Evil*. Oxford: Oxford University Press.
Szasz, T. (1976). The Myth of Mental Illness. In *Biomedical Ethics and the Law*, edited by James M. Humber and Robert F. Almeder, 113–122. Boston, MA: Springer US.
Tasioulas, J., and Vayena, E. (2020). Just Global Health: Integrating Human Rights and Common Goods. In *The Oxford Handbook of Global Justice*, edited by Thom Brooks, 139–162. Oxford: Oxford University Press.
Tedeschi, R. G., and Calhoun, L. G. (2004). Posttraumatic Growth: Conceptual Foundations and Empirical Evidence. *Psychological Inquiry* 15: 1–18.
Thurston, H. J., and Attwater, D. (Eds.). (1990). *Butler's Lives of the Saints*. Westminster, MD: Christian Classics.
Tillich, P. (1981). *The Meaning of Health: The Relation of Religion and Health*. Richmond, CA: North Atlantic Books.
Titus, C. S. (2017). Aquinas, Seligman, and Positive Psychology: A Christian Approach to the Use of the Virtues in Psychology. *Journal of Positive Psychology* 12(5): 447–458.
Tjeltveit, A. C. (2004). The Good, the Bad, the Obligatory, and the Virtuous: The Ethical Contexts of Psychotherapy. *Journal of Psychotherapy Integration* 14(2): 149–167.

Toussaint, L. L., Worthington, E. L., and Williams, D. R. (2015). *Forgiveness and Health: Scientific Evidence and Theories Relating Forgiveness to Better Health.* Dordrecht, Netherlands: Springer.

Trinitapoli, J., and Weinreb, A. (2012). *Religion and AIDS in Africa.* New York: Oxford University Press.

Trudel-Fitzgerald, C., Millstein, R. A., Von Hippel, C., Howe, C. J., Tomasso, L. P., Wagner, G. R., and VanderWeele, T. J. (2019). Psychological Well-Being as Part of the Public Health Debate? Insight into Dimensions, Interventions, and Policy. *BMC Public Health* 19(1): 1–11.

Tutu, D. (2000). *No Future without Forgiveness.* New York: Image.

Twenge, J. M., Haidt, J., Blake, A. B., McAllister, C., Lemon, H., and Le Roy, A. (2021). Worldwide Increases in Adolescent Loneliness. *Journal of Adolescence* 93: 257–269.

UNCESCR (United Nations Committee on Economic, Social and Cultural Rights). (2000). General Comment No. 14 (Twenty Second Session). The Right to the Highest Attainable Standard of Health. UN Document E/C.12/2000/4. United Nations Digital Library. https://digitallibrary.un.org/record/425041?ln=en.

Van Inwagen, P. (2008). *The Problem of Evil.* Oxford: Oxford University Press.

Van Ness, P. H. (1999). Religion and Public Health. *Journal of Religion and Health* 38: 15–26.

Van Nieuwenhove, R. (2005). "Bearing the Marks of Christ's Passion": Aquinas' Soteriology. In *The Theology of Thomas Aquinas*, edited by Rik Van Nieuwenhove and Joseph Wawryko, 277–302. Notre Dame, IN: University of Notre Dame Press.

Van Zeller, H. (2015). *The Mystery of Suffering.* Notre Dame, IN: Ave Maria Press.

VandeCreek, L., and Burton, L. (Eds.). (2001). Professional Chaplaincy: Its Role and Importance in Healthcare. *Journal of Pastoral Care* 55(1): 81–97.

VanderWeele, T. J. (2017a). On the Promotion of Human Flourishing. *Proceedings of the National Academy of Sciences, U.S.A.* 31: 8148–8156.

VanderWeele, T. J. (2017b). Outcome-Wide Epidemiology. *Epidemiology* 28(3): 399–402.

VanderWeele, T. J. (2017c). Religion and Health: A Synthesis. In *Spirituality and Religion within the Culture of Medicine: From Evidence to Practice*, edited by J. R. Peteet, and M. J. Balboni, 358–401. New York: Oxford University Press.

VanderWeele, T. J. (2017d). Religious Communities and Human Flourishing. *Current Directions in Psychological Science* 26: 476–481.

VanderWeele, T. J. (2017e). Knowledge Beyond Science? Assessing the Evidence for the Christian Faith. Lecture at Indiana University, October 29, 2017. Available at: https://hfh.fas.harvard.edu/sites/projects.iq.harvard.edu/files/pik/files/sciencechristianity.pdf

VanderWeele, T. J. (2018a). Is Forgiveness a Public Health Issue? *American Journal of Public Health* 108: 189–190.

VanderWeele, T. J. (2018b). Religious Communities. In *The Routledge International Handbook of Psychosocial Epidemiology*, edited by M. Kivimäki, D. G. Batty, I. Kawachi, and A. Steptoe. London: Routledge.

VanderWeele, T. J. (2019a). Measures of Community Well-Being: A Template. *International Journal of Community Well-Being* 2: 253–275.

VanderWeele, T. J. (2019b). Suffering and Response: Directions in Empirical Research. *Social Science & Medicine* 224: 58–66.

VanderWeele, T. J. (2020a). Activities for Flourishing: An Evidence-Based Guide. *Journal of Positive Psychology and Wellbeing* 4: 79–91.

VanderWeele, T. J. (2020b). Challenges Estimating Total Lives Lost in COVID-19 Decisions: Consideration of Mortality Related to Unemployment, Social Isolation, and Depression. *Journal of the American Medical Association* 324(5): 445–446.

VanderWeele, T. J. (2020c). Spiritual Well-Being and Human Flourishing: Conceptual, Causal, and Policy Relations. In *Religion and Human Flourishing*, edited by Adam B. Cohen, 43–54. Waco, TX: Baylor University Press.

VanderWeele, T. J. (2022a). The Importance, Opportunities, and Challenges of Empirically Assessing Character for the Promotion of Flourishing. *Journal of Education* 202(2). DOI: 10.1177/00220574211026905.

VanderWeele, T. J. (2022b). Virtues, Mental Health, and Human Flourishing. In *Virtues in Psychiatric Practice*, edited by J. R. Peteet. Oxford: Oxford University Press.

VanderWeele, T. J. (2023a). Abortion and Mental Health—Context and Common Ground. *Journal of the American Medical Association Psychiatry* 80(2): 105–106.

VanderWeele, T. J. (2023b). Moral Controversies and Academic Public Health: Notes on Navigating and Surviving Academic Freedom Challenges. *Global Epidemiology* 6: 10019.

VanderWeele, T. J. (2023c). On an analytic definition of love. *Journal of Ethics and Social Philosophy* 25: 105–135.

VanderWeele, T. J. (2024). Flourishing and the Proper Scope of Medicine and Public Health. *Journal of Epidemiology and Community Health*, doi: 10.1136/jech-2023-220553.

VanderWeele, T. J., and Lomas, T. (2023). Terminology and the Well-Being Literature. *Affective Science* 4: 36–40.

VanderWeele, T. J., Li, S., Tsai, A. C., and Kawachi, I. (2016). Association between Religious Service Attendance and Lower Suicide Rates among US Women. *Journal of the American Medical Association Psychiatry* 73(8): 845–851.

VanderWeele, T. J., Yu, J., Cozier, Y. C., Wise, L., Argentieri, M. A., Rosenberg, L., Palmer, J. R., and Shields, A. E. (2017). Attendance at Religious Services, Prayer, Religious Coping, and Religious/Spiritual Identity as Predictors of All-Cause Mortality in the Black Women's Health Study. *American Journal of Epidemiology* 185(7): 515–522.

VanderWeele, T. J., McNeely, E., and Koh, H. K. (2019a). Flourishing as a Definition of Health—Reply. *Journal of the American Medical Association* 322(10): 981–982.

VanderWeele, T. J., McNeely, E., and Koh, H. K. (2019b). Reimagining Health—Flourishing. *Journal of the American Medical Association* 321(17): 1667–1668.

VanderWeele, T. J., Trudel-Fitzgerald, C., Allin, P., Farrelly, C., Fletcher, G., Frederick, D. E., Hall, J., Helliwell, J. F., Kim, E. S., Lauinger, W. A., Lee, M. T., Lyubomirsky, S., Margolis, S., McNeely, E., Messer, N., Tay, L., Viswanath, V., Węziak-Białowolska, D., and Kubzansky, L. D. (2020a). Current Recommendations on the Selection of Measures for Well-Being. *Preventive Medicine*, 133: 106004.

VanderWeele, T. J., Mathur, M. B., and Chen, Y. (2020b). Outcome-Wide Longitudinal Designs for Causal Inference: A New Template for Empirical Studies. *Statistical Science* 35(3): 437–466.

VanderWeele, T. J., Long, K., and Balboni, M. J. (2021). On Tradition-Specific Measures of Spiritual Well-Being. In *Measuring Well-Being: Interdisciplinary Perspectives from the Social Sciences and the Humanities*, edited by M. Lee, L. D. Kubzansky, and T. J. VanderWeele, 482–498. Oxford: Oxford University Press.

VanderWeele, T. J., Balboni, T. A., and Koh, H. K. (2022). Religious Service Attendance and Implications for Clinical Care, Community Participation and Public Health. *American Journal of Epidemiology*, 191: 31–35.

Vermeule, A. (2022). *Common Good Constitutionalism*. Polity Press: Cambridge UK.

Vidal, M. (1987). Structural Sin: A New Category in Moral Theology. In *History and Conscience: Studies in Honor of Father Sean O'Riordan, CSsR*, edited by R. Gallagher and B. McConvery, 181–198. Dublin: Gill and Macmillan.

Vieten, C., and Lukoff, D. (2022). Spiritual and Religious Competencies in Psychology. *American Psychologist* 77(1): 26–38.

Volf, M. (2015). *Flourishing: Why We Need Religion in a Globalized World*. New Haven, CT: Yale University Press.

Von Schirnding, Y. E. R. (2015). Environmental Health Practice. In *Textbook of Global Public Health*, 6th ed., edited by R. Detels, M. Gulliford, Q. Abdool Karim, and Chorh Chuan Tan, 1523–1541. Oxford: Oxford University Press.

Wade, N. G., Hoyt, W. T., Kidwell, J. E., and Worthington Jr., E. L. (2014). Efficacy of Psychotherapeutic Interventions to Promote Forgiveness: A Meta-Analysis. *Journal of Consulting and Clinical Psychology* 82(1): 154–170.

Wakefield, J. C. (1992). Disorder as Harmful Dysfunction: A Conceptual Critique of DSM-III-R's Definition of Mental Disorder. *Psychological Review* 99(2): 232–247.

Wakefield, J. C. (2000). Aristotle as Sociobiologist: The "Function of a Human Being" Argument, Black Box Essentialism, and the Concept of Mental Disorder. *Philosophy, Psychiatry, & Psychology* 7(1): 17–44.

Waring, D. (2016). *The Healing Virtues: Character Ethics in Psychotherapy*. Oxford: Oxford University Press.

Wei, J., Hou, R., Zhang, X., Xu, H., Xie, L., Chandrasekar, E. K., Ying, M., and Goodman, M. (2019). The Association of Late-Life Depression with All-Cause and Cardiovascular Mortality among Community-Dwelling Older Adults: Systematic Review and Meta-Analysis. *British Journal of Psychiatry* 215(2): 449–455.

Weil, S. (1951). *Waiting on God: Religious and Philosophical Essays*. London: Routledge and Kegan Paul.

Westfall, C. L., and Dyer, B. R. (Eds.). (2016). *The Bible and Social Justice: Old Testament and New Testament Foundations for the Church's Urgent Call*. Eugene, OR: Pickwick Publications.

Westminster Assembly. (1647/2014). *Westminster Shorter Catechism*. Radford, VA: SMK Books.

Węziak-Białowolska, D., McNeely, E., and VanderWeele, T. J. (2019). Human Flourishing in Cross Cultural Settings: Evidence from the US, China, Sri Lanka, Cambodia and Mexico. *Frontiers in Psychology* 10: Article 1269.

Weziak-Bialowolska, D., Bialowolski, P., Sacco, P. L., VanderWeele, T. J., and McNeely, E. (2020). Well-Being in Life and Well-Being at Work: Which Comes First? Evidence from a Longitudinal Study. *Frontiers in Public Health* 8: 103.

Węziak-Białowolska, D., Białowolski, P., VanderWeele, T. J., and McNeely, E. (2021). Character Strengths Involving an Orientation to Promote Good Can Help Your Health and Well-Being. Evidence from Two Longitudinal Studies. *American Journal of Health Promotion* 35: 388–398.

Węziak-Bialowolska, D., Lee, M. T., Bialowolski, P., McNeely, E., Chen, Y., Cowden, R. G., and VanderWeele, T. J. (2023). Associations between the Importance of Well-Being Domains and the Subsequent Experience of Well-Being. *Sustainability* 15(1): 594.

WHO (World Health Organization). (1946). Constitution. https://www.who.int/about/accountability/governance/constitution.

Wiebel, D. T. (2007). A Loving-Kindness Intervention: Boosting Compassion for Self and Others. Ph.D. diss., Ohio University.

Wilcox, W. B. (2011). *Why Marriage Matters: 30 Conclusions from the Social Sciences*. 3rd. ed. New York: Institute for American Values/National Marriage Project.

Wilkinson, J. (1998). *The Bible and Healing*. Grand Rapids, MI: William B. Eerdmans Publishing.

Wittgenstein, L. (1953). *Philosophical Investigations*. Translated by G. E. M. Anscombe. New York: Macmillan.

Wright, T. (2012). *The Resurrection of the Son of God*. Spck.
Wolterstorff, N. (2015). *Justice in Love*. Grand Rapids, MI: William B. Eerdmans Publishing.
Wood, A. M., and Tarrier, N. (2010). Positive Clinical Psychology: A New Vision and Strategy for Integrated Research and Practice. *Clinical Psychology Review* 30(7): 819–829.
Wood, R. G., Goesling, B., and Avellar, S. (2007). *The Effects of Marriage on Health: A Synthesis of Recent Research Evidence*. Washington, DC: U.S. Department of Health and Human Services.
Woodward, A., and Macmillan, A. (2015). The Environment and Climate Change. In *Oxford Textbook of Global Public Health*, 6th ed., edited by R. Detels, M. Gulliford, Quarraisha Abdool Karim, and Chorh Chuan Tan. Oxford: Oxford University Press.
Woolfolk, R. L. (2012). Virtue and Psychotherapy. *Philosophy, Psychiatry, & Psychology* 19(1): 41–43.
Worthington, E. L. (2013). *Forgiveness and Reconciliation: Theory and Application*. New York: Taylor & Francis.
Worthington, E. L. (2021). Your Path to REACH Forgiveness. Everett Worthington website. https://evworthington.squarespace.com/diy-workbooks.
Wrzesniewski, A., and Dutton, J. E. (2001). Crafting a Job: Revisioning Employees as Active Crafters of Their Work. *Academy of Management Review* 26(2): 179–201.
Yeager, D., Glei, D. A., Au, M., Lin, H.-S., Sloan, R. P., and Weinstein, M. (2006). Religious Involvement and Health Outcomes among Older Persons in Taiwan. *Social Science & Medicine* 63(8): 2228–2241.
Young, J. (2014). *The Death of God and the Meaning of Life*. London: Routledge.
Zachar, P., First, M. B., and Kendler, K. S. (2017). The Bereavement Exclusion Debate in the DSM-5: A History. *Clinical Psychological Science* 5(5): 890–906.
Zachar, P., and Kendler, K. S. (2017). The Philosophy of Nosology. *Annual Review of Clinical Psychology* 13: 49–71.
Zinnbauer, B. J., and Pargament, K. I. (2000). Working with the Sacred: Four Approaches to Religious and Spiritual Issues in Counseling. *Journal of Counseling & Development* 78: 162–171.

INDEX

Page numbers with an n refer to footnotes.

A
abortion, 46, 177–180, 180n18, 180n19
abuse scandals, 253
accidents, ill health and, 152–153
aging
   bodily health and, 45, 97, 151, 156, 164, 226, 251, 305
   mental stimulation and, 84
   social isolation and, 84
alcohol use, 81, 82, 84
alms, 202. *See also* material resources
Ambrose, on cardinal virtues, 19n20
angels, 153
anger, suffering and, 164
anointing of the sick, 244
anxiety, 40n21. *See also* mental health; mental well-being
   bodily health and, 50
   forgiveness and, 236n14, 237n18, 279–280, 305
   relationships and, 48
   suffering and, 164
apostolate, 289–290
Aquinas, Thomas, 11n2
   on the common good, 55n11, 58n19, 177n13
   on evil, 167n9, 168n12
   on God's will, 238n19
   on happiness, 16–18, 16n2, 17n13

   on healing, 45n4
   on healthy habits, 82
   on hope, 256n6, 256n7
   hope vs. charity, 257n8
   on human flourishing, 22n28
   on the incarnation, 218n11
   on justice, 62n27
   on laws, 64n34
   life, intentionally ending, 46n8
   on love, 204–205n9
   on love of God, 206
   on murder, 178n14
   on punishment, 211n24, 223n26, 225n33
   on resurrection, 224n29
   on sin, 134, 134n5, 134–135n6, 135n7
   sin and death, 155n1
   on sin and free will, 167n9
   on spiritual well-being, 71
   on suffering of Jesus Christ, 219n15
   theology of, 11n1
   on virtue, 50n18
Aristotle
   on friendship, 59n22
   on happiness, 16, 16n2, 17n13
   on purpose, 60n25
   on virtue, 19, 245n31
association, freedom of, 291
atonement, 219n13, 221n19, 222–223n25

Augustine, St., 1, 6
  God as cause of health, 45n5
  on God's use of sin for good, 256n5
  on love of God, 206
  on restlessness, 131
  on sacrifice, 221n18
  on values, 91

B
baptism, 243
basic goods, 24–26, 24n35, 25n37, 25n38, 26n39. *See also* common good
beauty, bodily health and, 83n4
belonging, sense of, 60, 60n24
Benedict XVI, 209
bereavement, 35–36, 36n15
bodily health, 16, 28–43. *See also* physical well-being
  aging and, 45, 97, 151, 156, 164, 226, 251, 305
  beauty and, 83n4
  brain and, 32–34, 37
  character and, 49, 50n17
  community and, 93
  definitions of, 28–29
  depression and, 48, 50, 117
  disability perspectives, 30n3, 127, 127n58
  disease and injury, 30
  exclusive focus on and decision-making, 116–118
  fallenness and, 151
  fortitude and, 49, 49n17
  God's intent for, 28–29, 133–134
  vs. health of the person, 7, 33–34, 99–100, 293–294, 298
  human flourishing and, 31–32, 125–128
  lack of consideration of in psychological theories of well-being, 120–121
  limits of, 96–97
  medicine and, 100–102, 101n3
  mental illness and, 47–50
  normality, 29–30
  vs. physical well-being, 83, 83n3, 83n4
  purpose and, 49
  repair of, 81
  reproductive system, 30–31
  at resurrection of the dead, 262
  salvation and, 251
  sustaining practices, 81–83
  systems, functioning of, 29–30, 81–83
body
  health as natural state of, 44–45
  mind and, 40–41
  vs. person, 33–34
  as a temple, 50
brain
  bodily health and, 32–34, 37
  health of vs. mental health, 33–34
  mental illness and, 37–39
  vs. mind, 33–34, 33–34n10, 37
  psychiatry and, 102–106
brokenness, suffering and, 163
Buddhism
  meditative practices, 282n39
  spiritual well-being and, 23n34

C
Cain and Abel, story of, 53
calling, 75–76. *See also* purpose
capital punishment, 46, 46–47n8, 178n14
cardinal virtues, 19–20, 19n20
caregiving, 246–248
Catholic Church
  abuse scandals, 253
  on capital punishment, 46–47n8, 178n14
  common good and community, 60n23
  HIV/AIDS and, 271–272n10, 272n11
  on human rights, 63n32

on marriage, 66n38
moral theology of, 118
sacraments of, 242
social teaching, 111–112, 111n22, 230n4
theology and, 10–11n1
celibacy, 42
Centesimus annus (John Paul II), 182
character
bodily health and, 49, 50n17
communion with God and, 73–74
community life and, 233
development, promotion of, 277–279, 278n27
growth in, 74–76
growth in during ill health, 254–255
healing and, 245–246
in ill health, 254–255
importance of in maintaining health, 173–175
lack of consideration of in psychological theories of well-being, 119–120, 120n44
prayer and, 76
relationships and, 86–88
restoration of, 194
suffering and, 166, 246
valuing, 89
charity. *See also* love
communion with God and, 77–78
God's initiative and grace, 79, 212–214
grace and, 79, 212–214
vs. hope, 257n8
peace and, 78
children. *See also* family
marriage and, 67n42
Christianity
healing, call to bring, 231–232
moral teachings, 20
salvation, message of, 231–232
temporal vs. eternal flourishing, 287
theological virtues, 20, 78–79

Church. *See also* Catholic Church
abuse scandals, 253
communal life of, 230
discipline in, 253–254
healing, agent of, 253–254
healing and salvation, message of, 229–232
salvation and sin in, 252–254
as universal community of believers, 229n1
civil rights advocacy, 270–271
coherence, 18–19n16
common good
Aquinas on, 55n11, 58n19, 177n13
community and, 54–58, 54n9, 55n10, 56n14, 60n23, 61n26, 92
general vs. particular, 56n14
individual liberties and, 177n13
universal, 56n14
communal well-being, assessment of, 121–122
communion with God
approaching with faith, hope, and love, 73
character and, 73–74
charity and, 77–78
community, service, and purpose, 74–76
complete health and, 197
faith, 73
final, 225
fortitude and, 74
as friendship, 73, 74, 77, 78, 213–214
full, 265
God's initiation and grace, 78–79, 225
God's intent for, 70–72
during ill health, 255–256
ill health and, 255–256
justice and, 74
person, final end of, 70–72
prayer and contemplation, 76–77

communion with God (*cont.*)
  promise of, 259–266
  requirements of, 73–79
community
  belonging, sense of, 60, 60n24
  bodily health and, 93
  brought to wholeness by love, 208–209
  character and, 233
  common good and, 54–58, 54n9, 55n10, 56n14, 60n23, 61n26, 92
  corporate solidarity and, 53–54
  in creation narratives, 53
  family and, 66–68, 68n44
  features of, 58–61, 58n20, 61n26
  growth and, 74–76
  healing and, 232–234, 233n8
  health and, 91–93, 273–277, 273n12, 273n13, 276–277n22, 301–302
  human flourishing and, 15, 21, 52–69, 57n16, 61n26
  importance of, 296, 301–302
  Jesus on importance of, 53–54
  justice and, 62–65, 62n28
  lack of consideration of in psychological theories of well-being, 120
  leadership and, 59
  practices and structures of, 59–60
  purpose and, 60–61, 60n25
  relationships and, 59, 92–93
  unjust structures and, 145–148
  wholeness of a person and, 52–54
Compendium of the Social Doctrine of the Church
  on civilization of love, 209
  on common good, 54n9, 58n18, 60n23, 64n33, 65n35
  on disabilities, 127n58
  on human development, 111n22
  on human rights, 63n32
  integral humanism, 112n24
  on natural law, 6n15, 14–15n10
confirmation of faith, 243

contemplation, communion with God and, 76–77
contraception, 179n17
corporal alms, 202
corporate solidarity, 53–54
counseling
  health of the person and, 105–106
  tradition-specific practices, 109–110, 109n20
COVID-19 pandemic, 117, 177n13
creation. *See also* goodness of creation
  fallenness and, 152–153, 152n8
  healing and restoration of, 259–260
  transformation of, 264
creation narratives
  community, importance of, 53
  fallenness and, 149–150
  God's intent and, 11–12
  goodness and, 11–12, 11–12n4, 44
  love and relationships in, 42
  Scriptures, 11–12, 11–12n4
  sin and death, 155
  work in, 94

D
dark night of the soul experiences, 169–170
death
  fiction of overcoming, 183–185
  ill health and, 156–157
  of Jesus Christ, 219–221
  resurrection from, 262
  sin and, 155–158, 155n1
decisional forgiveness, 236, 236n16
depression
  abortion and, 180n18
  bereavement and, 36, 36n15
  bodily health and, 48, 50, 117
  forgiveness and, 236n14, 237n18, 279–280, 305
  negative mental experiences and, 40n21
  purpose, lack of, 49
  relationships and, 48

religious communities,
   participation in, 273, 273n12, 273n13
   suffering and, 164
desire-fulfillment theories, 17n13, 72n5
Diagnostic and Statistical Manual of Mental Disorders, 36n15
disability perspectives on health, 30n3, 127, 127n58
discipline, 253–254
discrimination
   addressing, 176–177, 176–177n12
   unjust structures, 143, 145, 147
disease
   bodily health and, 30
   definitions of, 133n1
   suffering and, 163–164
divorce, 67n41

E
economic inequality, 144
education, 86–87, 86n8
elderly people. *See* aging
emotional forgiveness, 236, 236n16
empathy, suffering and, 165–166
enemies, love of, 210–212, 211n24
environment, care for, 181–183. *See also* creation
eternal flourishing, 22, 22–23n29, 23, 70–72, 71n4, 72n5
eucharist, celebration of, 243
euthanasia, 46, 180–181, 180n19
evangelical counsels, 241n24
evangelism, 289–290
evil
   Aquinas on, 167n9, 168n12
   existence of, 166–167
   judgment of, 260–261
exercise, 81, 82

F
faith
   communion with God, 73
   confirmation of, 243
   God's initiative and grace, 78–79
   growth in, 75–76
   healing and, 198
   healing and restoration of creation, 260
   hope for full restoration, 256–257
   Jesus's life and death, 213
   salvation and, 226–228, 227n34
   as a virtue, 20, 227n36
fallenness. *See also* sin
   bodily health and, 151
   creation and, 152–153, 152n8
   in creation narratives, 149–150
   freedom and, 150–151
   humans' relationship to creation, 152–153, 152n8
   ill health and, 149–154
   mental health and, 151–152
   relationships and, 151–152
   stress and, 154
   wrongful acts and, 149–151
family
   community and, 66–68, 68n44
   human flourishing and, 66–68, 86n8
   marriage and, 67–68
fasting, healing and, 240–242
forgiveness, 211–212, 217
   anxiety and, 236n14, 237n18, 279–280, 305
   Aquinas on, 238n19
   decisional vs. emotional, 236, 236n16
   depression and, 236n14, 237n18, 279–280, 305
   healing and, 234–238
   health and, 236–237, 279–281, 280n32, 304–305
   interventions, 237n18, 279–281, 280n32
   justice and, 235–236, 281
   relationships and, 237
   Scriptures on, 235

fortitude
  bodily health and, 49, 49n17
  communion with God and, 74
  grit, 49n15
  as a virtue, 19–20
Francis, Pope, 46n8
freedom
  fallenness and, 150–151
  God's intent and, 153, 167
  sin and, 97, 134
  suffering and, 166–170
friendship
  Aristotle on, 59n22
  as a basic good, 26n39
  communion with God as, 73, 74, 77, 78, 213–214

G
generosity, 49n17, 138n3, 175
God. *See also* communion with God; God's intent
  as cause of health, 45, 45n5
  complete freedom from sin, 262–263
  final restoration by, 170–171
  healing, principal agent of, 215–216
  healing and restoration of creation, 259–260
  Jesus Christ and salvation, 217–226
  love of as integral to restoration to wholeness, 205–206, 206–207n15
  love of empowers love of neighbor, 206–208
  nature of in Jesus's life and teachings, 218–219
  relationship with, 21
  restoration of health and, 160–161
  separation from, 140, 159–160
  suffering, allowing, 166–170
  Trinity, 52–53
  union with, 42

God's intent
  for bodily health, 28–29, 133–134
  for communion with, 70–72
  completion of, 259–266
  in creation narratives, 11–12
  discerning, 10–12
  freedom and, 153, 167
  healing and restoration of wholeness, 195
  for human flourishing, 17n13, 18, 20–22
  injustice, contrary to, 145–146
  for love and relationship, 41–42
  love of neighbors and, 205
  relationships and, 41–42, 234
  for stewardship, 80–81
  for wholeness, 6–7, 6n15, 8n21, 18
good, judgment of, 260–261
goodness of creation, 11–12, 11–12n4
  human body and, 44
  person as integrated whole, 44–51
  wholeness and, 13–15
grace
  availability of, 261
  charity and, 79, 212–214
  communion with God and, 78–79
  salvation and, 227n35
gratitude, 85–86
grief, 35–36
gross domestic product (GDP), 115, 295–296
guilt, 140–141

H
habits, healthy, 82, 88
happiness
  Aquinas on, 16–18, 16n2, 17n13
  Aristotle on, 16, 16n2, 17n13
  human flourishing and, 15, 17n13
  mental well-being and, 16–17, 16n12, 17n13

hatred, cycles of, 210, 212
healing, 45
  Aquinas on, 45n4
  bodily, 193
  caregiving and, 246–248
  character, growth in, 245–246
  Christians called to bring, 231–232
  Church and, 229–232, 253–254
  community life and, 232–234, 233n8
  complete, 196
  of creation, 259–260
  faith and, 198
  fasting and, 240–242
  forgiveness and, 234–238
  God as principal agent of, 215–216
  during ill health, 254–255
  implications of, 267–292
  Jesus and, 215–228
  limits of, 251–258
  love as foundation for, 200–201
  love of neighbors and, 201–205, 206–208, 231–232
  marriage and, 244
  medicine and, 248–249, 248n34
  ordination to Christian ministry, 245
  pathways to, 300–305
  prayer and, 238–240, 239–240n20, 244
  religious communities, participation in, 273–276, 273n12, 273n13
  as restoration of wholeness, 193–195, 300
  sacraments and, 242–245
  salvation and, 191, 197–198
  from sin, 196–199
  theology of, 300
  through medicine, 248–249, 248n34

health. *See also* bodily health; mental health
  aspects of, interaction, 47–50
  of body vs. of person, 7, 33–34, 99–100, 293–294, 298
  causes, diversity of, 80
  character, importance of, 173–175
  character development and, 277–279, 278n27
  common understandings of, 287–290
  communion with God and, 197
  community and, 91–93, 273–277, 273n12, 273n13, 276–277n22, 301–302
  conceptions of, 4–5, 5n7
  definitions of, 3–4, 3n2, 5–6, 5n7, 5n8, 12
  etymology of, 3, 3n1
  forgiveness and, 236–237, 279–281, 280n32, 304–305
  God, and restoration of, 160–161
  God as cause of, 45, 45n5
  highest attainable standard of, 283–287, 284n41, 304
  as human flourishing, 13–15, 13n7, 13–14n8
  love, promotion of, 281–287, 282n39, 303–304
  marriage and, 67n41
  measurements of, 295–296
  as natural state of body, 44–45
  religious communities, participation in, 273–276, 273n12, 273n13, 302
  responsibility and, 80–98
  suffering and renewal of, 164–166
  virtue, importance of, 174–175, 174n4
health as wholeness. *See also* wholeness
  body vs. person, 7, 33–34, 99–100, 293–294, 298
  as an ideal, 8

health as wholeness (*cont.*)
  implications of, 99–129
  introduction to, 3–9
  overview of, 1
  as physical, mental, social, and spiritual well-being, 10–12
hedonism, 72n5
Hippocratic oath, 180n19
HIV/AIDS, 271, 271–272n10, 272n11
holiness, 7, 7n18
Holy Spirit, gifts of, 259n1
hope, 20
  Aquinas on, 256n6, 256n7
  vs. charity, 257n8
  communion with God and, 73
  empirical effects of, 257n12
  for full restoration, 256–257
  God's initiative and grace, 78–79
  growth in, 75–76
  as a virtue, 257n11
hospitals, 107n13
human flourishing, 13–15, 13n7, 13–14n8
  in all domains of life, 85–88
  alternative definition, 25n38
  Aquinas on, 22n28
  bodily health and, 31–32, 125–128
  community and, 15, 21, 52–69, 57n16, 61n26
  definitions of, 14n9
  domains of, 15–23, 24–26, 24n35, 24–25n36, 25n37, 26n39, 26n40
  family and, 66–68, 86n8
  God's intent for, 17n13, 18, 20–22
  happiness and, 15, 17n13
  health as, 13–15, 13n7, 13–14n8
  individuals affects societies, 96
  love and, 203n5
  multidimensionality, 125, 127
  natural law and, 14–15n10
  promotion of, 125–128
  relationships and, 15, 20–21
  societies affects individuals, 95–96
  theology of, 21–22
  unjust structures diminish opportunities for, 143–145
  values and, 89–91, 89n12, 91n16
  values shared across traditions, 23–27
  work and, 86–87, 86n8, 93–95, 95n30
human nature, 6, 15, 17n13, 52
human rights, 63, 63n30, 63n31, 63n32

I
ill health
  as absence of wholeness, 133–136
  causes of, 298–300
  character, growth in, 254–255
  communion with God and, 255–256
  death and, 156–157
  definitions of, 133n1
  fallenness and, 149–154
  fiction of ultimately overcoming, 183–185
  final restoration by God, 170–171
  guilt and, 140–141
  healing during, 254–255
  implications of, 172–189
  inevitability of, 96–97
  injustice and, 142–148
  natural disasters, accidents, and pollution, 152–153
  personal growth and healing during, 254–255
  poor habits, 139
  prevention of and public health, 248
  religious communities, participation in, 273n13
  sin and, 131, 134–136, 159–161, 298–300
  stress and, 154

suffering and, 162–171
wrongful acts and, 137–148, 172–173, 298–300
incapacity, 159–161
incarnation, 218n11. 225
individual liberties, 177n13
injury, 30
injustice
  addressing, 175–177
  contrary to God's intent, 145–146
  ill health and, 142–148
  Scriptures on, 145–146, 146n10
  unjust structures, 142–145
integral humanism, 111n22, 112n24, 114–115n31
intercessory prayer, 239–240n20

J
Jesus Christ
  anticipated return of, 259
  community, importance of, 53–54
  death of, 219–221
  on discipline, 254
  faith and restoration of creation, 260
  God, nature of in life and teachings, 218–219
  God and problem of sin, 217–226
  healing and, 215–228
  life and death of, 212–213
  on love, 21, 200, 201, 204–205
  on love of enemies, 210
  nature of God and God's love, 218–219
  as perfect exemplar, 218
  resurrection of, 224–225, 224n29
  sacrifice of, 221–222, 221n18
  salvation and, 215–228
  suffering of, 219n15
Jim Crow laws, 143
Job, book of, 164n4, 174n4
John Paul II, 42
  Centesimus annus, 182
  Salvifici doloris, 48, 163
  Sollicitudo rei solialis, 57

justice, 19–20. *See also* human rights; legal rights
  Aquinas on, 62n27
  communion with God and, 74
  community and, 62–65, 62n28
  forgiveness and, 235–236, 281
  love and, 235–236n12, 304
  love of enemies and, 211, 211n24
  restoration of creation and, 260–261
  Scriptures on, 145–146, 146n10

K
kindness, 85, 204. *See also* loving-kindness
knowledge
  communion with God and, 73–74
  experience or contemplation of God, 77
  of God's foregiveness, 238

L
laws, Aquinas on, 64n34
leadership, 59
legal rights, nations/states and, 64–65, 64n33, 65n35
legal systems, 144–145
life
  good of, 46–47
  intentionally ending, 46–47, 46n8
  respect for, 46–47, 177–181
life expectancy, 114
life satisfaction, assessments of, 114n30, 114–115n31
loneliness, 122
love, 20. *See also* charity
  Aquinas on, 204–205n9
  capacity for, 41–42
  centrality of, 21, 77–78, 200
  civilization of, 209
  communion with God and, 73–74
  communities brought to wholeness by, 208–209
  contagion of, 204, 204n6

love (*cont.*)
  in creation narratives, 42
  definitions of, 202n2
  discipline and punishment, 254
  of enemies, 210–212, 211n24
  of God and restoration to wholeness, 205–206, 206–207n15
  of God empowers love of neighbor, 206–208
  God's initiative and grace, 78–79
  God's intent for, 41–42
  growth in, 75–76
  healing, foundation for, 200–201
  health, highest attainable standard of, 283–287, 284n41, 304
  human flourishing and, 203n5
  importance and necessity of, 283–287
  interpersonal, 202n2
  Jesus on, 21, 200, 201, 204–205, 210
  justice and, 235–236n12, 304
  material resources and, 202–203
  of neighbors and healing, 201–205, 206–208, 231–232
  of perpetrators, 254
  promotion of and health, 281–287, 282n39, 303–304
  relationships and community, 21
loving-kindness, 203n5, 282n39

M
marriage, 42
  Catholic Church on, 66n38
  character, growth in, 86
  children, effect on, 67n42
  contraception and, 179n17
  family and, 67–68
  healing and, 244
  health and, 67n41
  purpose and, 86–87
  same-sex, 143n3

material resources
  abortion and, 178–179
  community responsibility for, 92
  love and, 202–203
  society and individual flourishing and, 95–96
  voluntarily giving up, 241–242, 241n24
meaning
  human flourishing and, 15, 18–19
  of life, 19n17
meaninglessness, 164
medical care, bodily health and, 81–82
medicine
  bodily health and health of the person, 100–102, 101n3
  healing and, 248–249, 248n34
  human well-being, assessment of, 113–116, 113n27
  individual wrongdoing and, 172–173, 173n2
  limits of, 183–184, 184n31, 184n32
  moral injury, attentiveness to, 186–188, 187n36
  other pathways to healing, 268–269
  proper purview of, 293
  religion, discussions of, 275–276, 275n18, 301
  religious communities, partnership with, 269–273, 269n2, 302–303
  spiritual well-being and, 123–125
  structural pluralism, 107–109, 107n13, 108–109n16
  suffering, attentiveness to, 185–186
  tradition-specific practices, 106–110, 107n13
men, in creation narratives, 42
mental health, 16. *See also* mental well-being
  abortion and, 180n18
  bereavement, 35–36, 36n15
  bodily health and, 47–50

vs. brain health, 33–34
character and virtue, 174n4
community life and, 234
conceptions of, 34–37, 37n17, 38–39n19
definitions of, 35n13
fallenness and, 151–152
health of the person and, 102–106
mind, wholeness of, 34–41
as part of bodily health, 32–34
relationships, effect on, 48
repair of, 84–85
stimulation and, 84
suffering and, 164
sustaining practices, 84–85
term, use of, 34n12
wholeness and, 103
mental illness
bodily health and, 47–50
brain and, 37–39
conceptions of, 39n20
definitions of, 37–38n18
negative mental experiences and, 37–39, 38–39n19, 40n21, 40–41n22
perspectives on, 35n14
term, use of, 34n12
treatment for, 40–41n22, 84–85
mental well-being, 23n31. *See also* mental health
happiness and, 16–17, 16n12, 17n13
term, use of, 34n12
understanding and knowledge, 18
mind
body and, 40–41
vs. brain, 33–34, 33–34n10, 37
wholeness of, 47–48
wholeness of and mental health, 34–41
moral injury, 186–188, 187n36
murder, Aquinas on, 178n14
mutuality, communion with God and, 78

N
narcotics, 81, 82, 84
nations/states, rights and, 64–65, 64n33, 65n35
natural disasters, 152–153
natural law, 6n15, 14–15n10
natural law theory, 25n36
natural rights, vs. human rights, 63n31
Nazi Holocaust, 143
negative mental experience, 37–39, 38–39n19, 40n21, 40–41n22
neighbors, love of, 201–205, 206–208, 231–232
nervous system, 32
nutrition, 81, 82

O
objective list theories, 24–25n36, 25n37, 72n5
ordination to Christian ministry, 245
original sin, 150–151

P
palliative care, 181, 181n21
Paul, St.
  on the body as a temple, 50
  on forgiveness, 235
  on Jesus's death, 220, 220n16
  on love, 21, 89, 205
  on love of enemies, 210–211
  on the resurrected body, 262
  sin and death, 155
  spiritual well-being and, 71
  on struggle with sin, 252, 255n4, 256
  on suffering, 165, 168, 246
Paul VI
  on civilization of love, 209
  Populorum progressio, 111
peace, charity and, 78
perfectionist theories, 72–73n5

person, health of. *See also* human flourishing
  bodily health, effect on, 100–102, 101n3
  vs. body, 7, 33–34, 99–100, 293–294, 298
  Catholic social teaching on, 111–112, 111n22
  community, and wholeness of, 52–54
  created as integrated whole, 44–51
  mental health and, 102–106
physical exercise, 81, 82
physical well-being, 23n31, 83, 83n3, 83n4. *See also* bodily health
Plato, 19n20, 245n31
pluralistic society
  public health in, 294–296
  well-being, understanding of, 287–290, 288n54
pollution, 152–153, 271
poor, preferential option for, 230, 230n4
poor habits, ill health and, 139
Populorum progressio (Paul VI), 111
pornography, 173n2
post-traumatic growth, 166n7
post-traumatic stress disorder (PTSD), 187–188
practical wisdom. *See* prudence
practices
  of good community, 59–60
  for healing, 232–245
  spiritual, 71
prayer
  character and, 76
  communion with God and, 76–77
  healing and, 238–240, 239–240n20, 244
  reciprocation in, 78
  suffering and, 168

prudence, 19–20, 74, 165, 175, 245, 255
psychiatry
  purview of, 102–106, 293
  tradition-specific practices, 106–110
psychology
  neglect of by medicine, 268–269
  well-being, theories of, 119–121, 120n44, 120n45
public health
  bodily health, exclusive focus on, 117–118
  human well-being, assessment of, 113–116, 113n27
  ill health, prevention of, 248
  individual wrongdoing and, 172–173, 173n2
  moral injury, attentiveness to, 186–188
  moral message of religious groups, 270–271
  other pathways to healing, 268–269
  in pluralistic society, 294–296
  purview of, 110–112
  religious communities, participation in, 274
  religious communities, partnership with, 269–273, 269n2, 302–303
  social well-being and, 121–122
  spiritual well-being and, 123–125
  suffering, attentiveness to, 185–186
public policy
  bodily health, exclusive focus on, 117–118
  human well-being, assessment of, 113–116, 113n27
  moral injury, attentiveness to, 186–188
  in pluralistic society, 294–296

purview of, 110–112
social well-being and, 121–122
spiritual well-being and, 123–125
suffering, attentiveness to, 185–186
punishment
  Aquinas on, 211n24, 223n26, 225n33
  love and, 235–236n12, 254
  love of enemies and, 211n24
purgatory, 251n1
purpose. *See also* calling
  Aristotle on, 60n25
  bodily health and, 49
  depression and, 49
  of good community, 60–61, 60n25
  relationships and, 86–88

R

REACH model, 280n32
reflection, health maintenance and, 87–88
relationships
  anxiety and, 48
  capacity for, 41–42
  character and, 86–88
  community and, 59, 92–93
  depression and, 48
  fallenness and, 151–152
  forgiveness and, 237
  with God, 21
  God's intent and, 41–42, 234
  human flourishing and, 15, 20–21
  importance of, 296
  lack of consideration of in psychological theories of well-being, 120
  love and healing, 203–204
  mental health, effect of, 48
  public policy consideration of, 121–122
  purpose and, 86–88
  restoration of, 194
  suffering and, 165–166
  temporal flourishing and, 86–88
  wrongful acts and, 138
religion
  freedom of, 63, 177, 291
  health and, 232
  in medicine, discussions of, 106–110, 275–276, 275n18, 301
  spiritual well-being and, 24n35, 123
religious community. *See also* community
  advocacy and, 270–271
  depression and, 273, 273n12, 273n13
  healing and, 273–276, 273n12, 273n13
  health, promotion of, 270
  human flourishing and, 86–87, 86n8
  participation in and health, 273–276, 273n12, 273n13, 302
  partnerships with medicine and public health, 269–273, 269n2, 302–303
  spiritual goals, freedom to pursue, 290–292
  temporal flourishing and, 86
religious services, health and, 233n7, 234n10
reproductive system, 30–31, 179n17
responsibility, health and, 80–98
  community, 91–97
  individual, 80–91, 96–97
rest, health maintenance and, 87
restlessness, 131
restoration of creation, 259–266
  complete freedom from sin, 262–263

restoration of creation (*cont.*)
   faith in Jesus Christ and, 260
   full communion with God, 265
   God's promise of, 259
   justice, establishment of, 260–261
   perfect bodily health, 262
   through Jesus Christ, 260
   transformation and, 264
resurrection of Jesus Christ, 224–225, 224n29
resurrection of the dead, 262–263

S
sacraments, 230, 242–245, 242n25
sacrifice, 221–222, 221n18
saints, lives of, 208
salvation
   bodily health and, 251
   Christians and message of, 231–232
   Church and, 229–232, 252–254
   grace and, 227n35
   healing and, 191, 197–198
   implications of, 267–292
   individual reception of, 226–228
   Jesus and, 215–228, 227n34
   mystery in, 226–228
   in Scriptures, 227n35
   sin and, 197–198, 251–254
Salvifici doloris (John Paul II), 48, 163
same-sex marriage, 143n3
Scriptures
   on caregiving, 246–248
   on community, 52–53, 232–233
   confession of sin, 243–244
   creation, transformation of, 264
   creation narratives, 11–12, 11–12n4
   on forgiveness, 235
   God as principal agent of healing, 215–216, 215–216n3
   healing accounts in, 198
   healing as restoration of wholeness, 193–194
   injustice, God's opposition to, 145–146, 146n10
   on justice, 145–146, 146n10
   love, centrality of, 77–78
   love of God empowers love of neighbor, 208
   on prayer and healing, 238–239
   on restoration of creation, 259
   resurrection of Jesus Christ, 224
   on salvation, 227n35
   sin and death, 155
   on sin and Jesus's death, 219–221
   on spiritual well-being, 71n4
   suffering and, 174n4
Second Vatican Council, 118
service toward others
   calling and, 75–76
   healing through care for others, 246–248
   character, growth in, 74–76
   as love for God, 74–75
sin. *See also* fallenness; wrongful acts
   Aquinas on, 134, 134n5, 134–135n6, 135n7, 155n1, 167n9
   complete freedom from, 262–263
   confession of, 243–244
   in creation narratives, 155
   death and, 155–158, 155n1
   freedom and, 97, 134
   grace and, 261
   healing from, 196–199
   human efforts to deal with, 216–217
   ill health and, 131, 134–136, 159–161, 298–300
   implications of, 172–189
   incapacity and, 159–161
   Jesus Christ and salvation, 217–226
   need to address, 159–161

resurrection and, 224–225
salvation and, 197–198,
   251–254
spiritual death and, 156
struggle with, 252
sleep, 82
social connection, 122
social isolation, 84
social well-being, 23n31, 121–122,
   268–269
society, 95–96, 142–145
solidarity, 57, 57n17
Sollicitudo rei solialis (John
   Paul II), 57
speech, freedom of, 291
Spe Salvi (Benedict XVI), 209
spiritual alms, 202
spiritual beings, 153
spiritual death, 156
spiritual well-being, 12, 12–13n6
   across traditions, 23, 24n34
   Aquinas on, 71
   assessment of, 123–125
   bodily health and, 50
   fasting and, 241
   freedom to pursue, 290–292
   God, relationship with, 23n31, 78
   God's initiative and grace, 79
   health and, 70–79
   human flourishing and, 15,
      22–23
   medicine and, 123–125
   neglect of by medicine, 268–269
   suffering and, 166–170
   values and, 89–91
stewardship, 80–81
stress, 84, 154
structural pluralism, 107–109,
   107n13, 108–109n16,
   287–292
structures, of good community,
   59–60
substitution, Jesus's death as,
   222–223, 223n28

suffering
   anxiety and, 164
   attentiveness to, 185–186
   brokenness and, 163
   character, growth in, 166,
      246
   dark night of the soul
      experiences, 169–170
   definitions of, 162
   depression and, 164
   disease and, 163–164
   final restoration by God,
      170–171
   freedom and, 166–170
   God allowing, 166–170
   ill health and, 162–171
   of Jesus Christ, 219n15
   Job, book of, 164n4, 174n4
   meaning of, 163, 170
   medicine and attentiveness to,
      185–186
   mental health and, 164
   prayer and, 168
   relationships and, 165–166
   renewed health and, 164–166
   transformation and, 164–166,
      166n7, 170–171
suicide, 46
Summa Theologica (Aquinas),
   11n1, 11n2, 58n19, 62n27,
   218n11
Sustainable Development Goals,
   112n25, 114
systems
   bodily health and, 29–30, 81–83
   health, maintaining, 80–81

T
temperance, 19–20
   bodily health and, 49, 82
   character and, 175, 245
   communion with God and, 74
   development of, 255
   fasting and, 241–242

temporal flourishing
  aspects of, 85–88
  definitions of, 22
  eternal flourishing and, 22–23n29, 72–73n5
  relationships and, 86–88
  religious community and, 86
  spiritual well-being and, 71–72
Ten Commandments, 137
theological virtues, 20, 78–79
theology
  Aquinas and, 11n1
  bodily health, 28–29
  Catholic Church and, 10–11n1
  challenges of, 10n1
  of healing, 300
  human flourishing and, 21–22
  on human nature, 6
  mental health, relationship with bodily health, 48
  mystery in, 11, 11n2
  role of, 10–11
  of wholeness, 300
Theology of the Body (John Paul II), 42
tobacco use, 81, 82
tradition-specific practices in healthcare, 102–106, 107n13, 124
transformation, suffering and, 164–166, 166n7, 170–171, 254–256
Trinity, 52–53, 60n24, 226
trust and Reconciliation Commission, 271

U
United Nations, Sustainable Development Goals, 112n25, 114
unjust structures
  addressing, 175–177
  community and, 145–148
  contrary to God's intent, 145–146
  human flourishing, diminished opportunities for, 143–145

V
values
  human flourishing and, 89–91, 89n12, 91n16
  shared across traditions, 23–27
vices, ill health and, 139
victim blaming, 172, 174
virtue
  Aquinas on, 50n18
  Aristotle on, 19, 245n31
  bodily health and, 49, 49–50n17
  cardinal virtues, 19–20, 19n20
  goodness and, 19–20
  health, importance of maintaining, 174–175, 174n4
  human flourishing and, 15, 19n20
  lack of consideration of in psychological theories of well-being, 119–120
  Plato on, 245n31
  theological, 20
  valuing, 89
vocation. *See* calling

W
war, 46
well-being. *See also* human flourishing
  aspects of, 296–297
  assessment of, 113–116, 113n27
  community, importance of, 296, 301
  vs. human flourishing, 13–14n8, 14n9
  indicators of, 113–116, 113n27, 114n30
  measurements of, 295–296

psychological theories of, 119–121, 120n45
relationships, importance of, 296
understanding of in a pluralistic society, 287–290, 288n54
wholeness. *See also* health as wholeness
  communities brought to by love, 208–209
  enemies, love of, 210–212, 211n24
  etymology of, 7n18
  fulfillment of, 259–266
  God's intent for, 6–7, 6n15, 8n21, 18
  goodness and, 13–15
  healing as restoration of, 193–195, 300
  ill health as absence of, 133–136
  loving God and, 205–206, 206–207n15
  restoration of and sin, 196–197
  theology of, 300
women, in creation narratives, 42
work
  in creation narratives, 94
  human flourishing and, 86–87, 86n8, 93–95, 95n30
World Happiness Report, 114n30, 114–115n31
World Health Organization, 3, 12, 283–285, 293, 297, 304
wrongful acts. *See also* sin
  fallenness and, 149–151
  God, separation from, 140
  guilt and, 140–141
  ill health and, 137–148, 172–173, 298–300
  relationships and, 138
  toward oneself, 138–139
  toward others, 137–138
  unjust structures, 142–145

Tyler J. VanderWeele is the John L. Loeb and Frances Lehman Loeb Professor of Epidemiology at the Harvard T. H. Chan School of Public Health, and director of the Human Flourishing Program and co-director of the Initiative on Health, Spirituality, and Religion at Harvard University.